Lecture Notes of the Institute for Computer Sciences, Social Informatics and Telecommunications Engineering 135

T0212822

More information about this series at http://www.springer.com/series/8197

Tegawendé F. Bissyandé · Gertjan van Stam (Eds.)

e-Infrastructure
and e-Services
for Developing Countries

5th International Conference, AFRICOMM 2013
Blantyre, Malawi, November 25–27, 2013
Revised Selected Papers

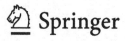 Springer

Editors
Tegawendé F. Bissyandé
University of Luxembourg
Luxembourg
Luxembourg

Gertjan van Stam
Scientific and Industrial Research
 and Development Centre
Harare
Zimbabwe

ISSN 1867-8211   ISSN 1867-822X (electronic)
ISBN 978-3-319-08367-4 ISBN 978-3-319-08368-1 (eBook)
DOI 10.1007/978-3-319-08368-1

Library of Congress Control Number: 2014944062

Springer Cham Heidelberg New York Dordrecht London

Printed on acid-free paper

Springer is part of Springer Science+Business Media (www.springer.com)

Preface

Africomm 2013, the 5th version of the EAI Conference on e-Infrastructure and e-Services for Developing Countries, held during November 25–28 in Blantyre, Malawi, proved to be a unique and truly African meeting place. Scientists, practitioners, students, and professionals met to discuss research and development of efficient and effective infrastructures and solutions in situations of limited resources. This work is of utmost importance as it constitutes a key-enabler for the diffusion of ICT in developing countries.

In a concerted effort, participants interacted to discuss issues and trends, recent research, innovation advances and in-the-field experiences related to e-Governance, e-Infrastructure, and e-Business with a focus on developing countries.

This volume of papers testifies of the exemplary efforts and sacrifices made by participants and the Organizing Committee. The excellent work supported an exciting program, and provides a unique insight in appropriate technology and practice. We thank the peer-reviewers and all involved for a job well done. Thanks to our Malawian colleagues for excellent arrangements.

The papers, the commitment to participate, the sending communities, and the representation of research, practise, and interaction, made Africomm 2013 a milestone event.

Special thanks to the program chair, Tegawendé Bissyandé, for the excellent preservation of academic ethics and value.

Let these conference proceedings of Africomm 2013 be a milestone of agency and empowerment for cultural aligned practices in e-Infrastructure and e-Services in developing countries.

May 2014   Gertjan van Stam

Organization

Steering Committee

Imrich Chlamtac (Chair)   CREATE-NET, Italy
Salomao Julio Manhica   UTICT, Mozambique
Fausto Giunchiglia   University of Trento, Italy
Paolo Traverso   FBK, Italy

Conference Organization Committee

General Chair

Gertjan van Stam   SIRDC, Zimbabwe

PC Chair

Tegawendé F. Bissyandé   University of Luxembourg, Luxembourg

Local Chair

Chomora Mikeka   University of Malawi, Malawi

Publicity Chair

Philip Lutaaya   MTAC-MTTI, Uganda

Student Affairs

Isaac Munyaradzi   GISP, Zimbabwe

Technical Program Committee

Bissyande F. Tegawendé   University of Luxembourg, Luxembourg
Chedom Fotso Donatien   University of Pau, France
Chikumba Patrick Albert   University of Malawi, Malawi

Contents

Exploiting IEEE802.11n MIMO Technology for Cost-Effective Broadband Back-Hauling

Michael Rademacher[✉], Mathias Kretschmer, and Karl Jonas

Fraunhofer FOKUS, Sankt Augustin, Germany
{michael.rademacher,mathias.kretschmer,karl.jonas}@fokus.fraunhofer.de

Abstract. The lack of affordable broadband Internet connectivity in rural areas, especially in emerging regions, is seen as a major barrier for access to knowledge, education or government services. In order to reduce the costs of back-hauling in rural regions, often without access to a stable power grid, alternative solutions are required to provide high-bandwidth back-hauling at minimal power consumption to allow solar-powered operation. In this paper, we show that cost-effective low-power IEEE802.11n (MIMO) hardware together with a single cross-polarized antenna can be a viable solution to the problem. Our study shows that up to 200 Mbps of actual throughput can be achieved over distances larger than 10 km while the power consumption of a typical forwarding node is well below 10 Watts (http://wiback.org/repeater) - suitable for a cost-effective solar-powered operation. Through theoretical analysis and extensive measurements we show that such a low-cost setup can be used to establish reliable long-distance links providing high-bandwidth connectivity at low latencies and consequently providing the capacity demanded by today's services - everywhere. Exploiting these findings we are in the process of extending existing fiber-based infrastructures in rural Africa with our Wireless Back-Haul (WiBACK) architecture.

Keywords: IEEE 802.11n · MIMO · Long-distance · Wireless back-haul

1 Introduction

Operators in rural areas often face the challenge to support the bandwidth and QoS demands of today's on-line service offerings. While in urban areas back-hauling capacity can be increased at relatively low costs via a wire-line infrastructure, in rural areas wireless technologies are often the only affordable means to establish back-hauling connectivity. Especially in emerging regions, the potential lack of access to a stable power grid is another crucial factor regarding the CAPEX and OPEX considerations of candidate technologies.

In such scenarios, back-hauling networks are often built based on commercial-of-the-shelf IEEE802.11 WiFi technology, to due its relatively high capacity and a low energy footprint. Managed by Wireless Mesh Network (WMN)-style protocols such architectures, for example our carrier-grade WiBACK[1] architecture,

---

[1] http://www.wiback.org

© Institute for Computer Sciences, Social Informatics and Telecommunications Engineering 2014
T.F. Bissyandé and G. van Stam (Eds.): AFRICOMM 2013, LNICST 135, pp. 1–11, 2014.
DOI: 10.1007/978-3-319-08368-1_1

offer the potential to reduce CAPEX and OPEX tremendously due to their self-configuration and self-management features, thus providing a resilient and fault-tolerant network [1–3].

Legacy IEEE802.11a technology typically supports a maximum effective data rate of approximately 30 Mbps [4], which can easily become a bottle neck in the network, especially if triple-play services are to be supported. The more recent IEEE802.11n standard [5] promises a tremendous increase of the actual throughput by introducing more efficient Modulation and Coding Schemes (MCSs), frame aggregation and Multiple Input Multiple Output (MIMO) support. The main focus of the IEEE 802.11n standard is rather short distance communication and many devices with the ability of using those advanced features can already be found in consumer electronic devices.

The topology of a typical WiBACK scenario, however, is based on point-to-point links with distances reaching from a few hundred meters up to several kilometers defining a completely different scenario as intended by the IEEE standard. In this paper we explore the applicability of IEEE 802.11n for long-distance WiFi links and therefore as an option to increase the overall capacity inside a WiBACK network. Our major focus is on exploiting the capacity gains introduced by the MIMO capabilities using a single cross-polarized antenna, which would allow to a very cost-effective design of multi-radio forwarding nodes.

The remainder of the paper is structured as follows. In Sect. 2 we introduce related work and briefly summarize the main concepts of IEEE802.11n and MIMO including upcoming challenges with long distance links. Section 3 describes our experiments with long distance 802.11n MIMO links and their results which we conclude in Sect. 4.

2   Related Work and Background

In [6] experiments with long distance MIMO links focusing on polarized antennas[2] are presented. Using .11n draft 2.0 and a maximum link distance of 700 m, they show that polarized antennas improve MIMO for long distance and a maximum throughput of 60 Mbps was reached. In [7] the authors show that even for long distance MIMO links high ranked channel matrices are possible. The focus in [8] is the definition of a model describing the coverage and capacity of a .11n cell based approach. In [9] similar considerations about 802.11n links were done however, their results differ from ours. The maximum throughput reached was 40 Mbps exploiting all 802.11n features over 1.8 km and they measured a significant gradual decrease over the link distance. This throughput decrease seems to be related to a low SNR rather than to the applicability of 802.11n features on long distance links. To the best of our knowledge, no prior research has investigated the maximum possible throughput of IEEE802.11n MIMO long-distance links (>10 km) using a single cross-polarized antenna while taking QoS considerations into account.

---

[2] And the influence of the "Keyhole Effect".

2.1 Technology Enhancements of IEEE802.11n

Rather than summarizing the standard in general the purpose of the following section is to theoretically identify the main difference between .11a and .11n so previous knowledge about the concepts of WiFi is desirable. All following information are taken from the current standard itself [5] as well as [10].

Physical Layer. Regarding the main concepts of the PHY layer .11a and .11n use the same principles to ensure interoperability. However, 802.11n extends the concepts in every parameterizable value aiming at a throughput increase of the current maximum 54 Mbps as described in the following.

Although IEEE802.11a allocated a channel width of 20 MHz only 16.56 MHz are used divided into 53 subcarriers (0.3125 MHz each) with 48 of them containing data bits. IEEE802.11n exploits the 20 MHz more efficiently by adding two *additional* data *sub-carriers* on each side increasing the maximum physical throughput to 54 Mbps $* \frac{52}{48} = 58.5$ Mbps.

To detect a limited number of errors after the transmission .11a use convolutional codes with a maximum coding rate of 3/4. With less redundancy, 802.11n introduces an *additional coding rate* of 5/6 increasing the maximum physical data rate to 58.5 Mbps $* \frac{4}{3} * \frac{5}{6} = 65$ Mbps.

Intersymbol interference is an unwanted phenomena in telecommunications where one symbol interferes with subsequent ones. For IEEE802.11a one OFDM symbol last 4 μs consisting of 3.2 μs data and a guard period of 0.8 μs, .11n introduced the optional feature of a *shortened guard-interval* lasting 0.4 μs and decreasing the overall symbol duration to 3.6 μs and therefore increase the maximum throughput to 65 Mbps $* \frac{4}{3.6} = 72.2$ Mbps.

To overcome the limits proposed by the Shannon-Hartley theorem, the most obvious move to increase the throughput is to use a wider communication channel, while .11a defines a maximum *channel width* of 20 MHz[3] .11n allows to double this capacity to 40 MHz. Two direct 20 MHz neighbor channels can be bundled to overall 116 OFDM sub-carriers (108 containing data) increasing the maximum physical data rate to 72.2 Mbps $* \frac{108}{52} = 150$ Mbps.

All introduced enhancements in this sections apply equally to all lower 802.11n modulations as well and are, for the 802.11n case, called Modulation and Coding Scheme (MCS) labeled from zero to seven.

Medium Access Control Layer. After applying the high throughput enhancements to the physical layer, changes on the MAC layer were mandatory due to the poor scaling of throughput at the MAC layer, especially when using high physical data rates [10]. Some of the following MAC enhancement were already introduced by the IEEE802.11e standard nevertheless they are consistently extended for .11n.

Between every transmission a small period of time (SIFS - 16 μs) is added to ensure the receiver has the chance to sent an acknowledgement or other stations

---

[3] With the exception of the Atheros proprietary "Super-G" mode.

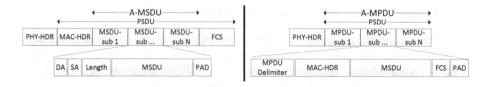

Fig. 1. Frame aggregation: A-MSDU and A-MPDU [11]

can apply for a transmission (back-off). Arbitration interframe spaces (AIFS) lead to the possibility of prioritizing traffic from different classes (i.e. voice over best effort) and Reduced Interframe spaces (RIFS - 2 μs) provide the possibility of a so called burst transmission (Fig. 1).

IEEE802.11n further increases the efficiency by surrendering inter-frame spaces between data frames leading to the main .11n MAC layer technique - *frame aggregation*. The standard distinguish between two different types of aggregation: the aggregate MAC protocol service unit (A-MSDU) and the aggregate MAC protocol data unit (A-MPDU) logically residing at the top (A-MSDU) or the bottom (A-MPDU) of the MAC layer [11]. The A-MPDU method aggregates completely formatted MAC frames including a MAC header for every sub-frame which consequently make the A-MSDU method more efficient. Both mechanisms share the same restriction that each sub-frame in one block has to share the same addresses and traffic class. For the A-MPDU case the *Block ACK protocol* efficiently confirms sub-frames through a bitmap to acknowledge or demand a retransmission.

Multiple Input Multiple Output. MIMO describes a system using a transmitter and receiver with multiple antennas communicating through a propagation environment [10]. Theoretically, MIMO promises an extraordinary increase in the capacity of wireless networks and has therefore drawn considerable attention in the last decade [7]. Although MIMO can be considered as a physical layer enhancements it is not limited to WiFi and a central issue in this report which justifies the approach in this separate section.

To understand the potential as well as the challenges of the MIMO signal transmission technique a further simplified communication channel model taken from [10] is given for a Single Input Single Output in Eq. 1 and for a 2×2 MIMO[4] system in Eq. 2.

$$y = h * x + z \tag{1}$$

$$\begin{pmatrix} y_1 \\ y_2 \end{pmatrix} = \begin{pmatrix} h_{11} & h_{12} \\ h_{21} & h_{22} \end{pmatrix} * \begin{pmatrix} x_1 \\ x_2 \end{pmatrix} + \begin{pmatrix} z_1 \\ z_2 \end{pmatrix} \tag{2}$$

These equations may be used to describe each OFDM sub-carrier in the frequency domain. Different approaches can be found in [7,10,12]. In this model x describes the transmitted, y the received signal and z is Additive White Gaussian

---

[4] Two transmitting and receiving antennas.

Noise (AWGN). Variable h is defined as the channel fading coefficient, a complex scalar element representing the gain and phase of the channel usually modeled as Rayleigh fading. A simplified but here still sufficient approach is to define fading as the attenuation deviation affecting the signal. Deviations occurs for example by geographical conditions, the used radio frequency or multi-path propagation. For the MIMO case (2) h_{ij} describes the fading coefficient occurring for the transmission from antenna i to j. To extract the wanted information x from the received signal y the receiver needs to challenge two main tasks. First the coefficients h_{ij} needs to be specified which is for .11n realized by the so called pilot based channel estimation where predefined symbols are attached in the beginning of every OFDM frame. The second task is rather mathematical but explains the main challenge for MIMO well. To extract the information, the matrix H needs to be inverted [10] which is only possible if the matrix is non-singular ($h_{ii} \neq h_{ij}$).

$$x = \widehat{x} - z * h^{-1} \tag{3}$$

$$\begin{pmatrix} x_1 \\ x_2 \end{pmatrix} = \widehat{\begin{pmatrix} x_1 \\ x_2 \end{pmatrix}} - z * \begin{pmatrix} h_{11} & h_{12} \\ h_{21} & h_{22} \end{pmatrix}^{-1} \tag{4}$$

This process is mathematical described through Eqs. 3 and 4 where $\widehat{X} = Y * H^{-1}$ describes the noisy estimate of the received signal[5]. From a practical point of view this means that the transmitted signal (x_1) needs to be received in a different way on every receiving antenna ($y_{1,2}$) to creat a non-singular channel matrix. This so called well conditioned matrix provides the possibility to distinguish between different streams from the MIMO transmission[6]. In an typical indoor environment this de-correlation of the signals mainly arise from rays bouncing from walls and obstacles as well as short distance between the antennas leading to randomly distributed coefficients [10].

To exploit the possibility of MIMO, different signal processing techniques are included in the latest WiFi standard [5] namely Maximal-Ratio Combining (MRC), Space-Time Bloc Coding (STBC) and Spatial Multiplexing where MRC and STBC offer a gain in diversity and only spatial multiplexing has the ability of increasing the maximum capacity of the channel, in theory, linear by the number of antennas located at transmitter and receiver. Spatial Multiplexing with two antennas leads to additional MCS numbered from 8 to 15 with modulations and codings accordingly to the SISO equivalent 0–7.

Long Distances. Following the theoretical considerations regarding MIMO, different options to exploit this technique for long distance WiFi links arise where the main challenge is the de-correlation of the streams to reach a throughput increase by spatial multiplexing. The first option is spatial antenna diversity in combination with high gain directional antennas. The disadvantage of this option is the large spacing needed between the two antennas which is relative to the

---

[5] We use capital letters to describe the SISO and MIMO case.
[6] We can describe Eqs. 2 and 4 as the solution to a system of linear equations.

distance between the receiver and the transmitter. In [7] a model predicting the spacing needed and in [6] practical examples are given but both conclude, that such a deployment is not practical also because of the need for long coaxial cable. The second option is the usage of two antennas where one points to a large obstacle to force a multi path propagation due to reflexions. The typical WiBACK use-case bar this option on the one hand due to the rural environment and on the other hand because of complex process of antenna pointing not suitable for untrained persons. The third option is the usage of a single antenna with the ability of sending two streams with different polarizations called *cross-polarized antennas*. Depending on the quality and kind of antenna, there is an attenuation *between* the two signals of approximately 20–30 dB. This attenuation should lead to sufficient de-correlation of the signals in a long-distance environment to enable MIMO operation to increase the maximum throughput. This option has no known practical disadvantage and only a minor affect on the costs of our network equipment (CAPEX)[7].

3   Measurements

To evaluate and compare the behavior of .11n techniques on long distances different test links have been set up and utilized. A short link in a laboratory environment using stubby antennas serves as reference to evaluate the long distance influence. Two different long distance links have been installed, both originating at the Fraunhofer Campus in Birlinghoven, Germany. The first link terminates with non-perfect[8] conditions and a distance of 5 km at tree nursery while the second ends with perfect propagation conditions 10.3 km away on a radio tower. All three links with exception of the radio tower[9] use the same hardware, a tailor-made embedded computer equipped with dual Intel Atom N2800 CPUs and three Ubiquity SR71 wireless cards based on the Atheros AR9280 chipset. Two different kinds of MIMO antennas were used - a Ubiquity Rocket Dish 5G30 offering enough gain for high modulations over 10.3 km and a Mars MA-WA56-DP25NB at both sides of the 5 km link. The operating System is Debian Squeeze using a modified kernel which is optimized for long distance links in terms of MAC layer timings, contention window sizes and transmission buffer to ensure that enough packets are available for A-MPDU aggregation. As wireless driver serves ath9k and the rate control algorithm is PID while most of the time a fixed rate is chosen to prevent instable performance as shown in [13]. Some test beforehand proofs that with two notable exception every 802.11n-enhancement is already implemented in the ath9k driver - short guard interval and A-MSDU aggregation are not available in ad hoc mode. All measurements were done using a tool called *80211Analyzer* developed at Fraunhofer FOKUS at the receiver and the *mgen* traffic generator at the transmitter. The *80211Analyzer* receives WiFi frames via the monitor device which is working parallel to the standard interface

---

[7] The price of the cross-polarized antenna is marginally higher.

[8] LOS with obstacles looming in the Fresnel Zone.

[9] Slower CPU: AMD Geode LX 800.

Table 1. Fixed parameters for all measurements

Parameter	Value (default)
Distance (ACK-Timeout and Slot)	5 km/10 km (0.3 km)
Chance to retry a packet	1(7)
Transport layer protocol	UDP
Payload	1450 Bytes
Packets per second	=Physical-rate/Payload

offering the ability to evaluate all lower packet headers as well as - after reordering - any possible retransmissions and losses. To ensure comparability Table 1 shows a fixed set of parameters used for all following measurements.

3.1 Results

Utilizing the three introduced test scenarios this section describes the performed experiments and their results. By stepwise enabling the .11n features introduced in Sect. 2.1 we are in the situation of evaluating their applicability for long distance links separately. Figure 2 shows the result for enabling the OFDM-enhancements as well as A-MPDU aggregation with a maximum size of 2^{16} byte. By stepwise increasing the Modulation and Coding Scheme (MCS) from 0–7 every minute the physical data rate increases to 65 Mbps. The MAC layer

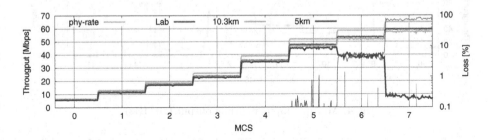

Fig. 2. OFDM-enhancements and A-MPDU

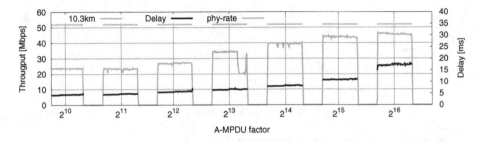

Fig. 3. Influence of the A-MPDU factor (fixed MCS 5)

aggregation successfully closes the gap between physical and real throughput induced in the .11a standard [14] by back-offs and inter-frame spaces so that the throughput for the laboratory and 10.3 km link raises simultaneously to 60 Mbps. A weak RSSI trough bad propagation conditions[10] causes that MCS 5 is the best rate for the 5 km link but the behavior for lower or equal to MCS 5 is identical to the other scenarios. To evaluate the inevitably increasing delay induced by aggregation we applied all available A-MPDU factors to the 10 km link as shown in Fig. 3. The first two A-MPDU factors have no difference in throughput and latency due to a large payload in combination with a MTU of 1470 byte. After that, the throughput increases with every doubling step of the A-MPDU factor. The increase is not linear, it is steep at the beginning and flattens at the end because of the fixed time for back-offs, IFS and block acknowledgments. As expected the latency rises with increasing A-MPDU factor which occurs due to the longer buffering of the packets before transmitting them in an aggregated way. While the relative throughput increase between the two highest A-MPDU factors is low, the increase in the latency is with 6 ms high in comparison, but also approximately computable[11]. Figure 4 pictures the applicability of cross polarized antennas to use .11n with spatial multiplexing. As described in Sect. 2.1 MIMO is a physical layer enhancement therefore loss is included in the plot instead of delay. It can be observed that the throughput

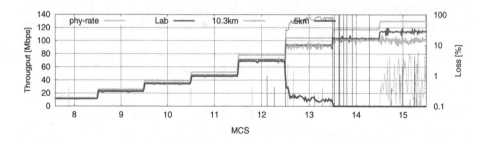

Fig. 4. Multiple input multiple output (20 MHz)

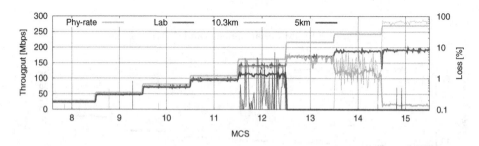

Fig. 5. 802.11n on long distance links

---

[10] This applies to all forthcoming measurements as well.

[11] $\frac{2^{15} byte}{40 Mbps} = 6.5\,ms.$

increased nearly by factor two using the aerials in the laboratory *as well as* the cross polarized antennas on the long distance links. This indicates that the cross polarized antennas are suitable for long distance .11n MIMO links. The attenuation between the two streams on different polarizations is sufficient to form a nearly perfect channel matrix, which is an unexpected result. By increasing the channel width to 40 MHz our last measurement provides a complete view using all available 802.11n enhancements at the same time. Figure 5 pictures that the throughput in the laboratory environment increases to nearly 200 Mbps. As mentioned, the hardware at the radio tower is older with less CPU power than the other systems. With the usage of MCS 14 the CPU was saturated and the *mgen* process failed creating the amount of packets needed for this data rate. Nevertheless, the throughput rises up to 170 Mbps over 10km using 802.11n and by evaluating the lower modulation there are no reasons to assume that 200 Mbps are not possible.

4   Conclusion

By exploiting the main features of the IEEE802.11n standard, the maximum actual throughput for a 10 km link inside our WiBACK network increases from 30 Mbps to 170 Mbps measured in a real scenario. Hence, our results indicate that, for our investigated use cases, the IEEE802.11n physical enhancements are also applicable to long-distance links. With such data rates we are able to provide a cost and energy efficient alternative to existing technologies, such as fixed microwave links, in wireless Back-Hauling. The main difference between the laboratory environment and the two real point-to-point links is the increased acknowledgement timeout, which results in a slightly lower throughput. Especially the usage of a single cross polarized antenna provides a very cost-effective solution for increasing the throughput by nearly 100 % without any changes to other QoS parameters such as latency. Doubling the bandwidth to 40 MHz would have the same effect, but is often discouraged due to possible interferences with other links within the scarce frequency spectrum. Additional key features are the newly introduced MAC layer using packet aggregation and selective block ACKs. Considering the latency, this feature has the disadvantage of increasing the airtime of an aggregated frame, which may cause medium access latencies for concurrent traffic. However, the queuing time is predictable and packet aggregation is controllable in several ways by setting the A-MPDU factor and by enabling this feature just for certain traffic classes.

4.1   Future Work

Optimizing parameters such as back-off timings, AIFS for traffic class separation as well as various queue lengths is the next important step to further increase the Quality of Service and thereby the user experience in our WiBACK network. This optimization should be based on a traffic mix including different packet sizes, acknowledgments and face challenges occurring with protocols like TCP. We plan to apply the findings of this paper to sub-GHz WiFi (i.e. TVWS, 802.11ah) to increase the efficiency of this high potential frequency ranges.

Analytical Model. To perform this optimization we are currently evaluating, exploiting and extending different analytical models describing the IEEE802.11 MAC layer such as the one by Bianchi [15]. Describing our point-to-point links with an accurate model will provide us besides the optimization with the opportunity of a centralized capacity estimation of our network.

Acknowledgment. This work has been funded by the Federal Ministry of Education and Research of the Federal Republic of Germany (Förderkennzeichen 01 BU 1116, SolarMesh - Energieeffizientes, autonomes großflächiges Sprach- und Datenfunknetz mit flacher IP- Architektur). The authors alone are responsible for the content of this paper.

References

1. Kretschmer, M., Batroff, P., Niephaus, C., Ghinea, G.: Topology discovery and maintenance for heterogeneous wireless Back-Haul networks supporting unidirectional technologies. In: 17th Asia-Pacific Conference on Communications (APCC 2011), Kota Kinabalu, Sabah, Malaysia, Oct 2011
2. Henkel, D., Englaender, S., Kretschmer, M., Niephaus, C.: Connecting the unconnected - economical constraints and technical requirements towards a Back-Haul network for rural areas. In: IEEE Globecom 2011 Workshop on Rural Communications-Technologies, Applications, Strategies and Policies (RuralComm 2011) (GC'11 Workshop - RuralComm), Houston, Texas, USA, Dec 2011
3. Kretschmer, M., Niephaus, C., Ghinea, G.: A wireless back-haul architecture supporting dynamic broadcast and white space coexistence. In: ICCCN 2012 Workshops: 6th International Workshop on Wireless Mesh and Ad Hoc Networks (WiMAN) (WiMAN 2012), Munich, Germany, July 2012
4. Xiao, Y., Rosdahl, J.: Throughput and delay limits of IEEE 802.11. IEEE Commun. Lett. **6**(8), 355–357 (2002)
5. IEEE Std 802.11-2012 (Revision of IEEE Std 802.11-2007), pp. 1–2793, Feb 2012
6. Vella, J., Zammit, S.: Performance improvement of long distance mimo links using cross polarized antennas. In: MELECON 2010–2010 15th IEEE Mediterranean Electrotechnical Conference, pp. 1287–1292 (2010)
7. Gesbert, D., Bolcskei, H., Gore, D., Paulraj, A.: Outdoor mimo wireless channels: models and performance prediction. IEEE Trans. Commun. **50**, 1926–1934 (2002)
8. Ting, A., Chieng, D., Kwong, K.-H.: Capacity and coverage analysis of rural multi-radio multi-hop network deployment using IEEE802.11n radios. In: 2011 IEEE 10th Malaysia International Conference on Communications (MICC), pp. 77–82 (2011)
9. Paul, U., Crepaldi, R., Lee, J., Lee, S.-J., Etkin, R.: Characterizing wifi link performance in open outdoor networks. In: 2011 8th Annual IEEE Communications Society Conference on Sensor, Mesh and Ad Hoc Communications and Networks (SECON), pp. 251–259 (2011)
10. Perahia, E., Stacey, R.: Next Generation Wireless LANs - Throughput, Robustness, and Reliability in 802.11n, 1st corrected edn. Cambridge University Press, Cambridge (2010)

11. Skordoulis, D., Ni, Q., Chen, H.-H., Stephens, A., Liu, C., Jamalipour, A.: IEEE 802.11n mac frame aggregation mechanisms for next-generation high-throughput wlans. IEEE Wirel. Commun. **15**, 40–47 (2008)
12. Tse, D., Viswanath, P.: Fundamentals of Wireless Communication. Cambridge University Press, New York (2005)
13. Kretschmer, M., Horstmann, T., Batroff, P., Rademacher, M., Ghinea, G.: Link calibration and property estimation in self-managed wireless back-haul networks. In: 2012 18th Asia-Pacific Conference on Communications (APCC), pp. 232–237 (2012)
14. IEEE Std 802.11-2007 (Revision of IEEE Std 802.11-1999), pp. C1–1184, Dec 2007
15. Bianchi, G.: Performance analysis of the IEEE 802.11 distributed coordination function. IEEE J. Sel. Areas Commun. **18**(3), 535–547 (2000)

Review of Power Line Communications Standards in Africa

A.R. Ndjiongue, A.J. Snyders, Hendrick C. Ferreira, and S. Rimer[✉]

Faculty of Engineering and the Built Environment, University of Johannesburg,
P.O. Box 524, Auckland Park, Johannesburg 2006, South Africa
{ndjiongue,ajsnyders,hcferreira,suvendic}@uj.ac.za

Abstract. The standards in power line communications (PLC) calibrate parameters such as frequencies allocation, signal level, security, topology of the network and many others parameters. The leap forward of power line communications technology is motivated by the willingness of the standardization organizations (SDO)s such as ITU, IEC, ISO, IEEE, CENELEC to define how the technologies are going to be deployed. This paper presents the different SDOs, Alliances and groups regulating the PLC sector. The interoperability and coexistence for some technologies are underlined. The process of developing PLC standards by ITU, IEEE 1901, CENELEC is described. The advantages and disadvantages of using PLC technology in Africa are discussed.

Keywords: Standards · SDOs · Alliances · Technologies · PLC · Communication · Frequency

1 Introduction

To provide efficient transparent communication over the power line network, standards are fundamental. A standard is a document providing rules requirements and guidelines for a product, process and services [1, 2]. The document is prepared and produced by the standardization organizations (SDOs). In power line communications (PLC), the SDOs focus on the physical (PHY) and on the data link (DLL) layers as shown on Fig. 1. The other layers are reserved for the application. The power line communications technology shares some regulations with the wired based communication technologies such as telephone wire.

Power line communications is characterized by two regulated segments named narrow band power line communications (NBPLC) and broad band power line communications (BBPLC). BBPLC deals with frequencies above 1 MHz while NBPLC deals with frequencies less than 500 kHz. The range of frequencies between 3 kHz and 145.8 kHz is regulated by the European committee for electrotechnical standardization (CENELEC) [3, 4]. It is suitable for low data transmission over power line. It is possible to deploy high data transmission over NBPLC in the range of frequencies between 145.3 kHz and 478.125 kHz, which corresponds to the second frequency band of the federal communication commission (FCC) [5]. This paper presents in Sect. 2 the repartition of the frequencies between SDOs. Forthwith, some applications of power line communications for both NBPLC and BBPLC are

© Institute for Computer Sciences, Social Informatics and Telecommunications Engineering 2014
T.F. Bissyandé and G. van Stam (Eds.): AFRICOMM 2013, LNICST 135, pp. 12–21, 2014.
DOI: 10.1007/978-3-319-08368-1_2

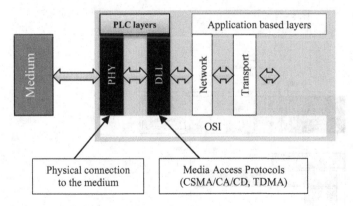

Fig. 1. Illustration of the PLC layers

presented in Sect. 3. The Sect. 4 talks about coexistence of standards and interoperability between technologies. Section 5 gives the advantages and disadvantages of PLC technology in African context.

2 Frequency Allocation Chart

The international telecommunication union (ITU), the international organization for standardization (ISO), the international electrotechnical commission (IEC), the institute of electrical and electronics engineers (IEEE) and CENELEC are the main SDOs that develop and propose standards in communication sector. G3-PLC, Powerline intelligent metering evolution (PRIME), the american national standards institute (ANSI), KNX and HOMEPLUG are some groups and alliances that develop and deploy standards and technologies in power line communications sector. These SDOs, groups and alliances are characterized by their frequency band. Some work on NBPLC while others are on BBPLC. SDOs such as IEEE and ITU are proposing standards and technologies for both NBPLC and BBPLC. The authors analyzed the frequency band of each SDO and alliance and the summary of the bands occupied are presented on Fig. 2. The IEEE organization proposes for NBPLC to work in the range of frequencies between 9 kHz and 500 kHz [6]. The ITU organization works on the range of frequencies from 3 kHz to 490 kHz, while CENELEC proposes the frequencies between 3 kHz and 148.5 kHz. Over BBPLC, IEEE works on the range of frequencies between 2 MHz and 50 MHz while the ITU organization proposes a wider range of frequencies: from 2 MHz to 100 MHz [7, 8]. The CENELEC organization does not work on BBPLC [2, 9]. G3-PLC, PRIME, ANSI and KNX propose technologies using the CENELEC's frequency bands. G3-PLC works on the range between 35 kHz–90 kHz while PRIME alliance uses the frequency band 42 kHz–90 kHz. ANSI proposes technologies for the frequencies from 86 kHz–131 kHz and KNX works with the band of frequencies between 125 kHz to 140 kHz [10]. HomePlug is present over the whole PLC's frequency band. It proposes HomePlug Green PHY (HPGH NB), standards and technologies over narrow band occupying the

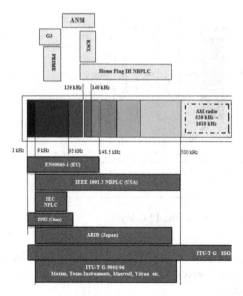

a Frequencies between 3 kHzand 2 MHz

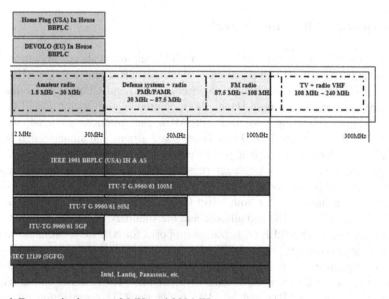

b Frequencies between 2 MHzand 300 MHz

Fig. 2. Power line communications frequencies allocation by SDOs, alliances and groups

range of frequencies between 120 kHz and 400 kHz. HomePlug also proposes HomePlug Green PHY (HPGP BB) and HomePlug AV (HPAV) using the frequency band 1.8 MHz to 30 MHz [11]. HomePlug AV2 technologies extends the HPAV's frequencies to 86 MHz [10, 12]. HPGP BB differs from HPAV on the modulation schemes used, the forward error correction (FEC) methods and the access modes [10].

The IEEE 1901-2010 standard uses the frequencies between 2 MHz and 50 MHz. The IEEE 1901.2 provides standards for low frequency, less than 500 kHz, narrow band power line communications for smart grid applications. Its uses the frequency band 10 kHz–490 kHz for low and high data transmission [6]. The ITU organization separates standards for the physical layer (PHY) and for the data link layer (DLL). It proposes a technology named ITU-T G.hnem for NBPLC. The ITU-T G.9955 standard specifies the regulations for PHY while the ITU-T G.9956 standard gives rules for DLL [8]. The technology proposed by the ITU organization on BBPLC is ITU-T G.hnem. The ITU-T G.hnem complies with two different standards: The ITU-T G.9960 standard developed for PHY layer and the ITU-T G.9961 standard proposed for DLL. The ITU organization on BBPLC specifies a platform for smart grid (2 MHz to 30 MHz), it also gives specifications to differentiate between two cases: when the distance between two modules is greater than 50 m (2 MHz to 50 MHz) and when the distance is greater than 100 m (2 MHz to 100 MHz) [8]. The CENELEC organization is composed of many technical bodies. One of them is in charge of developing EN50065-1 standard (Signaling on low-voltage electrical installations in the frequency range 3 kHz to 148.5 kHz - Part 1: General requirements, frequency bands and elec-tromagnetic disturbances) [3, 4]. The EN50065-1 standard divides its frequency band in 4 sub-bands [3, 4]: CENELEC-A (3 kHz–95 kHz), reserved exclusively for energy providers, and respectively CENELEC B-C-D (95 kHz–125 kHz; 125 kHz–140 kHz and 140 kHz–148.5 kHz). The CENELEC B-C-D sub-bands are opened for end user applications. The 2010's version of the EN50065-1 is superseded by the EN50065-1: 2011. The EN50065-1: 2011 standard was ratified on 2011-03-21; it was available on 2011-04-22, announced on 2011-09-21 and published on 2012-03-21 [13].

The CENELEC organization shares some information with the international electrotechnical commission (IEC), with the european committee for standardization (CEN) and with the european telecommunication standards institute (ETSI). Some PLC's projects under IEC are developed in collaboration with the international organization for standardization (ISO).

The IEC NBPLC's standards propose to work between 3 kHz and 76 kHz [6]. The special international committee on radio interference (CISPR) acting under IEC gives the limits of the interferences. The disturbances limits for PLC systems are defined by the CISPR22 standard. The electric power research institute (EPRI) organization in China prefers the range between 3 kHz and 90 kHz while the FCC organization in USA works over the range from 10 kHz to 490 kHz [14]. The association of radio industries and businesses (ARIB) organization in Japan proposes the ARIB STD – TB4 standard, using the range between 10 kHz and 450 kHz. In Canada, the inter-ference causing equipment standard (ICES) proposes ICES – 006 standards working in the range of frequencies between 0 and 535 kHz [15]. The transmission level for all the standards is compatible with the graph proposed on Fig. 3. It is proposed by the CENELEC and the FCC organizations [3, 4]. In NBPLC frequency bands, the ITU-T G.hnem and the IEEE P1901.2 technologies, ANSI, HomePlug, PRIME, ISO and IEC use the signal level proposed in EN50065-1 by the CENELEC organization, they use FCC's signal level when the frequency is out of the CENELEC's range of fre-quencies. In certain applications, the IEC standards use exclusively the CENELEC's

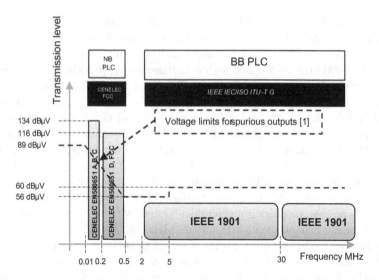

Fig. 3. Transmission level spurious output [3, 4]

transmission level. The standards' elaboration methods within the main IDOs were analysed by the authors and the summary is presented on Fig. 4.

3 Applications of Power Line Communications

The applications of power line communications technologies cover the whole axis of frequencies proposed in Fig. 2. In accordance with the application, the axis is divided into three portions as indicated in Fig. 5. Any portion is suitable for some specific applications.

The broad band PLC uses the frequency band between 1 MHz and 300 MHz. It is suitable for high data rate transmission, more than 10 Mbps. The NBPLC's portion uses the CENELEC bands for low data rate transmission, less than 50 kbps. Over the frequencies from 145.3 kHz to 500 kHz, the NBPLC's technologies are used to perform high data rate transmission between 50 kbps and 1 Mbps. Thereby, the applications of the power line communications technology are related to the frequency band used. The applications of BBPLC can not be deployed over NBPLC frequencies. The deployment of the technology over each range of frequencies is supported by many companies and organisations. Table 1 gives some specifications on the application of the power line communications technology. It shows the frequency band, some modulation schemes proposed by the SDOs for both NBPLC and BBPLC. The complexity of the forward error correction (FEC), the access method and some companies and organisations supporting the standards are also mentioned.

The NBPLC frequency bands are used for metering, lighting, energy and grid management.

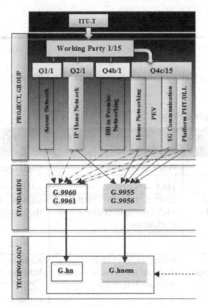

a: Building up for ITU-T G.hn and G.hnem

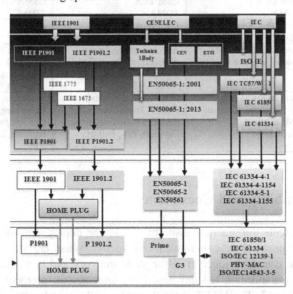

b: Building up for IEEE1901, CENELEC and IEC

Fig. 4. PLC standards building up

The BBPLC frequency band is used for applications such as last mile telecom, voice over IP and high definition television. Companies such as Gorlitz and alliances such as G3-PLC, PRIME are specialised in meter manufacturing. The KNX organisation is the standard for home and building control.

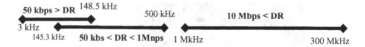

Fig. 5. Data rate (DR) repartition over PLC frequencies

Table 1. Applications of PLC [6, 9, 12, 15, 16]

	NBPLC		BBPLC
	Low data rate	High data rate	High data rate
frequency	3 – 148.5 kHz	145.3 – 478.125kHz	1 MHz–300 MHz
Modulation and coding	FSK , BPSK, FFH (Fast frequency hopping), SFSK (dual ch/spread FSK), DCSK diff chirp shift keying	DBPSK, DQPSK, OFDM MCM multiple carrier modulation	MCM/COFDM Bit loading
FEC	Low complexity and reliability *(RS + Convolutional)*	Strong, high reliability designed *(RS + Convolutional, Differential coding)*	Medium Maximum throughput *(Convolutional Turbo Code CTC for FFT Concatenated Reed-Solomon and Convolutional code for WAVELET)*
Access	CSMA/CA TDMA	CSMA/CA TDMA	CSMA/CA TDMA
Transport layer	IPv6, IPv4, Ethernet I EC62056	IPv6, IPv4, Ethernet I EC62056	IPv6
Application	Automatic Meter AMR Power Line Area Network	Airfield lighting, Energy management, Smart Grid application and metering, AMR/AMR	Last Mile Telecom (LMT}, Internet, VoIP, IH networking, High definition TV (HDTV) ...
Companies and organisations	Bush Jaeger, Echelon, Gorlitz, Ytran, Renesos, AMI solution, Landis&Gyr ...	ADD Grup, iAd, Maxim, PRIME, landis&Gyr, G3, ANSY, STMicroelectronic, Usyscom, Ziv , Philips KNX...	Amperiom, Current, DS2, Home plug, Mitsubishi, OPERA, Panasonic, Spidcom, Devolo...

4 Interoperability and Coexistence

This section presents the practical issue related to the deployment of standards and technologies in power line communications sector. What are the standards and technologies that can work together in the same network and in the same frequency band? The ITU organisation has developed the inter system protocol (ISP) scheme named ITU-T G.9972. The ITU-T G.9972 standard allows at least four technologies simultaneously [10]. The recommendations of ITU were accepted by some other organisations such as IEEE. The IEEE organisation has developed the IEEE 2030 standard for smart grid interoperability. The IEEE 1901.2 devices integrate the interoperability option for PRIME and G3 legacy specifications. Those devices must implement CENELEC A band [16].

The coexistence must be seen as the ability of more than one technology, network, system or device to exchange data and to be able to use the information exchanged.

In NBPLC frequency bands, technologies must develop mechanism to coexist with other narrow band technologies. The ITU-T G.9972 standard developed by the ITU organisation is in compliance with the coexistence as defined above. Within the IEEE organisation, the compliance and interoperability working group work (C & I WG) discusses the same issue. HomePlug alliance complies with the rules and regulations of coexistence and interoperability defined by C & IWG. It produces technologies and products that coexist and interoperate with other standards. This shows that the IEEE organisation complies with the recommendation acts G.9972 of the ITU organisation.

5   PLC Technology in African Context

The ITU organisation divides the world's communication by regions. Africa falls under ITU region I. Therefore, african countries align their frequency allocations with those specified for ITU region I [17]. In South Africa, the radio communication regulations are required by the electrical contractors association (ECA). It is compulsory for the companies proposing services to comply with the telecommunication laws. They must also comply with the rules and regulations of the independent communications authority of South Africa (ICASA). The african organisations look at a PLC's cost effective networking for the grid. Most of the devices are based on the Homeplug PLC standards, allowing different devices from different manufacturers to talk to each other. Companies such as INOVATECH are proposing high speed power line communications (HSPLC) services. They propose solutions for energy management such as real time monitoring, detection, measurement and waveform capture, remote automation and support for prepaid. Nexans proposes solutions for smart grid applications. In Ghana, CACTEL, the United Kingdom PLC's company carried out a series of communication demonstration over power lines. The tests were performed in collaboration with the telecommunication company and the electricity company of Ghana. CACTEL has successfully demonstrated the use of an automated meter reading (AMR) technology [18]. Goal technology solutions (GTS) is spreading power line communications technologies over the african countries such as South Africa, Uganda and Kenya. This shows that PLC in Africa is under way.

6   Conclusion

The description and the presentation of the standards governing power line communications technology was the purpose of this paper. The main SDOs were presented for both NBPLC and BBPLC frequency bands. The standard building up was also presented for the main SDOs. Some lines were written on the applications of power line communications technology. One point discussed the coexistence and the interoperability of several technologies. It is important to emphasise the fact that, even with the plethora of standards leading power line communications, there is still a gap. The effectiveness of the coexistence and the interoperability between technologies needs to be taken into serious consideration by the standardisation organisations and alliances. It is also very important for the manufacturers to comply with the CISPR limits. Africa was presented as the late comer in the power line communications area. The products proposed to the african countries are usually developed under others countries' regulations given the fact that the manufacturers are not based in Africa. It is then fundamental to rise in Africa organisations such as the south african radio league (SARL) to adapt international regulations to the african context.

Acknowledgment. This work is based on research supported in part by NRF and by the ESKOM Tertiary Education Support Programme (TESP), reference number 264030.

References

1. Tietje, E.D., III: International standards for the appraisal of wave energy converters. MTS/ IEEE Biloxi-Marine Technology for Our Future: Global and Local Challenges, OCEANS'09, pp. 1–5, 26–29 October 2009
2. Draft Standard for PoweRline Intelligent Metering Evolution (PRIME), 1.3A ed., PRIME Alliance Technical Working Group, May 2010. http://www.prime-alliance.org/portals/0/specs/PRIME-spec_v1%203%20E_201005.pdf
3. CENELEC.: Signaling on low voltage installations in frequency range 3 kHz to 148.5 kHz - Part 1, General requirements, frequency-bands and Electromagnetic Disturbance. IHS, CENELEC FPREN 50056-1, September 2010
4. Boraboi, B.: Narrow Band Power Line Communication, Applications and Challenges. Ariane Controls Inc, Québec (2013)
5. Encyclopedia Radio Spectrum. http://www.fcc.gov/encyclopedia/radio-spectrum-allocation
6. IEEE P1901 Working Group. Official web site. IEEE Standards Association. Retrieved 21 July 2011
7. Pokrzywa, J., Reidy, M.: SAE's J1772 'combo connector' for AC and DC changing advances with IEEE's help. SAE International. Retrieved 12 August 2011
8. G.9972, Coexistence mechanism for wire line home networking transceivers. ITU-T, November 2011
9. Hoch, M.: Comparison of PLC G3 and PRIME. 15th IEEE Symposium on Power Line Communications and Its Applications, pp. 165–169, Udine, Italy, 3–6 April 2011
10. Logvinov, O.: Netricity PLC and the IEEE P1901.2 Standard. HomePlug Power Line Alliance
11. Jordan Cordova, C.E.P., Asare-Bediako, B., Vanalme, G.M.A., Kling, W.L.: Overview and comparison of leading communication standard technologies for smart home area networks enabling energy management systems. 46th International Universities' Power Engineering Conference (UPEC'11), Soest, Germany, 5–8 September 2011
12. HomePlug/Panasonic Merged Proposal Takes the First Step in Becoming a Worldwide Standard through the Efforts of the IEEE P1901 Work Group. News release (HomePlug Powerline Alliance). 30 October 2007. Retrieved 23 July 2011
13. Standard Evolution Forcast. http://www.cenelec.eu/dyn/www/f?p=104:74:3282435438878299
14. Ferreira, H.C., Lampe, L., Newbury, J., Swart, T.G. (eds.): Power Line Communications. Wiley, Chichester (2010)
15. De Lima Fernandes, A., Dave, P.: Power Line Communications in Energy Markets. Cypress Semiconductor Corporation. Industrial Control Design Line August 2011

16. Galli, S.: G.hnem status update. IEEE ISPLC 2011. PLC Standardization Panel, Udine, Italy, 5 April 2011
17. ICASA.: Government Gazette, 22 July 2008, No 31264
18. Balancing Act Africa. http://www.balancingact-africa.com/news/en/issue-no-273/internet/cactel-successfully/en

Simulation of Wireless Sensor Node Transmission Over a Multiple Access Channel

Katleho Kanyane, Babu Sean Paul, Suvendi Rimer$^{(\boxtimes)}$, and Khmaies Ouahada

Department of Electrical Engineering, University of Johannesburg,
Johannesburg, South Africa
kkanyane@gmail.com, suvendic@uj.ac.za

Abstract. Smart Grids are emerging as a sustainable technology that can greatly improve the quality, cost and efficiency of electrical power distribution. Wireless communication technology, in particular wireless sensor networks, are being considered as a viable solution to Smart Grid communication requirements. Homes have multiple electrical appliances that may communicate concurrently. In addition, electrical appliances induce white noise that can interfere with the wireless signal. In this paper an indoor wireless sensor multiple access communication environment is simulated based on the IEEE 802.15.4 wireless communication standard. An indoor wireless propagation model is implemented and the effects of signal interference on the wireless signal are examined.

Keywords: Smart Grid · Wireless sensor networks · IEEE 802.15.4 · Wireless channel · Wireless interference · Indoor path loss model

1 Introduction

An electric grid having smart capability allows the power providers, distributors, and consumers to maintain a near real-time awareness of one anothers operating requirements and capabilities. Through this awareness, the Smart Grid is able to produce, distribute, and consume power in the most efficient and intelligent way. Two-way digital communication is an important enabling technology to Smart Grids [1].

Currently, most residential energy usage is from appliances used for lighting, cooking, indoor temperature control (such as heating or cooling systems), washing, and drying and entertainment purposes. Wireless sensor nodes connect equipment such as television, washing machines, etc., to a home are network (HAN) gateway (or coordinator), which in turn communicates with a larger smart grid network infrastructure. Wireless sensor nodes in a HAN would be used to collect user data and relay it to a local coordinator node [2]. The gateway node would gather the data from different wireless nodes and forward it to the power utility company for processing. In this environment several wireless sensors and gateways would be deployed.

© Institute for Computer Sciences, Social Informatics and Telecommunications Engineering 2014
T.F. Bissyandé and G. van Stam (Eds.): AFRICOMM 2013, LNICST 135, pp. 22–26, 2014.
DOI: 10.1007/978-3-319-08368-1_3

The wireless signal between the sensor node and the gateway will experience fading and interference as well as attenuation due to transmission through multiple inner walls. In addition, wireless nodes from closely spaced homes (such as apartment buildings), may be communicating simultaneously to their respective gateway node. A suitable channel access method must be selected to ensure reliable real-time communication between then nodes.

In this paper a Matlab simulation is used to investigate the propagation effects of an unmanaged multiple access channel to further understand the constraints imposed on the selection of the multiple access technique to use in wireless sensor networks deployed in Smart Grids.

Section 2 explains the design of the Matlab simulation of the wireless sensor network. The results and analysis of the results are documented in Sect. 3. The paper ends with a Conclusion in Sect. 4.

2   Algorithm Design

The scenario simulated consists of a group of nodes, where each node is located in a different room and 8 m apart from its nearest neighbour. The simulation considers the case where all the nodes are transmitting at the same time. A situation where each node in the network transmits to a single node may occur where each node transmits directly to a single sink node during the contention period in TDMA. The communication between two nodes in this environment is simulated and analysed. Only the physical layer baseband communication is considered. It is assumed that each node is transmitting at the same frequency. The simulation is developed for 2×6 residential apartment with each node located at the centre of each room.

The simulation is based on the IEEE 802.15.4 specification in the Industrial, Medical and Scientific (ISM) 2.4 GHz frequency band. The minimum transmit power is set to 33 dB according to the Texas Instruments data sheet for a 2.4 GHz IEEE 802.15.4 ZigBee RF transceiver [3]. The channel access method used is TDMA.

The simulation begins by generating a binary signal with bit values of -1 and 1. The gain of the transmitter is then applied to the signal and transmitted over the channel.

The signal power at the receiver P in dB, is calculated by taking the transmitter power P over the path loss L The power loss over the transmitted distance is computed using the ITU Indoor Path Loss model in the 2.4 GHz frequency band shown in Eq. (1) [4].

$$L_{total} = 20 \log_{10} f + N \log_{10} d + L_f(n) - 28. \tag{1}$$

$$P_{r(dB)} = \frac{P_{t(dB)}}{L_{total}}. \tag{2}$$

The simulation first calculates the bit error rate of the received signal as a function of the signal to noise ratio at node 1 when node 2 is only transmitting with the path loss and noise being computed at the receiver. Then the signals from 6 adjacent nodes, at the same distance as the transmitter node are factored in by using Eq. (1) and increasing the power of the interfering signal by the same signal power as the single node interfering power.

3   Results and Discussion

1000 messages with 1000 bits were generated as the input message. Each message was compared with its corresponding received message and the bit error rate was computed. The bit error rate was calculated for signal to noise ratios from 1 to 30 dB. Figures 1 and 2 are the plots of the bit error rate (BER) versus the

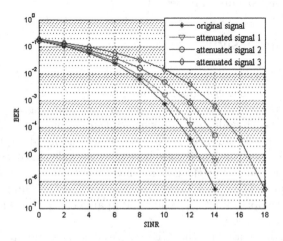

Fig. 1. Bit error rate versus SINR for increasing interfering signal strength

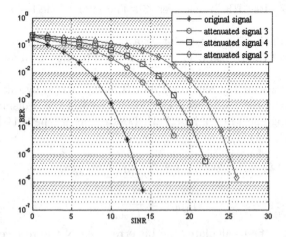

Fig. 2. BER vs SINR

signal to noise ratio at the receiver for the signal at the receiver for the different interference powers.

In Figs. 1 and 2 the bit error rate improved as a function of the signal to noise ratio. Even at very low SINR, the effect of interfering signal is noticeable Fig. 1, where the probability of error increases from 0.15 for no interference to 0.2 for 6 interfering signals at 0 dB. A plot of the bit error rate versus the number of

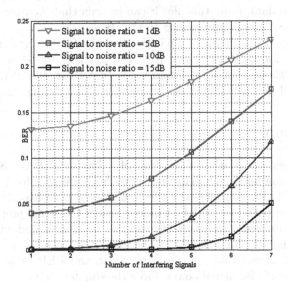

Fig. 3. Bit error rate versus number of interfering signals with plot for signal to noise ratios 1 dB, 5 dB, 10 dB and 15 dB

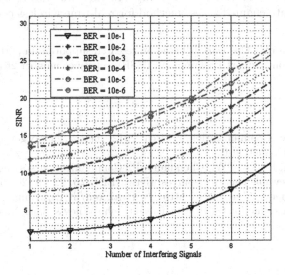

Fig. 4. Change in the SINR versus the number of interfering signals

interfering signals was generated from the experimental data to investigate the effect of increasing interference on the bit error rate. Figure 3 shows the bit error rate deteriorates as more interfering signals are present. It can also be seen that the rate at which the BER deteriorates increases non-linearly with the number of interfering signals. Figure 4 is the plot of the change in the SINR versus the number of interfering signals. This plot was generated by setting the BER to a fixed value and computing the SNR values for different interfering signals from the experimental data. From this plot it can be seen that increases to the signal to noise ratio yield less improvements to the BER.

There is only a maximum of 1.65 dB difference for bit error rates of 10^{-4} and 10^{-5} while for BER 10^{-2} and 10^{-3} the maximum difference is 2.95 dB. The graph also shows that to maintain a constant BER, the SNR increase per interfering signal becomes higher as the number of interfering signals increases.

4 Conclusion

This paper presents a Matlab simulation of a baseband IEEE 802.15.4 wireless communication between wireless nodes with interference from neighbouring nodes. The simulation considers the effects of indoor path loss through the use of the ITU indoor path loss model for indoor residential signal propagation. The effects of the interference from adjacent nodes are investigated with respect to the signal to noise ratio and the bit error rate at the receiver.

The analysis shows that the degradation to the BER is non-linear with respect to the interfering signal power. From the simulation it can be seen that to maintain a required BER, the increase in the signal to noise ratio was non-linear.

From the Matlab simulation it is shown that for a small 7 node wireless network, the effects of interference are large, further illustrating the requirement for an appropriate channel access method for real-time wireless communication.

Acknowledgement. This work is based on research supported in part by the Eskom Tertiary Education Support Programme (TESP), reference number 264030.

References

1. Litos Stategic Communication, March 2012. http://energy.gov/oe/downloads/smart-grid-introduction-0
2. Yu, F., Zhang, P., Xiao, W., Choudhury, P.: Communication systems for grid integration of renewable energy resources. Netw. IEEE **25**, 22–29 (2011)
3. Texas Instruments, March 2013. http://www.ti.com/lit/ds/symlink/cc2420.pdf
4. Seybold, J.: Introduction to RF Propagation. John Wiley & Sons, New Jersey (2005)

Communication Costs and Trade
in Sub Saharan Africa: A Gravity Approach

Evans Mupela[1](✉) and Adam Szirmai[2]

[1] HSRC, 134 Pretorius Street, Pretoria 0002, South Africa
emupela@yahoo.com, emupela@hsrc.ac.za
[2] UNU-MEIT, 19 Keizer Kareplein, Maastricht, The Netherlands
szirmai@merit.unu.edu

Abstract. This paper investigates the effects of connectivity charges (communication costs) on bilateral exports in Sub Saharan Africa (SSA). Data from 19 exporter countries was used together with communication costs data in a gravity model of trade setup. The export data derive from the IMF Direction of Trade and the COMTRADE databases, while the communication cost data was collated from a variety of sources including direct contact with service providers. We find that communication cost is an important factor in bilateral trade in the region. Communications have a significant negative effect on export intensity. The study also reveals that countries with high communication costs generally have lower export intensity than countries with low communication costs. The results suggest that investment in ICT infrastructure that brings down international communication costs will have a positive effect on regional trade in the long run.

Keywords: Trade · Gravity equation · Communication cost · Connectivity · Export

1 Introduction

Communication costs are an important aspect of the barriers to trade often referred to as trade costs. These are costs that have to be overcome in order to actualize a trade transaction or more formally stated: Trade costs are "all costs incurred in getting a good to a final user other than the cost of producing the good itself" [1] The higher these costs are, the more difficult it is to carry out trade and the smaller the volume of trade. Some of the more often researched barriers to trade are transport costs, exchange rates, freight charges and border related trade barriers. The impact of the cost of information gathering and transmission of messages has often been neglected or has been subsumed under transport costs or border related trade barriers. It is however important to model these costs separately as the share of services in world trade has increased dramatically over the last two decades and advances in information and communication technology (ICT) have made distance less important in the setup of trade transactions. A steady reduction in communication costs has resulted in a dramatic shrinkage of the time and space barriers which inhibit economic exchange over vast distances [2, 3].

© Institute for Computer Sciences, Social Informatics and Telecommunications Engineering 2014
T.F. Bissyandé and G. van Stam (Eds.): AFRICOMM 2013, LNICST 135, pp. 27–38, 2014.
DOI: 10.1007/978-3-319-08368-1_4

These developments have led researchers to take communication costs more seriously and treat them differently from transportation costs, which largely constitute the costs involved in getting a finished product from point A to point B.

Harris (1995) points out three reasons why communication costs are different from transport costs and why they should be treated differently [4]. One of the major differences according to Harris, is that from a supply point of view, communication costs, as opposed to transport costs are almost always a fixed cost, because the marginal cost of transmitting a message once the network is in place is zero. This is in contrast to Samuelson's iceberg model [5] used for transport costs, where part of the good is assumed to 'melt away' in the course of transportation. However, It is important to take cognizance of the fact that this refers to the supply side of the equation and that from the demand side communication costs are still a variable cost. While suppliers of communication infrastructure may not necessarily incur marginal costs for transmitting messages between users, they charge users for using the infrastructure based on either time or the amount of bandwidth transmitted.

Secondly, the natural monopoly and public good properties present in communication networks are another reason to consider these costs separately. Although the non-rivalry aspect of public goods is present in most communication networks, excludability is easily enforced by data encryption technologies and passwords that limit access to only these that are authorized or that have paid to do so. Harris (1995) also points to the presence of network externalities in communication networks as a defining difference between transport and communication [4] The concept of a network as a growing pool of links between a growing number of connected users makes it very distinct from a transport link between two points.

The new economic geography literature driven by Krugman [6] and Venables [7] has attributed the emergence of internationally distributed production networks to improvements in communication technologies that have made coordination of geographically dispersed production processes possible in more developed countries. SSA has seen very little of these dispersed production processes with most of the investments in the region heavily falling into extraction of primary resources and erection of retail outlets for finished products from more developed countries.

While earlier studies focused on the effect of country specific communication infrastructure on trade, they did not offer much evidence on how international communication costs affect trade flows. Fink et al. [8] take an early lead in expressly investigating the effect of international communication costs on trade flows by assuming that communication costs affect trade primarily by influencing variable trade costs between nations. More recent literature has studied variations of the problem in relation to specific markets and products [2, 9]. We follow Fink, Mattoo and Neagu and investigate the effect of bilateral communication costs on trade flows in SSA by employing bilateral cost of communication between countries in an augmented gravity model setting.

The contribution to this literature is that communication costs in SSA are linked to international gateways dominated by private foreign owned and operated satellites and show the effect of this on trade. The paper examines whether the cost of communications is an important variable in the realization of higher volumes of trade between SSA countries. The affordability of communications facilities and services for both the corporate world and the general population in SSA has become an imperative for participation in the new global world order.[1]

The objective of this paper is to empirically investigate whether bilateral communication costs matter for trade among SSA countries. It empirically tests the hypothesis that high communication costs in SSA have a negative impact on the volume of trade between countries. International communication costs in SSA are heavily influenced by the cost of access to international gateways dominated by foreign privately owned satellites (i.e. the foreign privately owned 'public infrastructure'). If the hypothesis is confirmed this would imply that having a privately owned foreign 'public' infrastructure has negative economic effects on SSA countries and that a publicly owned infrastructure would be more beneficial for economic development, reducing trade costs and enabling more trade, as argued in van Zon and Mupela [10].

Communication cost cuts across all phases of the life cycle of a product, from initial product design to marketing and after sales services. This aspect of communication is almost always neglected in studies of trade costs in a bid to compartmentalize costs to broader categories that make them easier to study. An example of this is the study by Anderson and Wincoop [11] that finds that 44 % of trade costs in developed countries are due to border related barriers, a broad category that includes communication costs. We isolate communication costs in this study and look at the cost of gathering, transmitting and receiving information across international barriers through international telephone and internet services. These are represented by cost of broadband and the cost of making international phone calls. These are the communication costs that are likely to affect international trade. So in general we argue that international communication costs are a function of international calling rates and internet broadband costs. International calling rates are measured in US dollars per minute while internet bandwidth is measured in dollars per Megabit per second (Mbps). This represents the variable cost aspect of communication.

The gravity model predicts that SSA countries will trade more with nearer countries in the region. The gravity tendency is likely to weaken when trade with bigger economies outside Africa is taken into account. For instance former colonial ties will result in trade relations with distant countries. The paper concentrates on effects among SSA countries so as to eliminate the effects of former colonial ties as much as possible.

An example of politically moderated trade relations with distant countries is the American government's bold policy initiative to support and promote export-led economic growth on the continent through the African Growth and Opportunity Act (AGOA) of 2000 under President Bill Clinton. The act seeks to promote growth on the African continent by promoting trade between the world's biggest economy and the African continent. AGOA allows SSA countries to export products to the USA duty free among other benefits. During the period 2001 to 2008 exports from the continent

---

[1] Whether increased intra African trade and trade openness indeed have positive effects on growth in Sub-Saharan Africa is not addressed in the present paper. This remains an important avenue for future research.

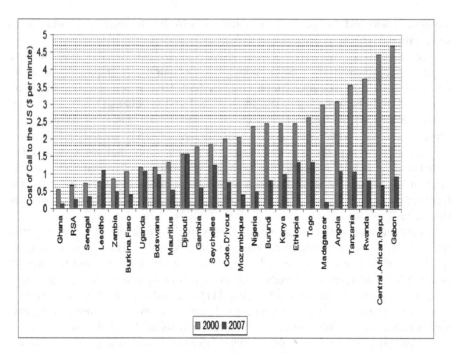

Fig. 1. International call charges between USA and AGOA African countries

to the US increased fourfold. It is interesting to note that call charges between the AGOA participating countries and the US also dropped dramatically during this period, in most cases by more than 50 % (see Fig. 1). The figure shows a dramatic drop in call charges to the USA between 2000 and 2007 in all countries except Djibouti where they remained the same. This does not necessarily mean that the drop in call charges led to higher exports but rather gives us further incentive to study whether this drop in communication costs could in any way have had a bearing on the increase in trade volumes between the US and the AGOA countries.

The rest of the paper is organized as follows: Sect. 2 gives a brief overview of the gravity model of trade. The empirical model and the variables in the analysis are discussed in Sect. 3. Section 4 follows with a description of the data, which is followed by a discussion of the results in Sect. 5. The paper closes with some concluding remarks and recommendations in Sect. 6.

2   The Gravity Model of Trade

The gravity equation of international trade tries to predict international trade flows based on the size of the economy and the distance between trading partners (see [3, 11–14] for details of the gravity model of trade).

Simply stated the model posits that the amount of trade between two countries is directly proportional to the product of their economic sizes (GDP) and inversely proportional to the physical distance between them. The empirical use of this form is accredited to Walter Isard in his work on Regional Science although lots of other sources credit first use of the equation in economics to Jan Tinbergen [13].

Despite the wide empirical success that this formulation has had in predicting bilateral trade flows between countries, the early literature criticized the gravity equation for not having any theoretical foundation in economics. This criticism led various authors to try and provide this justification. In 1979 James Anderson wrote "A Theoretical Foundation of the Gravity Equation" specifically to address some of these theoretical concerns. He demonstrated that the gravity equation could be derived from the properties of expenditure systems especially in countries where the structure of traded goods preferences is very similar. There were more theoretical justifications to follow. In a series of publications on the subject, Bergstrand developed a general equilibrium model of world trade, from which he derived the gravity equation under the assumption of perfect international product substitutability [15, 16]. He then followed this up with models based on monopolistic competition thus bringing together the two strands of literature on the matter, the product differentiation based literature and the monopolistic competition based models. Deardorf in proposing his two theories of frictionless and impeded trade notes:

"I suspect that any plausible model of trade would yield something very like the gravity equation, whose empirical success is therefore not evidence of anything, but just a fact of life"[2]

It is interesting to note the implications of the gravity formulation for SSA countries. Figure 2 shows strong gravity tendencies for trade amongst SSA countries.[3] The figure shows the total volume of trade from South Africa and from Zambia decreasing with distance from the exporting country. With a few exceptions, we see this trend in other countries as well to varying degrees (See Annex 3 for more examples).

The figure shows that distance seems to matter for trade in SSA. Even South Africa, which seems to have easier and relatively cheaper access to international connectivity, seems to keep the gravity trend (falling exports with increased distance) for trade with other African countries, although with much higher levels of exports than Zambia. South Africa has direct access to the sea and undersea fiber cable, which until recently was not available to most countries in SSA, which had to rely on expensive satellite capacity for their international connectivity. In spite of this South Africa still exhibits the gravity tendency in trade with other African countries. Communication has the capacity to make trade easier between far away countries. But if this communication is not affordable or is not easily accessible, then the problems of distance are compounded by the inability to communicate, which may affect trade intensity volumes downwards.

---

[2] page 12 in Chapter "Determinants of Bilateral Trade: Does Gravity Work in a Neoclassical World?" appearing in Volume entitled "The Regionalization of the World Economy" from the from the National Bureau of Economic Research

[3] As mentioned in the previous section, only SSA countries are included in the analysis, in order to avoid the confounding effects of strong trade ties to former colonial countries. The focus is on intra-African trade.

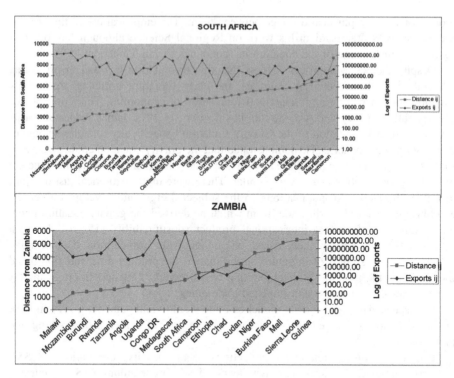

Fig. 2. Distance from RSA (top), Zambia (bottom) to other African countries and level of exports

3 The Empirical Model

We model the effects of communication costs on trade using an augmented version of the basic empirical gravity formulation (1)

$$\ln X_{ij} = \beta_0 + \beta_1 \ln Y_i + \beta_2 \ln Y_j + \sum_m \beta_{ij}^m \ln Z_{ij}^m + \varepsilon_{ij} \qquad (1)$$

where X_{ij} is the volume of exports from country i to country j, Y_i and Y_j and the economic masses of the trading partners and Z are all the barriers to trade between the pair including distance. The following is the multiplicative form of our empirical model:

$$X_{ij} = A \cdot \frac{GDP_j^{\beta_1} \bullet GDP_i^{\beta_2}}{Dist_{ij}^{\beta_3}} \cdot Fixed_{ij}^{\beta_4} \cdot Bband_i^{\beta_5} \cdot MA\_OTRI_i^{\beta_6} \cdot OTRI_j^{\beta_{76}} \cdot Outgoing_i^{\beta_8}$$
$$\cdot Landlocked_i^{\beta_9} \cdot ComBorder_{ij}^{\beta_{10}} \cdot Satellite_i^{\beta_{11}}$$

$$(2)$$

Table 1. Variable descriptions and expected signs

Variable	Description	Expected sign
Xintensity$_{ij}$	Intensity of exports from country i to country j in current dollar values for the year 2007	Dependent variable
X$_{ij}$	Level of exports between country i and country j	
GDP$_i$	GDP of country i in current 2007 dollars	
GDP$_j$	GDP of country j in current 2007 dollars	+ positive
Dist$_{ij}$	Geographic distance between capital cities of exporter country i and importer country in km	− negative
Fixed$_{ij}$	Cost of an international call from a fixed landline telephone from country i to country j in PPP $ per minute	− negative
InBband$_i$	Cost of entry level broadband connection, PPP $ per month	− negative
ComBorder$_{ij}$	A dummy variable signifying whether countries i and j share a common border or not	− negative
Outgoing$_i$	Total number of outgoing international calls made in 2007	+ positive
Landlocked$_i$	A dummy variable indicating whether a country is landlocked or not	− negative
Satellite$_i$	An infrastructure dummy indicating whether country is dependent on satellite connectivity	− negative
MAOTRI$_i$	The Market Access Trade Restrictiveness Index for country i	− negative
OTRI$_j$	The Overall Trade Restrictiveness Index in country j	− negative

GDP$_i$ and GDP$_j$ take the place of Y_i and Y_j. GDP is measured in measured in current 2007 dollars[4].

Dividing both sides of Eq. (2) by GDP$_i$ and then taking logs gives us an intensity version of the dependent variable X$_{ij}$,

$$\ln X\ \text{int}\ ensity_{ij} = \beta_0 + \beta_1 \ln GDP_j + (\beta_2 - 1)GDP_i - \beta_3 \ln Dist_{ij} + \beta_4 \ln Fixed_{ij}$$
$$+ \beta_5 \ln Bband_i + \beta_6 \ln MA\_OTRI_i + \beta_7 \ln OTRI_j + \beta_8 \ln Outgoing_i \quad (3)$$
$$+ \beta_9 Landlocked_i + \beta_{10} ComBorder_{ij} + \beta_{11} Satellite_i$$

The variables and expectations with regard to the signs of the coefficients are summarized in Table 1.

Normally the cost of satellite connectivity is very much higher than the cost of fiber connectivity. We expect the effect of communication costs on trade to be more pronounced in landlocked countries than in coastal countries due to their dependence on more expensive satellite international connectivity. The alternative scenario is the imperfect market scenario, where we have monopolistic rents being charged on fiber connectivity as well, due to the presence of monopolies along the SAT3 fiber cable operation. If the alternative scenario obtains, we should find no significant differences between the effect of communication costs in landlocked countries and in coastal countries.

---

[4] We tested the results using PPP Dollar GDP figures and found similar results. We show the results obtained using current dollar figures because these were more readily available in a consistent format than the PPP Dollar GDP figures.

Things are further complicated by the fact that not all countries along the coastline have access to undersea optical fiber cable. Countries along the coast without a fiber landing point also use satellite or buy capacity from neighboring countries that do have a landing point. In the latter case they have no control over how much they pay. If the countries with landing points are able to charge monopoly rents in the alternative scenario, being on the coast does not necessarily guarantee cheaper access to the international backbone. Again this should lead to no significant differences between coastal and landlocked countries.

It remains to be seen, however whether the continuing roll out of more fiber optic cable along the East and West African coastline will change this dynamic in the near future in response to more competition.

4 The Data

Several data sources were used to construct the main matrix of country pairs. Bilateral exports data was sourced from the IMF Direction of Trade database and the United Nations COMTRADE database. Distance data between countries' capitals was sourced from John Byers site chemical ecology[5].

Another important source of data was the World Development Indicators database of the World Bank. Publications of the International Telecommunications Union (ITU) provided most of the data for ICT indicators particularly the broadband cost in SSA countries. These included the 2009 publication "Africa Telecommunications Indicators 2008" and "Measuring The Information Society 2008 ITU". GDP figures were sourced from the Word Development Indicators database of the World Bank for the year 2007. These figures were matched with the corresponding 2007 levels of export and international calling prices. Various sources were used for this data depending on availability. Most of it was sourced directly from different countries national telecommunications web sites, directories and Communications Authorities.

A cross section of 2007 data for 19 exporting countries in SSA was used mainly due to the fact that it was difficult to construct a time series data set because fixed telephony tariff data was difficult to collect retrospectively. In countries where time series data was available like Zambia, Togo, and Malawi, there was very little fluctuation, if any, in the price of international calls charged by the fixed service providers between successive years. In certain countries like Nigeria, the incumbent fixed telephone operator had been recently privatized and the ensuing state of transition made it difficult to collect any meaningful series of retrospective data. Massive movements were evident in local call tariffs, mainly due to competition from cheaper local mobile cellular providers, but international call charges did not change much for successive years.

The implication of using a cross sectional data set for this study is that it is not possible to carry out explicit causality tests on the data.

---

[5] http://www.chemical-ecology.net/java/lat-long.htm

Of the nineteen exporter countries thirteen were landlocked and thirty pairs of trading partners had common borders. All landlocked countries depended on satellite infrastructure for their international connectivity.

5 Results and Discussion

Ordinary Least Squares (OLS) regressions show that distance and communication costs matter for trade in SSA. OLS was applied to the dataset for all countries and then to two sub-samples of landlocked countries and coastal countries. Though some variables change signs and lose significance when more variables are added to the regression, the overall result seems to be that distance affects export intensity negatively as does the cost of fixed line and broadband communication in both coastal and landlocked countries.

The results reveal the expected signs on most of the variables. $lnDist_{ij}$ is negative and significant at the 1 % level. $lnGDP_i$ and $lnGDP_j$ both come out positive and significant at the 1 % level as well. These variables all keep their signs and significance after more variables are added to the model. Although $lnOutgoing_i$ enters the model significantly with the expected positive sign, it drops its significance when $lnBband_i$ and $lnFixed_{ij}$ are added to the model. This was not expected. The volume of outgoing calls was expected to be positively correlated with export intensity and negatively correlated with the cost of making a fixed. The sub samples of coastal and landlocked countries also yielded erratic results for $lnOutgoing$ and $lnfixed$, which is not significant in the coastal sub sample. Whereas $lnOutgoing$ comes out with a negative sign (not expected) in the coastal countries, it keeps the positive expected sign in the landlocked sample. This is difficult to explain as the volume of outgoing calls was expected to affect export intensity positively in both samples. This is an area where further research will be required.

$lnMAOTRI_i$ and $lnOTRI_j$ are both negative and significant. The common border dummy is positive and significant as expected because sharing a common order in most cases also means sharing communication channels and other natural resources that facilitate trade between neighboring countries. The landlocked and satellite dummies also turn out with the expected signs in both regressions.

Most important for the study is the result that cost of international fixed line calling and cost of broadband seem to be negatively associated with the intensity of exports from country of origin (See Table 2). Further research will be required to verify this result. The costs of international calling in Africa are associated with the use of foreign operated satellite and fiber gateways. This result would imply that any reorganization of these international gateways to bring down the cost of international calling and broadband connections should have a positive effect on exports within SSA.

There seems to be a negative effect of cost of broadband on coastal regions in spite of the presence of fiber optic cable on the west coast of Africa. This would indicate that although the fiber optic cable is present it may not be as accessible as it is meant to be, leaving coastal countries with no option but to connect via satellite. The satellite dummy turns up negative and significant. It will be interesting to note how this

Table 2. Determinants of export intensity. All countries

lnXintensity	OLS All										
	(1)	(2)	(3)	(4)	(5)	(6)	(7)	(8)	(9)	(10)	(11)
$lnDist_{ij}$	-1.435***	-1.332***	-1.868***	-1.876***	-1.915***	-1.895***	-2.041***	-2.426***	-2.153***	-2.148***	-2.141***
	(0.216)	(0.206)	(0.186)	(0.187)	(0.184)	(0.184)	(0.185)	(0.254)	(0.287)	(0.287)	(0.287)
$lnGDP_j$		0.706***	0.704***	0.704***	0.678***	0.683***	0.664***	0.823***	0.803***	0.806***	0.814***
		(0.106)	(0.0920)	(0.0921)	(0.0909)	(0.0906)	(0.0894)	(0.121)	(0.120)	(0.120)	(0.120)
$lnGDP_i$			1.212***	1.160***	1.257***	1.133***	1.105***	1.021***	0.998***	0.924***	0.893***
			(0.104)	(0.164)	(0.164)	(0.176)	(0.174)	(0.228)	(0.227)	(0.242)	(0.243)
$lnOutgoing_i$				0.0689	-0.0577	0.0266	0.304	0.367	0.380	0.394	0.418*
				(0.106)	(0.167)	(0.172)	(0.185)	(0.240)	(0.238)	(0.239)	(0.240)
$lnBband_i$					-0.409***	-0.381***	-0.156	-0.174	-0.174	-0.126	-0.107
					(0.105)	(0.106)	(0.120)	(0.156)	(0.155)	(0.165)	(0.165)
$lnFixed_{ij}$						-0.352*	-0.584***	-0.755***	-0.697***	-0.726***	-0.715***
						(0.188)	(0.195)	(0.258)	(0.258)	(0.260)	(0.260)
$lnMAOTRI_i$							-0.854***	-0.728***	-0.684**	-0.678**	-0.715**
							(0.228)	(0.275)	(0.274)	(0.274)	(0.276)
$OTRI_j$								-3.897**	-3.554**	-3.611**	-3.616**
								(1.517)	(1.517)	(1.519)	(1.518)
$Comborder_{ij}$									1.149**	1.202**	1.210**
									(0.574)	(0.577)	(0.577)
$landlocked_i$										-0.432	-0.0884*
										(0.483)	(0.641)
$Satellite_i$											-0.679*
											(0.550)
Constant	2.192	17.41***	-6.742**	-6.646**	-4.846	-3.617	-6.725**	-0.158	-2.592	-1.258	-0.746
	(1.679)	(2.784)	(3.194)	(3.205)	(3.186)	(3.244)	(3.301)	(4.254)	(4.399)	(4.647)	(4.661)
Observations	641	641	641	641	641	641	421	421	421	421	421
R-squared	0.094	0.181	0.380	0.380	0.402	0.407	0.426	0.482	0.490	0.490	0.495

Standard errors in parentheses*** $p<0.01$, ** $p<0.05$, * $p<0.1$

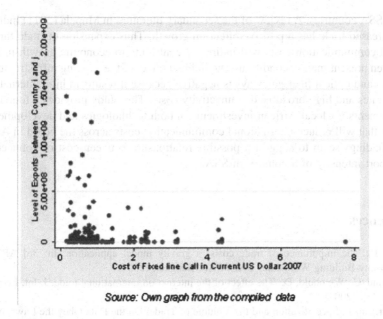

Source: Own graph from the compiled data

Fig. 3. Level of exports and international calling charges in SSA (2007)

dynamic will change with the arrival of more competition in the fiber business on the coast and the rollout of inland fiber networks in SSA.

Figure 3 shows the scatter plot for SSA. Exports are generally very low in countries with high calling rates per minute. The scatter plot shows a clear pattern of high bilateral call charges and low exports and a general trend of low bilateral calling charges and high exports. Although we have a lot of countries in the low cost/low export area of the plot, we do not have a single country in the high cost/high export area of the plot. This pattern is consistent with the regression results in the preceding table, which show a negative significant coefficient for communication costs generally.

Care should however be taken to note the low R-squared values of the regressions, 0.49 for all countries in the sample. This means that only about 49 % of the variations in export intensity can be explained by the independent variables, all things being equal. It is therefore advisable to take the results as indicative findings warranting further research and analysis rather than conclusive findings.

6 Concluding Remarks

Adding variables representing the cost of international connectivity to a traditional gravity equation, we find that international communication costs have a significant negative effect on the volume of trade in SSA. This implies that efforts aimed at reducing the cost of international communications in Africa may contribute to the reduction of trade friction between SSA countries and the increase in export intensity among SSA countries. A review of the secondary literature in Mupela (2011) indicates that increased trade has a positive effect on growth. Thus expansion of trade through reduced communication costs will indirectly contribute to economic growth in SSA.

Given present market conditions, the indirect effect of the existing infrastructure of satellites and optical fiber gateways is negative because it results in high international calling rates and high broadband connectivity costs. This study provides a foundation for arguments for local African investments in both technologies and development of policies that will reduce international communication costs across the board in Africa. These findings seem to suggest a possible relationship between cost of connectivity and export intensity of a country in SSA.

References

1. De, P.: The importance of trade costs: a gravity model application. In: 3rd ARTNeT Capacity Building Workshop: UNESCAP, Bangkok (2007)
2. Freund, C., Weinhold, D.: The effect of the internet on international trade. J. Int. Econ. **62**, 171–189 (2004)
3. Harrigan, J.: Specialization and the Volume of Trade: Do the Data Obey the Laws, NBER Working Paper 8675, December 2001 (2002)
4. Harris, R.: Trade and communication costs. Can. J. Econ. **28**, 46–75 (1995)
5. Samuelson, P.: The transfer problem and the transport costs: analysis of effects of trade impediments. Econ. J. **64**(254), 264–289 (1952)
6. Brezis, E., Krugman, P.: Technology and the life cycle of cities. J. Econ. Growth **2**(4), 369–383 (1997). (Springer)
7. Venables, A.: Spatial disparities in developing countries: Cities, regions and international trade. CEP Discussion Papers dp0593, Centre for Economic Performance, LSE (2003)
8. Fink C., Matoo A., Neagu I.: Assessing the impact of communication costs on international trade. World Bank, Development Research Group, Trade: Washington, D.C. (2002)
9. Tang, L.: Communication costs and trade of differentiated goods. Rev. Int. Econ. **14**(1), 54–68 (2006)
10. van Zon, A., Mupela, E.: Endogenous economic growth through connectivity. UNU-MERIT Working Paper Series 001, United Nations University (2010). (Unpublished)
11. Anderson, J., van Wincoop, E.: Trade costs. J. Econ. Lit. **42**(3), 691–751 (2004)
12. Anderson, J., van Wincoop, E.: Gravity and gravitas: a solution to the border puzzle. Am. Econ. Rev. **93**, 170–192 (2003)
13. Tinbergen, J.: An Analysis of World Trade Flows. Shaping the World Economy. Twentieth Century Fund, New York (1962)
14. Baldwin, R., Taglioni D.: Gravity for Dummies and Dummies for Gravity Equations. *NBER Working Papers 12516, National Bureau of Economic Research, Inc.* (2006)
15. Bergstrand, J.: The gravity equation in international trade: some microeconomic foundations and empirical evidence. Rev. Econ. Stat. **67**(3), 474–481 (1985). (MIT Press)
16. Bergstrand, J.: The generalized gravity equation, monopolistic competition, and the factor-proportions theory in international trade. Rev. Econ. Stat. **71**(1), 143–153 (1989). (MIT Press)

On Software-Defined Networking for Rural Areas: Controlling Wireless Networks with OpenFlow

Sami Ruponen[(⊠)]

VTT Technical Research Centre of Finland, Communication Networks,
Vuorimiehentie 3, 02150 Espoo, Finland
`sami.ruponen@vtt.fi`

Abstract. Software-defined networking (SDN) is gaining interest among the traditional vendors of networking devices and network operators. Promises such as simplified network control and resource management are valuable features for network operators. However, the SDN paradigm cannot suddenly bring more bandwidth to existing networks; it merely offers tools for more efficient use of available resources. Together, these benefits could provide means for network providers in rural areas to gain cost-efficiency. To this day, less research has been done on how to utilise SDN in practice in wireless rural area networking. This paper presents an on-going work on utilising SDN capabilities in wireless networks. It describes some design ideas and evaluates basic building blocks that enable SDN in low-cost wireless networks.

Keywords: SDN · OpenFlow · Open vSwitch · WiFi · Wireless mesh

1 Introduction

For many years, academic research has been done on software-defined networking (SDN). During the last years, it has also become increasingly popular among the network operators and equipment vendors. However, the research and business interests have mostly been on fixed networks and less on wireless networks.

SDN offers many promises such as simplified network control and resource management. Operators are keen on seeking means to reduce the costs of building, maintaining and operating networks. This is especially true for operators of rural communication networks, where the revenues and user density are low. For network device vendors, SDN can offer simplified software design inside the devices, because much of the control plane functionalities are run centralised in a remote controller. This also reduces the need for software updates in network devices and prolongs their service life.

While the networks are facing problems carrying the growing amounts of traffic, SDN cannot suddenly bring more bandwidth to the networks; it merely offers tools for more efficient use of available resources. SDN does not solve all

© Institute for Computer Sciences, Social Informatics and Telecommunications Engineering 2014
T.F. Bissyandé and G. van Stam (Eds.): AFRICOMM 2013, LNICST 135, pp. 39–48, 2014.
DOI: 10.1007/978-3-319-08368-1_5

the problems yet, but it seems to offer a viable solution towards enhancing the networking in emerging regions.

In [1] the authors argue that SDN is a promising technology for rural wireless networks and has an important role in offering people an Internet access worldwide. They further identify that SDN offers an approach to separate the physical construction and the actual operation of a network, thus offering new opportunities to reduce costs and lower technical and business barriers.

Current tools and methods for SDN are developed with a focus on wired high-speed networks. Wired and low-cost wireless networks have fundamentally different characteristics and indicators for evaluating their performance. For wired networks and devices, throughput is the often used performance metric, whereas in wireless networks, especially in case of rural area networking, this is not the most relevant metric. From experience, the speed or the quality of communication are not the most important issues for people living in rural areas. For them, it is often enough that it works – though slowly. For the operators in such areas, the simplicity and costs of building and management are the key issues.

This paper presents a practical solution towards bringing SDN concept into wireless networks based on low-cost WiFi technology and long-distance links. It describes some design ideas and concepts of an on-going work to enhance a wireless mesh testbed [2] with SDN capabilities. Further, it discusses some challenges and required functionality.

The rest of this paper is organised as follows. Section 2 presents related work in SDN applied to wireless networks. Section 3 introduces the background and components used in this work. Section 4 gives an overview on architecture of the SDN-capable wireless network under development. Section 5 presents the test configurations and measurement results of some key components using a small scale deployment. Finally, Sect. 6 concludes the paper.

2   Related Work

SDN applied in practice to wireless networks have been studied and demonstrated previously giving valuable references. In [8,9], the authors present two OpenFlow-based wireless mesh network architectures. The former is deployed over a 802.11 s standard mesh network, while the latter uses the traditional OLSR mesh routing protocol for the control, and OpenFlow for the data traffic. However, both seem to experience some bandwidth bottlenecks and require rather complex configuration to work.

In [10], the authors propose OpenFlow Wireless, a mobile wireless platform for experimental research of networks and services. It concentrates mostly on virtualising a network of switches and access points. Further, in [11], the authors introduce a concept of cloud-based, centralised MAC processing using virtual access points and an OpenFlow switch and controller. It inherently relies on wired network making it unsuitable for wireless backhauls. Last, in [12], the authors present a prototype SDN framework for enterprise WLANs based on an idea of a virtual access point abstraction. Each of these highlights the benefits of SDN in wireless networks and introduces interesting ideas but as such lack certain features that would allow their feasible use in rural area communication, or uses hardware that is not suitable.

3   Background

SDN is about making networks flexible and programmable. It enables high-level abstraction of network resources by hiding the complexity of the networking hardware. Essentially, this means decoupling the control tasks from forwarding tasks, i.e., separating the control plane and data plane functionalities.

The adoption of new features in networking are hindered by the complexity and the closed nature of existing architectures. Therefore, various new open architectures are being developed and taken into use. The next sections introduce some of the tools and architectures that can be used to build such an open SDN-capable network.[1]

3.1   OpenFlow

OpenFlow was originally proposed as a way to run experimental protocols in production networks [3]. Today, OpenFlow is a standard designed for SDN that enables the communication between the control plane and the data plane on supported devices and is defined by the Open Networking Foundation [4].

The OpenFlow standard describes the requirements for an OpenFlow-capable switch and the messaging between such a switch and a controller. Version 1.0.0 of the standard [5] is well supported and tested on OpenFlow devices while the more recent versions are not yet widely adopted or have only experimental support.

OpenFlow switches get instructions from a centralised controller regarding packet handling. A stream of packets with a set of matching characteristics, i.e., certain header values, are referred to as a flow and are applied with the same actions. Figure 1 depicts an overall OpenFlow architecture specified in the OpenFlow standard [5].

An OpenFlow-capable switch consists of a *flow table* and a *secure channel* to a controller. The *secure channel* is a TCP/IP connection between a controller and a switch that can be secured with Transport Layer Security (TLS). It is used by the controller, e.g., to set or delete flow entries in the flow table or to receive events or packets from the switch.

The *flow table* performs packet lookup and forwarding. It contains entries each composed of *header fields* to match against packets, *counters* for flow statistics, and *actions* that are applied to matching packets.

Header fields entry contains specific values (or a wildcard) for ingress port and header values, such as Ethernet addresses and IP addresses. A packet matches a

---

[1] It should be noted that SDN-like functionality can also be accomplished in existing networks with traditional methods and tools.

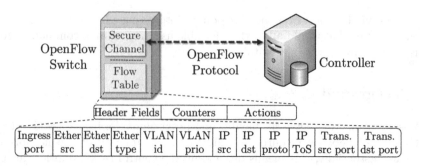

Fig. 1. OpenFlow architecture and flow Table components (v.1.0.0).

flow entry if all the header values of the incoming packet match those defined in the *header fields*. The flow entries are tested one by one until a match is found. If no match is found, the packet is to be sent to the controller.[2]

The flow entries are associated with zero or more actions that instruct how the matching packet should be handled. There are certain actions required to be supported and some optional actions. The mandatory ones include actions *drop* and *forward* either out from a physical port or to a virtual port (e.g. forwarding to the controller or for local processing). Optional actions include modifying a field (changing a header value) in the packet and forwarding a packet through the traditional forwarding path (e.g. normal L2 processing in a switch).

3.2   Open vSwitch

Open vSwitch [6] is a portable open source software switch that can run on a number of different operating systems and hardware platforms. It is designed to be used in virtualised server environments connecting virtual machines and physical networks together. However, it can still be used as a programmable stand-alone software switch similar to a dedicated hardware switch.

Simple software switches can be implemented in many ways. In Linux, one option is to use the Ethernet bridging support included in kernel. Together with the packet filtering and traffic control frameworks, and VLAN tagging support, very flexible packet handling can be achieved, but the configuration process and management can be a challenging task and subject to errors. With Open vSwitch, the above functionality[3] can be achieved using a single framework that additionally supports a centralised control using OpenFlow.

Figure 2 depicts a simplified architecture of Open vSwitch running in Linux. It consists of userspace daemons and a kernel datapath. Together, these implement the *flow table* and the *secure channel* in OpenFlow context. The core of

---

[2] This is a required behaviour, although others may be supported as a vendor extension.

[3] Open vSwitch offers additional features that are useful for network monitoring and managing the switch, although some of them might not be suitable for low-speed networks due to extra bandwidth requirements.

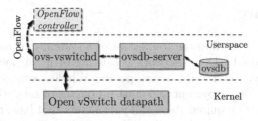

Fig. 2. Open vSwitch core components.

the switch is the *ovs-vswitchd* daemon. It controls the datapath and handles the communication with the OpenFlow controller. The database server (*ovsdb-server*) maintains the configuration details and statistics of the switch in a persistent database (*ovsdb*). In addition, several command line utilities can be used to configure the switch.

3.3   OpenFlow Controller

OpenFlow protocol is used to control and configure how packets are handled in individual network devices. However, it does not define the network-wide operation, e.g., how packets are carried between the ingress and the egress points. That is the responsibility of the application(s) running in the controller. The application executes the functionalities and policies that the operator has defined for its network.

Several open source software platforms are available to assist in building an OpenFlow controller. These platforms hide the low-level functions of OpenFlow and the communication with the network devices letting the developer to focus on the essentials, i.e., programming how the network operates.

POX [7] is one alternative for an OpenFlow controller platform, implemented with Python programming language. It offers interfaces to OpenFlow protocol and also sample components which the programmer can use as a basis for building more complicated controller functions. The sample components include functionalities such as L2 learning switch and topology discovery.

3.4   Hardware

OpenFlow is developed with the focus on wired high-speed networks. However, usually in rural areas, networks are constrained in many respects. First, due to the fact that the devices must be low-cost and have to operate on alternative power sources such as solar power and batteries, the processing power becomes limited. Secondly, the communication often relies on wireless links. Hence, to get realistic results on how OpenFlow would work in rural area networking, devices suited for such use are used throughout the development process and experiments.

4   Architecture

This section briefly describes the framework of a system that adds programmability into a wireless backhaul network consisting of mesh nodes with (point-to-point) WiFi links, and WiFi access points. Wireless connections introduce challenges during the deployment and start-up phases of network nodes because there are a number of required steps and parameters that have to be configured before the communication with a peer node is possible. The goal is to make this process as autonomic as possible.

The main components and their relations are shown in Fig. 3. The core components are the OpenFlow controller application and Open vSwitch. Since OpenFlow does not provide means to configure the underlying hardware, additional functionalities are required. Open vSwitch includes an OVSDB management protocol [13], that is one alternative for configuring the switch instances as well as the queues and the queuing discipline. However, before the previous steps can be remotely accomplished, the network interfaces, especially wireless, have to be properly configured to enable the connectivity to the neighbouring nodes and further towards the controller. Thus, additional methods are required to locally and remotely configure the physical layers of network interfaces.

The physical layer (*PHY*) management is handled by a *PHY agent* that configures the wireless interface parameters, such as frequency, transmission power, and operation mode. The agent is also used by a *PHY manager* running in the controller to tune the parameters and to monitor the status of the interfaces.

The most challenging tasks are related to the bootstrap process and handling of fault situations with non-existing connection to the controller. A special component (*Bootstrapping/Discontinuity manager*) is responsible of the initial configuration of the device, discovering its neighbouring nodes, and creating a connection to the controller.

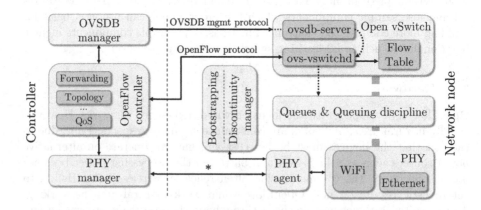

Fig. 3. Overall system architecture and main components.

Challenges. Due to the early state of the work, there are still open issues in details of how certain management and monitoring aspects of the physical interfaces are handled. Certain functionalities in the controller and in the nodes need to be implemented to support both self- and centralised configuration. *Peer and topology discovery* are essential functionalities that enable the node to form an initial route to the controller and the controller to efficiently handle packet forwarding. Equally important are the *Resiliency and fault recovery* in case of a node losing the connection to its peer node(s) or network partitioning.

Traffic prioritisation, shaping and policing contribute to the efficient and optimised use of network resources and enable to maintain certain quality of service. Due to the centralised control and decision making, certain traffic types, such as the management and control, must be given the priority over other traffic. The *link status and quality monitoring* are related to both resiliency and QoS. The controller must be able to monitor the current link status, bandwidth, and utilisation to be able to maintain proper connectivity and QoS levels, or even predict imminent link failures.

5 Testing and Measurements

This section briefly describes the setup that is used during the development and evaluation phases. It is a small scale hardware deployment in a laboratory environment that consists of a set of devices, with wired and wireless connections. The backhaul consists of nodes with directional antennas. Here, one node is actually built from multiple independent devices that are connected to each other either with a direct Ethernet link or through a switch. The access points connect to these nodes similarly.

5.1 Test Setup and Configurations

The setup depicted in Fig. 4 is used to test the OpenFlow functionalities of Open vSwitch and POX. Open vSwitch is running in each node and is configured to use POX as the OpenFlow controller. POX is started with a minimal setup using the stock components *openflow.of_01* and *forwarding.l2_learning*. This enables POX to configure the switches to act as one big logical L2 switch.

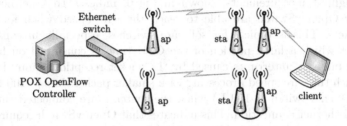

Fig. 4. Laboratory setup used for development and evaluation.

For a throughput test, a subset of the previous setup is used (Fig. 5). In this setup, the performance of both Linux bridge and Open vSwitch using wired and wireless connections between the two nodes in different combinations are measured. Here, the Open vSwitch instances in each node are running stand-alone, without a controller, because the throughput tests interfere the in-band communication between the controller and the nodes, thus interrupting the flow learning process.

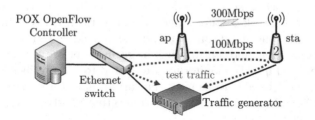

Fig. 5. Test setup for throughput measurements for Open vSwitch and Linux bridge using wired and wireless connections.

The testbed is currently deployed using Ubiquiti AirMAX devices that offer a simple and robust design with an 802.11n radio and one or two Ethernet interfaces. All the wireless connections are unencrypted and use 5 GHz frequency band with 40 MHz channel width and 2×2 MIMO. Also, the 4-address frame format is used on WiFi links between the backhaul nodes to enable transparent bridging [14]. Since OpenFlow has no support for setting up the wireless links, they are manually configured.

The wireless point-to-point links between the mesh nodes offer a theoretical maximum bandwidth of 300 Mbps. The wired Ethernet uses 100 Mbps full-duplex connections. A separate embedded PC is used to host the OpenFlow controller.

All the nodes are running OpenWrt 12.09 which uses Linux kernel version 3.3.8. Wireless interfaces use *ath9k* kernel driver. Open vSwitch is built using the latest available version 1.10.0. For POX, the git branch *carp* is used.

5.2   Measurement Results

The throughput measurements, shown in Fig. 6, indicate that neither Linux bridge nor Open vSwitch are able to reach the wire speed when forwarding small packets. This is typical for software switches, especially in constrained devices, for which a large portion of the CPU time is consumed on handling the high number of interrupts caused by the packet reception. Linux bridge is able to reach the wire speed processing with smaller packet sizes ($\sim$100 B) compared to Open vSwitch ($\sim$150 B) when the switches are connected through a 100 Mbps Ethernet connection. This indicates that Open vSwitch requires more CPU cycles per packet, probably resulting from the more complex matching process compared to simple Linux bridging.

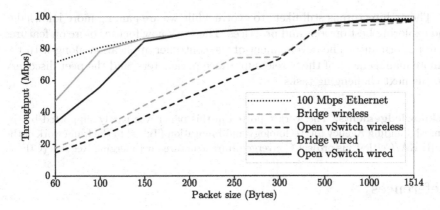

Fig. 6. Throughput results of Open vSwitch and Linux bridge with wired and wireless connections. Packet size includes the Ethernet header and the payload. The results indicate a near lossless situation.

The same trend is seen when the switches are connected through the wireless interface. In this case, the achieved throughput is significantly lower and wire speed forwarding is achieved when the packet size is increased to ∼500 Bytes. The bottleneck comes from the extra processing cycles required when sending the packet out from the wireless interface rather than from the bandwidth of the wireless link[4]. However, at the same time, on the receiver side, the CPU load was significantly lower with the same packet rate.

Although the wireless connection performs worse, especially with small packet sizes, the long link spans between the wireless nodes usually limit the achievable bandwidth to few tens of megabits per second. Also, situations where the traffic consists only of small packets can be considered quite exceptional. Hence, the wireless connections and software switches remain useful given their target use case.

6   Conclusion and Future Work

This paper has evaluated some openly available applications that can be used as a base for building an OpenFlow-controlled wireless mesh network. The results seemed promising and indicate that it is indeed feasible to use those applications, even on low-cost and low-performance devices, to build a programmable network for rural areas. As such, they don't yet provide all the required functionalities. Therefore, this paper also presented an architecture, based on an on-going work, that tries to fulfil the gap in required features and provide a wireless backhaul with simplified management and flexibility using OpenFlow along with other management protocols. The actual packet forwarding relies heavily on Open vSwitch, unlike other previous work proposed so far.

---

[4] The bandwidth during the test varied from 240 Mbps to 300 Mbps.

The architecture is still likely to evolve while we are gaining more knowledge and exploring best options and practices. The work now focuses more on features than performance. The development of the controller application along with the remote management of the wireless interface parameters, and the peer discovery are the next challenging tasks.

Acknowledgements. The work reported in this paper was partly supported by the Finnish Funding Agency for Technology and Innovation (Tekes) in the framework of the EUREKA/Celtic-Plus project Converged Infrastructure for Emerging Regions (CIER).

References

1. Hasan, S., et al.: Enhancing rural connectivity with software defined networks. In: Proceedings of the 3rd ACM Symposium on Computing for Development (ACM DEV '13). ACM, New York (2013)
2. Ruponen, S., Zidbeck, J.: Testbed for rural area networking – first steps towards a solution. In: Jonas, K., Rai, I.A., Tchuente, M. (eds.) AFRICOMM 2012. LNICST, vol. 119, pp. 14–23. Springer, Heidelberg (2013)
3. McKeown, N., et al.: OpenFlow: enabling innovation in campus networks. SIG-COMM Comput. Commun. **38**, 69–74 (2008)
4. Open Networking Foundation. https://www.opennetworking.org/
5. OpenFlow Switch Specification, version 1.0.0 (2009). https://www.opennetworking.org/sdn-resources/onf-specifications
6. Open vSwitch. http://openvswitch.org
7. POX. http://www.noxrepo.org/pox/about-pox/
8. Chung, J., et al.: Experiences and challenges in deploying OpenFlow over a real wireless mesh network. In: Fourth IEEE Latin-American Conference on Communications (LATINCOM), Cuenca, Ecuador (2012)
9. Dely, P., et al.: OpenFlow for wireless mesh networks. In: Proceedings of 20th International Conference on Computer Communications and Networks (ICCCN), Maui, Hawaii (2011)
10. Yap, K-K., et al.: Blueprint for introducing innovation into wireless mobile networks. In: Proceedings of the Second ACM SIGCOMM Workshop on Virtualized Infrastructure Systems and Architectures, New Delhi, India (2010)
11. Dely, P., et al.: CloudMAC - An OpenFlow based Architecture for 802.11 MAC Layer Processing in the Cloud. In: 8th IEEE Broadband Wireless Access workshop (BWA2012), Anaheim, California (2012)
12. Suresh, L., et al.: Towards programmable enterprise WLANS with Odin. In: Proceedings of the First Workshop on Hot Topics in Software Defined Networks (HotSDN '12), Helsinki, Finland (2012)
13. Pfaff, B., et al.: The Open vSwitch Database Management Protocol. IETF, I-D, draft-pfaff-ovsdb-proto-02 (2013)
14. Client Mode Wireless - OpenWrt Wiki. http://wiki.openwrt.org/doc/howto/clientmode#solution.using.wds

Thought Leadership in e-Governance, e-Infrastructure, and e-Business in Africa

Gertjan van Stam(⊠)

Scientific and Industrial Research and Development Centre (SIRDC),
Harare, Zimbabwe
gertjan.vanstam@worksgroup.org

Abstract. This paper positions Thought Leadership in e-Governance, e-Infrastructure, and e-Business in Africa, in the context of Social Innovation. It discusses the various perspectives on Thought Leadership, the components of Thought Leadership, its relevance in Africa and its targets. Further, the paper expands on the issues of vision, values and context.

Keywords: e-services · Thought leadership · Social innovation · Africa

1 Introduction

The field of e-Governance, e-Infrastructure, and e-Business in Africa is one ideally positioned for Social Innovation. This paper endeavors to provide inputs to the approach of Thought Leadership, including its definitions and African embedding. It presents a perspective on Though Leadership from the context of Africa. The work is based upon the author's studies and experience in e-Governance, e-Infrastructure, and e-Business in Africa since 1987. The paper unearths principles for a thought leadership by which methods and activities in Social Innovation can be designed and evaluated. Further, it considers how these principles could be outworked in practice to interact especially in Communities of Practice in Africa. The paper identifies practical components that the professionals in the World-of-Things need to contemplate and coordinate in order to support the World-of-Humans effectively in their respective communities [1]. These components are inputs for building out of Community of Practice gearing towards an African positioning of e-Governance, e-Infrastructure, and e-Business.

Social Innovation concerns innovative activities and services motivated by the goal of meeting a social need [2]. A Community of Practice is a network of people who share a theme, craft and/or a profession, often with the aim to learn from each other, and leading to development, standardization, and dissemination of knowledge [3].

© Institute for Computer Sciences, Social Informatics and Telecommunications Engineering 2014
T.F. Bissyandé and G. van Stam (Eds.): AFRICOMM 2013, LNICST 135, pp. 49–58, 2014.
DOI: 10.1007/978-3-319-08368-1_6

> *Social Innovation, a Vision*
>
> Our collective future needs innovation that takes
> place within the context of communities,
> experiments to find alternative strategies to address
> social needs,
> with people, and user-centric,
> questioning the status-quo,
> unearth the potential of all people,
> with technology as enabler,
> and collaboration to learn from different worlds.
> Social Innovation is not concerned with
> opportunities for competition only, but rather in
> enabling people in communities to improve
> activities for tasks they are part of,
> and for introduction of new tasks as they become
> necessary in a changing world,
> all within a context of shared values, norms and
> motivation.

2 Positioning Thought Leadership

Thought leadership serves to enhance engagement of professionals with the subject of e-Governance, e-Infrastructure, and e-Business. It spurs migration of the current transactional relationship of Africa with the West towards fellowship and interactions sharing common interests. Thought leadership aims to foster sustainable and indigenous capacity through inspiration, enabling and empowering, and engaging with a wide range of knowledge. Thought leadership supports and engenders skills and character development in professionals to be effective in the local, regional, and international context, and champions indigenous human capital and institutions, also in Africa.

3 Perspectives on Thought Leadership

Wikipedia defines Thought Leadership as '*content that is recognized by others as innovative, covering trends and topics that influence an industry*' A thought leader is 'a person or firm that is not only recognized but also who profits from the recognition of authority' [4]. 'Thought leadership should be an entry point to a relationship. Thought leadership should intrigue, challenge, and inspire even people already familiar with a company. It should help start a relationship where none exists, and it should enhance existing relationships' [5].

Thought Leadership influences the thinking in an area or subject. Its effectiveness is measured by the *amount of followers*. Leadership is distinct from 'management' and is not measured by position, rank, or title. Leadership explicitly deals with issues of vision, values, and motivation. Management deals with the process of assuring that the (resulting) programs and objectives are implemented [6]. Leadership requires progression through

1. careful positioning, attaining explicit rights to influence others
2. expressed permission, grounded in lasting relationships
3. tangible production, with sustainable achievements through commendable actions
4. capacity development, building abilities in individuals and organizations
5. honorable representation, through recognition of *wholesome being*

Migrating through these phases takes time and effort. They diligently harnass the most important ingredient for leadership: *integrity*. Integrity is the basis for credibility and trust.

In this paper, Thought Leadership is about 'establishing an authority on relevant topics by delivering guidance to the biggest questions on the minds of stakeholders'. Thought Leadership exposes authoritative perspectives on topics relevant for the professions involved in e-Governance, e-Infrastructure, and e-Business. The key for effectiveness is alignment with the agenda set by stakeholders [7]. The audience - in their specific context and culture - determines what the questions are, and these issues are thus specific and often highly diverse. The level of authority is determined by how well Thought Leadership facilitates interaction with these important issues.

Thought leadership content aims to provide guidance on relevant issues. Thought Leadership defines positions aligned with - or translated into - the context and culture of the audience. Table 1 gives an example of the diverse landscape of context and culture, when comparing Western and African tradition.

Thought Leadership is important for the Community of Practice and all stakeholders interacting with e-Governance, e-Infrastructure, and e-Business in the world. It is especially relevant for governance, education, and research entities. This is because of the complexity and length of the decision-making process in these bodies and the large number of people involved.

By exercising Thought Leadership, a Community of Practice becomes part of crucial conversations. Ultimately, Thought Leadership can be a tangible outcome of African Renaissance and pivotal part of its execution.

Exposure of thought leaders is the start of social engagement, where real people talk about real issues with real powers. However, thought leaders often introduce disruptive forces through which new ideas can flourish. It involves motion that challenges assumptions and chews away at the status quo. Politically savvy, thought leaders present *truth to power*, engender creativity, address social needs, work with people, are user centric, utilize the potential of people, utilize technology as key enabler, and upholds collaboration of different worlds.

Table 1. Example of different traditions in Western countries and sub-Saharan Countries [1]

Western Tradition	African Tradition
Ratio	Relatio
What	Who
Individual	Community
Rights	Responsibilities
Goods	Relationships
Credentials	Character
Actor	Member
Future	History
Short Term	Long Term
Abundancy	Scarcity
Literacy	Orality
Power	Authority
Emerging	Proven
Concise	Elaborate
Proactive	Reactive
Consistency	Paradox
Essential	Existence

3.1   Functional Components

The issues of capacity development and definition of progress are huge and complex. They have been dealt with elsewhere (e.g [8,9]). Further, this complexity grows continuously as in the networked world previously independent systems are increasingly interacting. Thus, risks continue to grow, with chances of system failures increasing in frequency and severity, even in synchronisation; It becomes progressively more difficult to predict outcomes of interventions or course of action [10].

Through Thought Leadership, the Community of Practice can strengthen its service innovation and develop a skill set that supports the promoting of the underlying technology and engineering to the general public. This involves engagement with the (engineering) communities on wider issues through

- adaption to global constraints and local environments
- options for functioning in areas of high complexity and low predictability
- awareness of actions of other stakeholders in shaping global properties that affect e-Governance, e-Infrastructure, and e-Business
- values and behaviours that serve as a guide in making governance and technology choices in the face of complexity

The challenges are huge in the setting of diverse histories, geographies, and policies. Various level of infrastructures and sustenance complicate comparisons.

The divergence of speeds of progress challenges *peace*. There are huge *inequalities* between the disenfranchised and others, between urban and rural,

and within the social strata of societies [11]. In practice, there are growing disparities in income and quality of living worldwide. Further, there are many cultures
and many models of development that require dedicated study for comprehen-
sion. Involving professionals who do not reside in the top-league and most affluent
areas in the world involves specific knowledge and particular skills. These skills
are in short supply [12].

Different context and cultures necessitate different ways of networking and
facilitating meetings of professionals to support fruitful interactions. Also, the
spread of economic activities varies per region, for instance in agriculture, mining
and services.

Interactions with Africa involve a complex array of issues and challenges, like

- infrastructure
- stability and resource governance
- food security
- national and regional capacity for progress
- generating jobs for the bulging youth population

Further challenges are the roles of - and in - regional integration, with its physical,
(geo-)political, economic and professional components.

With its global span and relevance, the Community of Practice in
e-Governance, e-Infrastructure, and e-Business must rely on opportunities for
partnerships. Thought Leadership involves thoughtfulness and engendering of
innovative activities. Opportunities exist with public sector institutions, policy
units, think tanks, businesses, regional institutes, universities, applied research
and training institutes. Evolving and new opportunities open opportunities for
'leapfrogging', for instance because of the growing interconnectedness in the
world and opportunities for self-directed learning (MOOCs) [13].

Disenfranchised environments are often faced with

- Science and Technology education without facilities for experimentation, labs
  and/or access to information
- non alignment of education with the local society [8]
- absence of a culture of innovation in the formal sector, with most innovation
  taking place in the informal sector
- an array of unaligned strategies and goals

One option to approach this setting is 'scenario analysis'. This helps to define
the strategy and actions that can be utilized to adapt as the outcomes approach
pre-defined patterns [10]. They include analysis of leverage points, significant
trade-offs, adaptive strategies, avoidance zones, and selection approaches. In
this dynamic and complex environment, addressing and measuring *long term
processes* is at least as important as measuring of *short term outcomes* [9].

Probabilistic models and dynamic complex system models can be used to
select most appropriate set of actions for each of the possible scenarios through
Social Innovation that involves community engagement for transformative change
in communities [14]. An action example is to establish partnerships for connecting resource rich but capacity poor countries with middle income countries

through regional and global integration [10]. This necessitates the rise of significant local leaders. Such is possible through cultural appropriate mentorship and the presentation of contextualized role-models [15]. These leaders drive the change for sustainable progress, skills building within ethics and integrity, leadership and technical skills development in the sphere of accountable governance, economic policy and management, science and technology, and agricultural and mining activities.

3.2   Realities on the Ground

Societies are split in a disenfranchised environment, mostly in the informal sectors, and a (thin) layer of wealth in the formal sectors. Currently, many African technologists may suffer from neglect and paternalism. For example, recently a Zambian engineer posted on his Facebook: "How can we change the perception that Zambian engineers are trained to repair and maintain? I for one have designed and modified many components".

Most e-Governance, e-Infrastructure, and e-Business feature a Western-centric worldview and mind frame [16]. This mind frame can be far removed from the mind frames - or the expressed memes - of other societies, especially from those in the 'developing world'. e-Governance, e-Infrastructure, and e-Business's services and often target Western or affluent consumers only. In Africa, implementation of e-Governance, e-Infrastructure, and e-Business involves interaction in complex and segregated societies, many languages and cultures. At present, many potential members of Communities of Practice do not know how to stay involved or miss the invitations to do so. Often, Western-based products and services are difficult to understand or use in the African setting. Therefore, Thought leadership involves sensitization on issues of *transculturality*. For example, thought Leadership in disenfranchised communities can involve interaction within oral traditions through creating space and opportunity for members who's voices are often absent in discourse [15]. Such leadership empowers and enables local professionals and Communities of Practice to be agents of their own change. Capacity building includes issues of

- capacity 'to do'
- use of local resources, skills and knowledge
- expanding channels to express African organizational capabilities and achievements
- addressing the roles of politics, power, and incentives

In disenfranchised communities, effectiveness is often hampered by a lack of knowledge sharing, limited mentoring due to few experienced mentors, and insufficient education facilities. The risks involved contain the dissatisfier of poor achievements in capacity development, a short term focus, low levels of legitimacy of development strategies, paternalism, weak or non-existent dialogue mechanisms, and the low effectiveness of formal institutions [10].

4   Targets for Thought Leadership

Thought Leadership targets the creation and effectiveness of professionals. A knowledge economy needs engineers with good vocational skills [17,18].

4.1   The End in Mind

Imagine, a time between 5 and 8 years from now, in e-Governance, e-Infrastructure, and e-Business, thought leaders inspire and drive growth of professional capacity in underserved and developing regions of the world. This growth comes from a wave of hundreds of thousands of young people, 18–23 years old, that enter the national workforces and future-shape their nations. Imagine them as professionals of outstanding ability, already experienced in managing the World-of-Things congruent with the local context and culture, ready to take on any local challenge, with diligence and skill for sustainable progress in local industries and institutes.

Imagine them as businessmen and women, as entrepreneurs at small and great level, who show integrity, who have the best interest of their communities and customers at heart and who have learned to progress without abusing or exploiting their communities or their environment. Imagine them as electricians, computer experts, operators, planners, and researchers who offer a high quality service at a fair price, and who steward their own and others' resources wisely. Imagine them as service-providers of their nations: teachers, council members, civil servants, and experts all passionate about uplifting the lives of others, all playing their part in building the nation without taking advantage of their positions. Imagine them as politicians who truly understand what it is to be a servant-leader. Imagine them as a generation of young people full of health and vigour, because they have understood their own value. Imagine them as being mindful, even passionate, about caring for the needy, contributing generously and wisely of their time, talents and finances to the needs of the disenfranchised in their communities. Imagine them having an understanding and appreciation of the great sweep peoples, cultures, languages and lifestyles and worldviews.

Imagine the sustainable progress they instill to their nation.

This could be the 'end-product' of thought leadership - people of character, skills, integrity, abilities and service who impact the World-of-Humans through the World-of-Things.

4.2   Shared Values

The development of shared values is a key factor for effective collaboration, and the first item on the Thought Leadership agenda. Developing shared values benefits from integral thinking on interior human development [14]. It involves fundamental views on society, governance, and more [19]. The translation of the shared values into daily practice depends on the expressed memes in society [20]. Shared values inform an integral approach and also incorporate inputs from a relational basis complementary to rational inputs, with the balancing of individualistic and collectivistic perspectives, in order to find a way how to align with local values [15].

4.3 The Context

Many African communities lack the opportunity to meet economic, social and other standards of well-being. This manifests through the inability to earn enough income, to meet material needs, to speak up for oneself, to maintain health and continuous education, and to maintain a sense of social and cultural affiliation. Lots of African professionals experience the equivalent of a poverty trap, involving

- low productivity, well below optimum
- lack of (access to) relevant information and education, affecting employability and access to opportunities
- gender issues
- lack of quality employment
- health issues (e.g. HIV)

4.4 Social Innovation

Social Innovation in line with the cultural and contextual environment aims for

- a holistic approach and focus on the priorities set by the environment itself
- aligning education with local realities
- assuring engineering activities focused on essential activities and structural progress
- growing opportunities through empowering the potential of local engineers
- peace and social cohesion, with equitable growth in jobs both in urban and rural areas

It strives to bring and keep the environment together, cherishes strong social bonds, lets people lead, focuses on priorities of the people, aims for sustainable impact, and makes use of available capabilities.

Thought Leadership supports to promote equitable growth across the various divides (e.g. urban/rural, and class), sustainable progress, and reduction of poverty through social change and effective adaptation to changing circumstances involving

- dialogue and establishment of relationships
- technology-relevant information
- locally produced and locally relevant knowledge
- empirical evidence to inform all stakeholders, supporting engineering policy and practice

In practice, this could take the forms of

- African and international conferences like Africomm, multi-stakeholder seminars, round tables, in-house seminars, and face-to-face meetings
- dissemination and celebration of good practice
- engineering and wellbeing assessment, commissioned local research, and case studies

– production of books, reports, and policy dialogue briefs
– target programs in priority areas like information, education, and innovation

  Therefore, thought leadership is bound to

– identify opportunities for the engagement of local professionals in development
– build community and establish alliances for social innovation
– involve government, industry, academia, NGOs, Foundations, social entrepreneurs, philanthropists, and professional bodies
– curate and disseminate new and existing content, and enhance dissemination of locally generated content
– bring about alternative platforms for content delivery
– stimulate and facilitate debate among key players
– adapt and reposition of standards
– participation of all stakeholders to fuel growth of professional capacity
– create infrastructure to facilitate social innovation
– exposing local capacity and methods to interact with local content
– identify topics for debate and local presence at relevant influential forums

For professionals in disenfranchised situations, Thought Leadership aims to break through the circle of poverty, dependency, and addresses the issues of peace, despair, ignorance, thinking, and choices. This needs a holistic approach instilling understanding, character, peace, sound thinking and choices, transformation and hope.

5 Conclusions

Thought Leadership is an opportunity for e-Governance, e-Infrastructure, and e-Business in Africa. Through Thought Leadership, Communities of Practice contribute to the global debate, influence public policy and avail relevant expertise and knowledge of professionals. Thought Leadership involves many aspects in a complex, multicultural environment.

References

1. van Stam, G.: Is technology the solution to the worlds major social challenges? In: IEEE Global Humanitarian Technology Conference, Seattle, USA. IEEE (2012)
2. Mulgan, G., Tucker, S., Ali, R., Sanders, B.: Social Innovation. University of Oxford, Oxford (2007)
3. Lave, J., Wenger, E.: Situated Learning: Legitimate Peripheral Participation (Learning in Doing: Social, Cognitive and Computational Perspectives). Cambridge University Press, Cambridge (1991)
4. Brenner, M.: What Is Thought Leadership? 5 Steps To Get It Right (2013)
5. Rasmus, D.W.: The Golden Rules of Creating Thoughtful Thought Leadership (2012)
6. Maxwell, J.C.: Developing the Leader Within You. Thomas Nelson, Nashville (2005)

7. Kroczek, A., van Stam, G., Mweetwa, F.: Stakeholder theory and ICT in rural Macha, Zambia. In: International Conference on ICT for Africa 2013, Harare, Zimbabwe (2013)
8. van Stam, G.: Towards an africanised expression of ICT (keynote speech). In: Jonas, K., Rai, I.A., Tchuente, M. (eds.) AFRICOMM 2012. LNICST, vol. 119, pp. 1–13. Springer, Heidelberg (2013)
9. van Stam, G.: Towards an IEEE Strategy in Social Innovation. In: 2012 IEEE Global Humanitarian Technology Conference (2012)
10. Leautier, F.A.: Unleashing Innovation and Learning for Capacity Development. In: eLearning Africa, Dar Es Salaam, Tanzania (2011)
11. Unwin, T.: Ensuring that we create an internet for all. In: Stockholm Internet Forum 2013 (2013)
12. Trompenaars, F., Hampden-Turner, C.: Riding the Waves of Culture: Understanding Cultural Diversity in Business, 2nd edn. Nicholas Brealey Publishing, London (2011)
13. van Stam, G.: MOOCs, an opportunity for african influence in western civilisation?. In: eLearning Africa, Windhoek, Namibia (2013)
14. van Stam, G.: Inclusive community engagement in social innovation, case Africa (Manuscript Submitted). In: IEEE Global Humanitarian Technology Conference, San Jose, CA (2013)
15. Bets, J., van Stam, G., Voorhoeve, A.-M.: Modeling and practise of integral development in Rural Zambia: Case Macha. In: Jonas, K., Rai, I.A., Tchuente, M. (eds.) AFRICOMM 2012. LNICST, vol. 119, pp. 211–220. Springer, Heidelberg (2013)
16. Dourish, P., Mainwaring, S.D.: Ubicomps Colonial Impulse. In: UbiComp'12, Pittsburg, USA (2012)
17. Kabanda, G.: African context for technological futures for digital learning and the endogenous growth of a knowledge economy (2013)
18. UNESCO. Engineering: Issues Challenges and Opportunities for Development. UNESCO Publishing, Paris (2010)
19. Porter, M.E., Kramer, M.R.: Strategy and society: the link between competitive advantage and corporate social responsibility. harvard Bus. Rev. **84**, 78–92 (2006)
20. Don Beck, E., Cowan, C.: Spiral Dynamics: Mastering Values, Leadership and Change. Wiley-Blackwell, New York (2005)

Towards Securing Communications in Infrastructure-Poor Areas

Daouda Ahmat[1]($\boxtimes$), Tegawendé F. Bissyandé[2,3], and Damien Magoni[1]

[1] LaBRI - CNRS, University of Bordeaux, Talence, France
{adaouda,magoni}@labri.fr
[2] SnT, University of Luxembourg, Luxembourg, Luxembourg
tegawende.bissyande@uni.lu
[3] FasoLabs, Ouagadougou, Burkina Faso

Abstract. Structured P2P networks have proven to be effective in the exchange of data between nodes whose identity and content are generally indexed in a DHT. For years, such DHT networks have allowed, among other users, third world inhabitants, such as African people, to exchange information among them and with the rest of the world without relying on a centralized infrastructure. Unfortunately, more than ever, reliability of communication across the Internet is threatened by various attacks, including usurpation of identity, eavesdropping or traffic modification. Thus, in order to overcome these security issues and allow peers to securely exchange data, we propose a new key management scheme that enables to handle public keys in the absence of a central coordination which would be required in a traditional PKI.

Keywords: P2P · Security · DHT · Key management · Distributed systems

1 Introduction

Opportunities of development are countless in a connected world. Unfortunately, participating to the information society remains a challenging endeavour for developing countries whose priorities lie elsewhere. Indeed, the lack of health care centers, schools, and practicable roads has pressing and damaging impact on the communities, outranking the need for investing in telecommunication infrastructures. In such contexts, opportunistic networking remains a prime choice to provide affordable means for sharing data, exchanging information and attempting to keep in touch with the rest of the world through internet [14].

Opportunistic networks are ideal for infrastructure-poor areas, where, contrary to traditional networking (1) all nodes of the network are not deployed together, (2) the size of the network cannot be approximately predicted, and (3) even the locations of the nodes are not pre-designed [10]. They constitute a special category of P2P networks where peers cannot rely on an 'observing' and 'mighty' central infrastructure whose existence is paramount. Instead, most

© Institute for Computer Sciences, Social Informatics and Telecommunications Engineering 2014
T.F. Bissyandé and G. van Stam (Eds.): AFRICOMM 2013, LNICST 135, pp. 59–69, 2014.
DOI: 10.1007/978-3-319-08368-1_7

implementations of P2P networks rely on a Distributed Hash Table (DHT) that provides a lookup service that each node in the network can use to map a given *key* with its corresponding *value*. Maintenance of the database of key/value mappings is obviously distributed among the nodes so as to avoid the use of a single point of failure that a central infrastructure would represent. Previous work has shown that it was possible to make DHTs scalable and reliable [16,23]. Consequently, in the absence of a central infrastructure, structured P2P networks can still benefit from the properties of DHTs to allow scalable interaction among connected nodes. Nonetheless, in the context of such setups, security and privacy remains challenging to implement and maintain.

Without guarantee of provision of a central infrastructure, P2P networks are bound to face security and reliability issues that existing common policies and techniques fail to take into account in their implementations. For example, standard securization measures for communication involve the use of key-based encryption which is often implemented with public-key cryptography. However, a central problem with the use of such type of cryptography lies in confidence that a given public key is authentic, i.e., that it is correct and belongs to the entity claimed, that it has not been tampered with or that is has not been replaced by a malicious third party. Usually, this confidence is guaranteed by a central Public-Key Infrastructure (PKI), in which one or several certificate authorities certify ownership of key pairs. There is therefore a requirement for a strong centralization to manage cryptography keys, a luxury that P2P networks cannot practically afford [24].

We propose in this paper to take into account the specificities of P2P networks and the security and reliability requirements for exchanging information in this era, to design a new approach for the management of public keys. Contrary to the traditional PKI, the management of public keys in our scheme is *decentralized*. Indeed, this management is distributed among the peers that form the P2P system. In practice, we rely on the "hyperbolic plane"-based topology where each node can select his parent accordingly in a distributed process. Public keys can then be forwarded safely for use by peers to ensure communication security. In previous work [1], we have proposed an approach to address the security issues of the communication sessions when users are mobile across the network of nodes. This approach targetting user-level applications is complementary to the approach developed in this paper which targets the security of the underlying network nodes.

The main contributions of this paper are:

- We first discuss the opportunities of P2P networks for developing regions: where and how they can be harnessed to deliver connectivity in a truely beneficial way. We then discuss the challenges that arise in such networks, focusing on the safety and reliability of communications.
- We then discuss the challenges for implementing authentication of sources in a P2P network. We emphasize on why traditional PKI which are currently successful on the Internet appear to be inadequate for P2P systems.

– We detail our approach for distributing the management of public keys across the different nodes. The novelty of this approach is that it leverages existing principles in a state-of-the art topology, to provide a reliable and secure way to manage public keys.

The remainder of this paper is organized as follows. Section 2 discusses P2P networking in the context of African developing regions. Section 3 enumerates the challenges that must be overcome to secure communications in P2P networks. Section 4.2 presents our approach. Section 6 discusses related work and Sect. 7 concludes.

2 P2P and Developing Areas

The network environment in developing regions, in particular Africa, is challenged. Networks in such areas are often characterized by frequent, lengthy, and unpredictable link outages, as well as congested usage of an already limited bandwidth [4]. A recent comparison of bandwidth available and its costs in developed and developing regions showed that the discrepancy reaches an order of magnitude. Saif *et al.* have reported that while a 2 Mbps ADSL link in the United States costs around US$40/month, a 2 Mbps broadband connection in Pakistan costs close to US$400/month [18]. Mainly three reasons explain such differences: (1) the cost of incoming bandwidth on links between developed and developing countries; (2) the lack of performant and adequate ISPs at the right scale; and (3) inadequate provisioning for "pre-paid" users who account for most internet users but whose base is harder to anticipate.

To address these issues, researchers and practitioners have relied on alternative paradigms involving Delay Tolerant Networks [4] and Opportunistic Networks [10,11,14,15] which appeared to suit the requirements of developing regions. In this context, Peer-to-peer systems have been proposed to support the enhancement of connectivity across developing areas. Researchers have thus proposed to apply P2P technologies to networking needs that are more urgent than simple (and often illegal ?) file sharing. For instance, P2P was found suitable for offline internet access [17,19].

3 Challenges

Securing communication in P2P networks is a challenging endeavor, especially with regards to the standard practice of crypting information. In this section, we precisely detail some obvious and non-obvious challenges to highlight the constraints of finding a solution for P2P systems.

Key distribution. The first challenge that we encounter is the mode of distributing cryptographic keys in infrastructure-poor or infrastructure-less areas. Indeed, traditionally, a management-friendly central infrastructure, called PKI, is relied upon for this task. In absence of infrastructure we propose a fully distributed approach to spread keys. To this end, we benefit from the distributed features of existing "hyperbolic plane" overlay networks, in particular self-organization.

Use of alternate infrastructure. Relying on the hyperbolic tree to assure the forwarding of cryptographic keys also comes with problems that traditional PKI was able to easily handled. Indeed, there is a new need to ensure in a distributed system that the construction of the overlay network where each peer is properly identified will guarantee the robustness of the exchange scenario with little possibility of corruption by any intermediate peer.

Exchange of keys. When initiating a communication in a P2P network, there will be a need for the peers to agree on the generation of a session key that the two peers will shared. A challenge in this requirement lies in the negotiation which should also be secured. Since usage of cryptography asymmetric algorithm to secure information is expensive, we propose to only rely on it in the key negotiation phase.

Detection of attacks. The last but note least issue is to provide a mechanism for detecting corrupted keys. Indeed, when a corrupted cryptographic key is detected, it should be revoked by peers who are aware of the corruption. The information must also be broadcasted in the network through a notification message that should assure that all corrupted keys are flushed out of the memory of connected peers. Similarly, a challenging endeavor will be to prevent the Man-in-the-middle attacks during session key negotiation phase.

4   System Design

In this section we discuss the different roadmaps that could be used to secure communications in P2P networks. We then detail our approach and the involved algorithms and heuristics.

4.1   Roadmap

In the absence of the traditional PKI for a central management of public keys, different schemes have been implemented to allow two peers to share a key (i.e., a secret) in a reliable way. We propose to go over those methods so as to highlight their limitations. We build our approach on top of these schemes, aiming at adressing with a DHT the different issues that we encounter in them:

- **Diffie-Hellman (DH) protocol** [5]

  The DH protocol is a strong cryptographic algorithm that enables sharing a secret between two nodes. Indeed, the proposed key exchange method allows two parties that have no prior knowledge of each other to jointly establish a shared secret. The strong point of the algorithm proposed by Diffie and Hellman also lies in the fact that the key exchange can be performed over an insecure communication channel. This protocol has been demonstrated to be secure against eavesdropping, and an extended version of the DH protocol has been implemented by Steiner *et al.* to share a secret in a group of n participating nodes [21].

Unfortunately, the DH scheme has been demonstrated to be opened to Man-in-the-middle (MITM) attacks, a category of attacks that should be ruled out in P2P networks.

- **DH-based multipath key exchange method** [22]
  To address the MITM attacks with the DH protocol, Takano *et al.* have proposed a multipath key exchange scheme that enables to forward different components of an encryption key through separate paths, in order to prevent MITM attacks. Their approach is focused on P2P networks using a ring topology, such as Chord [13] and Symphony [12], and uses clockwise/anti-clockwise routing technique. Nevertheless, despite its interesting features, this approach still suffers a few issues:

- it is restricted to a specific category of P2P networks (Chord and Symphony), and the ring topology does not appear to be realistic in the scenario of opportunistic networking where P2P connections are ad-hoc.
- it makes various assumptions that cannot be guaranteed in a truely P2P opportunistic network.

4.2   An Enhanced Multipath DH-Based Key Management

In this section, we propose an improvement (extension) of the model designed by Y. Takano et al. [22]. Scalable, decentralized and self-organized networks such as DHT-based P2P systems enable many users to join them. Thus, each node can be connected to a lot of other nodes; there can be then several paths between two endpoints of the network. For the above reasons, network topology can be transformed into a graph: each node represents an edge of the graph and each link indicates a connection between two nodes. Considering that P2P networks consist of a large number of peers that have multiple connections with several peers, network topology could be represented by a p-connected graph.

Hyperbolic Addressing Tree. Our approach leverages previous work [3] where the authors have demonstrated that hyperbolic geometry can be efficiently used for characterizing the overlay in a P2P network. Figure 1 thus illustrates the hyperbolic plane where the area is subdivided in disjoint zones allowing for each node to be positionned in a unique way while being able to be connected to a finite number of other nodes. This number corresponds to the degree q of the spanning tree that is thus built.

In the hyperbolic plane, a node of the tree can independantly compute the addresses corresponding to its children in the tree, and the degree of the tree determines how many addresses each peer in the network will be able to give.

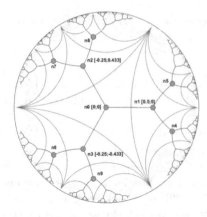

Algorithm 1: Dispatching, at source peer, for subkeys accross separate paths

Input: sourcePeer, listKeyComponents
Output: success / failure
degree ← getPeerDegree(sourcePeer);
list ← listKeyComponents;
if *degree* ≤ *0* || *list* = ∅ **then**
  | **return** failure;

foreach *subKey* ∈ *list* **do**
  | path ← selectSeparatePath();
  | routeSubKey(subKey, path);

return success;

Fig. 1. A regular tree in the hyperbolic plane where each node has a degree 3 (Image credit: Cassagnes *et al.* [3])

Thus by fixing the degree of the tree at the birth of the overlay, and by allowing each peer to connect to any peer at any time, the network can scale. In their work, Cassagnes *et al.* have proposed a distributed algorithm which ensures that the peers are contained in distinct spaces and have unique coordinates. As the global knowledge of the overlay is not necessary in their approach, "a new peer can obtain coordinates simply by asking an existing peer to be its parent and to give it an address for itself. If the asked peer has already given all its addresses, the new peer must ask an address to another existing peer. When a new peer obtains an address, it computes the addresses (i.e. hyperbolic coordinates) of its future children. The addressing tree is thus incrementally built at the same time than the overlay" [3]. For more details on the creation of the addressing tree, we refer the user to the work of Cassagnes *et al.* [3].

We modify the integration of a new peer to the overlay to allow:

– a more careful selection of the parents so as to allow the existence of redundants paths that do not immediately interset at a parent node of a given source node.
– a flexible construction of a P2P network that takes into account the security priorities of each connecting peer.

In our approch explicited by Algorithm 2, since every peer can connect to any other peer, a new peer can be forced to pick parents with specific properties when security is an important requirement for him. In our scheme, each peer must have at least two parents when it is concerned with security issues. Thus, while the redundant paths will allow to protect communication against eavesdropping, a selective connection will mitigate MITM attacks. Indeed, during the connection of a peer, each contacted potential parent will reply with the address it offers to a child as well as the addresses of the peers to whom it is already connected. Thus, the new peer can realise if this potential parent is also linked to his already selected other parent. In such cases, if the new peer requires very secure communications that will be MITM attack-proof, it must contact a different parent.

Algorithm 2: Attempt a connection to a parent node p

```
Input: p, alreadyConnectedParentAddrs
       allAddrLinkedToParent
Output: newAddr
newAddr ← ⊥;
(proposedChildAddr,allAddrLinkedToParent) ←
   requestAddrToParent(p);
foreach addr ∈ alreadyConnectedParentAddrs do
   if ∃ p_a ∈ allAddrLinkedToParent | p_a = addr
   then
       return ⊥; /* try to connect to a
                    different parent */

newAddr ← proposedChildAddr;
allAddrLinkedToParent ← allAddrLinkedToParent ∪ {p};
return newAddr;
```

Algorithm 3: Paths selection

```
Input: keyToTransmit, nodeNeighbours
nodeNeighbours ← sortConnectedNodes(nodeNeighbours);
keyComponents ← splitKey(keyToTransmit);
usedNode ← lastOf(nodeNeighbours);
while keyComponents ≠ ∅ do
   if usedNode = lastOf(nodeNeighbours) then
       usedNode ← firstOf(nodeNeighbours)
   else
       usedNode ← nextOf(nodeNeighbours)
   component ← firstOf(keyComponents);
   transmitViaSeparatePath(component, usedNode);
   ;
   keyComponents ← keyComponents \ {component};
```

Key Exchange Method. Although the DH crytographic algorithm [5] has been widely used to share secrets on unsecure communication channels, it is MITM attacks. In order to overcome this limitation of DH-based scenarios, we propose to use a multipath key exchange scheme.

Building upon a scalable P2P overlay [3] which uses virtual coordinates taken from the hyperbolic plane that is indifferent to underlying P2P network topology, our key exchange mechanism is based on multipath key negotiation as described in Algorithm 4. Takano *et al.* [22] have previously proposed a similar key negotiation mechanism. However, unlike our approach, their method is restricted only to Symphony and Chord P2P networks with a ring topology.

Algorithm 4: Key negotiation mechanism

p : a prime number

g : a generator

1. **Alice** selects a random number n, and computes $Key_a = g^n (mod\ p)$.
2. **Alice** selects q random numbers $ka_0, ..., ka_{q-1}$, such that $Key_a = \sum_{k=0}^{q-1} ka_k$ $(mod\ p)$.
3. **Alice** routes all ka_k to **Bob** via q potential separate paths[1].
4. **Bob** receives q Key_a's components $ka_0, ..., ka_{q-1}$ sended by **Alice** and computes $Key_a = \sum_{k=0}^{q-1} ka_k (mod\ p)$.
5. **Bob** selects a random number m, and computes $Key_b = g^m (mod\ p)$.
6. **Bob** chooses q random numbers $kb_0, ..., kb_{q-1}$, such that $Key_b = \sum_{k=0}^{q-1} kb_k$ $(mod\ p)$.
7. **Bob** sends all kb_k to **Alice** via q potential separate paths[1].
8. **Alice** receives q Key_b's components $kb_0, ..., kb_{q-1}$ from **Alice** and computes $Key_b = \sum_{k=0}^{q-1} kb_k (mod\ p)$.
9. **Alice** computes $Key = Key_b^n = g^{n \cdot m} (mod\ p)$.
10. **Bob** computes $Key = Key_a^m = g^{n \cdot m} (mod\ p)$.

---

[1] see **Algorithm 1** and next section for more details on the dispatching technique.

Method for Dispatching Splitted Key Components. When a source node s is attempting to exchange a key with a destination node d, it splits this key into several subkey components that must be dispatched through separate channels. Algorithm 1 illustrates how the dispatching of key components is implemented. We propose a straightforward technique to overcome the challenge of selecting the different paths that are necessary to route separately the each subkey towards the destination node.

As described previously, in the tree representing the nodes of our overlay network, the tree degree is set and known from start, and each connected node has a degree that may be less or equal to the tree degree. Thus, given n the tree degree, each node wishing to forward a key must split it into $n-1$ components that will be routed in separate paths. However, the selection of paths is iterative to account for the possibility that a few nodes may have less connections than the maximum possible. Thus, each node numbers the different nodes it is connected to and considers each of these nodes as the begining of a different path. Thus when a node has a degree k, it sends the first component to its first connected node (whether a parent or a child), and the second component to the second connected node, and so on until all connected nodes are used, and then it comes back to the first node to send the $(n-1-k)th$ component. We formally describe this path selection in Algorithm 3.

5   Security Analysis

In a multipath key exchange scheme, a malicious node that wishes to compromise a key being exchanged must be able to collect each and all subkey components routed in the network. Formally, when paths $\mathcal{P}_0, ..., \mathcal{P}_{q-1}$ are used to send several distinct keys from source $\mathcal{S}$ to destination $\mathcal{D}$, the only malicious nodes that could compromise the key should be located at the intersection of all paths, i.e. $M = \mathcal{P}_0 \cap ... \cap \mathcal{P}_{q-1}$. $\mathcal{S}$ and $\mathcal{D}$ are obviously ignored in this set. Thus, when $\mathcal{P}_0 \cap ... \cap \mathcal{P}_{q-1} = \{\mathcal{S}, \mathcal{D}\}$ (*bigon criterion* is respected [6, Lemma 2.5]) then all paths are disjoint and any MITM attack attempt cannot succeed. In such a desirable case, there exists a q-connected subgrah between $\mathcal{S}$ and $\mathcal{D}$ in the network topology. Consequently, the probability to have a MITM attack is estimated by $\sigma = \frac{|\mathcal{P}_0 \cap ... \cap \mathcal{P}_{q-1}| - 2}{|\mathcal{P}_0 \cup ... \cup \mathcal{P}_{q-1}| - 2}$ (where each path $\mathcal{P}_i$ is constituted of a set of consecutive hops from source to destination, and 2 represents the source and destination nodes, i.e. $|\{\mathcal{S}\}| + |\{\mathcal{D}\}|$).

The number of distinct paths is dependant on the source node degree. Thus, for a given *q-regular tree*, if q is a large number, then there is a very high probalitiy to have several disjoint transmission channels. Nonetheless, despite the robustness of our multipath negocation approach, cooperative MITM attacks, where several nodes maliciously cooperate to compromise a key, are possible. However, it is very hard, and excessively costly to execute such an attack in a real environment, especially in infrastructure poor areas.

6 Related Work

Previous work have proposed to use DHT infrastructure to manage cryptographic keys with more or less success and mostly with many caveats [8,25]. Wen et al. [26] have proposed a key management mechanism for DHT networks that transforms DHT table entries into a tree structure [7,9]. Srivasta and Liu have relied on the Diffie-Hellman algorithm to deliver a solution that prevents threats in DHT networks [20]. Their scheme, however, remained sensitive to Man-in-the-middle attacks.

Wang et al. have built a distributed PKI on top of the Chord structured overlay network [2]. They have used threshold cryptography to distribute the fonctionnality of the PKI across the nodes of the DHT network. This Chord-PKI provides traditional PKI features such as certification, revocation, storage and retrieval.

Takano et al. have proposed a Multipath Key Exchange similar to that proposed in our work [22]. Their techniques however were designed to fit the Symphony and Chord P2P systems and their ring topologies.

7 Conclusion

Scalable P2P networks are self-organizing, autonomous systems that accept any peer without the need of resorting to a central coordination. Each peer alternatively plays the role of a router in order to relay traffic to other peers. The flexibility of such settings thus allows them to operate effectively in infrastructure poor-areas. Unfortunately, the features that make them desirable also make them vulnerable to eavesdropping and modification attacks.

In order to address the security challenges of P2P networks, we propose an improvement of P2P paradigms devised in previous work [3,23] and a new approach for key exchange that generalizes a model proposed by Takano et al. [22]. On the one hand, we can still benefit from a truly scalable P2P overlay using hyperbolic coordinates where each node can decide on the strategy for accepting a parent node depending on its security priorities. On the other hand, we do not restrict our security scheme to a specific P2P topology, thus allowing our approach to be implemented in any P2P setup without any organization constraint.

In future work, we plan to implement a prototype of our system and assess it with simulation tools as well as with real-world experiments.

References

1. Ahmat, D., Magoni, D.: Muses: Mobile user secured session. In: Wireless Days (WD), 2012 IFIP, pp. 1–6 (2012)
2. Avramidis, A., Kotzanikolaou, P., Douligeris, C., Burmester, M.: Chord-pki: a distributed trust infrastructure based on p2p networks. Comput. Netw. 56(1), 378–398 (2012)

3. Cassagnes, C., Tiendrebeogo, T., Bromberg, D., Magoni, D.: Overlay addressing and routing system based on hyperbolic geometry. In: ISCC'11 - IEEE International Symposium on Computers and Communications, pp. 294–301, 28 June–1 July 2011

4. Demmer, M.J.: A Delay Tolerant Networking and System Architecture for Developing Regions. Ph.D. thesis, University of California, Berkeley (2008)

5. Diffie, W., Hellman, M.: New directions in cryptography. IEEE Trans. Inf. Theory **22**(6), 644–654 (1976)

6. Epstein, D.B.A.: Curves on 2-manifolds and isotopies. Acta Math. **115**(1), 15–16 (1966)

7. Kim, Y., Perrig, A., Tsudik, G.: Simple and fault-tolerant key agreement for dynamic collaborative groups (2000)

8. Kwon, H., Koh, S., Nah, J., Jang, J.: The secure routing mechanism for dht-based overlay network. In: 10th International Conference on Advanced Communication Technology, ICACT 2008, vol. 2, pp. 1300–1303 (2008)

9. Lee, P.P.C., Lui, J.C.S., Member, S., Yau, D.K.Y.: Distributed collaborative key agreement and authentication protocols for dynamic peer groups. IEEE/ACM Trans. Networking **14**, 263–276 (2006)

10. Lilien, L., Kamal, Z., Gupta, A.: Opportunistic networks: challenges in specializing the p2p paradigm. In: 17th International Workshop on Database and Expert Systems Applications, DEXA '06, pp. 722–726 (2006)

11. Lindgren, A., Hui, P.: The quest for a killer app for opportunistic and delay tolerant networks (invited paper). In: CHANTS, pp. 59–66 (2009)

12. Manku, G.S., Bawa, M., Raghavan, P.: Symphony: Distributed hashing in a small world. In: Proceedings of the 4th USENIX Symposium on Internet Technologies and Systems, pp. 127–140 (2003)

13. Morris, R., Karger, D., Kaashoek, F., Balakrishnan, H.: Chord: a scalable Peer-to-Peer lookup service for internet applications. In: ACM SIGCOMM 2001, San Diego, CA, September 2001

14. Ouoba, J., Bissyandé, T.F.: Leveraging the cultural model for opportunistic networking in Sub-Saharan Africa. In: Jonas, K., Rai, I.A., Tchuente, M. (eds.) AFRICOMM 2012. LNICST, vol. 119, pp. 163–173. Springer, Heidelberg (2013)

15. Reich, J., Chaintreau, A.: The age of impatience: optimal replication schemes for opportunistic networks. In: CoNEXT, pp. 85–96 (2009)

16. Risson, J., Moors, T.: Survey of research towards robust peer-to-peer networks: search methods. Comput. Netw. **50**(17), 3485–3521 (2006)

17. Saif, U., Chudhary, A.L., Butt, S., Butt, N.S., Murtaza, G.: Internet for the developing world: offline internet access at modem-speed dialup connections. In: International Conference on Information and Communication Technologies and Development, ICTD 2007, pp. 1–13 (2007)

18. Saif, U., Chudhary, A.L., Butt, S., Butt, N.F., Murtaza, G.: A peer-to-peer internet for the developing world. Inf. Technol. Int. Dev. **5**(1), 31–47 (2009)

19. Saif, U., Chudhary, A.L., Butt, S., Butt, N.F., Rodriguez, P., Saif, U., Chudhary, A.L.: Poor man's broadband: peer-to-peer dialup networking. ACM SIGCOMM Comput. Comm. Rev. **37**, 5–16 (2007)

20. Srivatsa, M., Liu, L.: Vulnerabilities and security threats in structured overlay networks: a quantitative analysis. In: 20th Annual Computer Security Applications Conference, pp. 252–261 (2004)

21. Steiner, M., Tsudik, G., Waidner, M.: Diffie-hellman key distribution extended to group communication. pp. 31–37. ACM Press (1996)

22. Takano, Y., Isozaki, N., Shinoda, Y.: Multipath key exchange on p2p networks. In: The First International Conference on Availability, Reliability and Security, ARES 2006, p. 8 (2006)
23. Tiendrebeogo, T., Ahmat, D., Magoni, D.: Reliable and scalable distributed hash tables harnessing hyperbolic coordinates. In: 2012 5th International Conference on New Technologies, Mobility and Security (NTMS), pp. 1–6 (2012)
24. Urdaneta, V., Pierre, G., Steen, M.V.: A survey of dht security techniques. ACM Comput. Surv. **43**(2), 8:1–8:49 (2011)
25. Wang, P., Osipkov, I., Kim, Y.: Myrmic: Secure and robust dht routing. Technical report (2007)
26. Wen, V., Shao-Zhang, N., Jian-Cheng, Z.: A key management mechanism for dht networks. In: 2012 Eighth International Conference on Intelligent Information Hiding and Multimedia Signal Processing (IIH-MSP), pp. 339–342 (2012)

A Pairing-Free Public Key Encryption with Keyword Searching for Cloud Storage Services

Thokozani Felix Vallent[1] and Hyunsung Kim[2(✉)]

[1] Department of Mathematics, Chancellor College,
University of Malawi, Zomba, Malawi
tfvallent@gmail.com
[2] Department of Cyber Security, Kyungil University,
Kyungsansi, Kyungbuk Province 712-701, Korea
secueye@gmail.com

Abstract. Although cloud computing provides a platform for numerous adorable applications, users are still detracts from fully utilizing its services, for fear of jeopardizing data confidentiality and privacy by surrendering maintenance and management roles in the hands of cloud service providers (CSPs). A natural resolution to users' concern is employing cryptographic measures which allow searching for a particular keyword flexibly stored in the cloud without divulging data privacy to any unwanted party even the CSP itself. Already there has been many keyword searchable encryption researches done, but they mostly bear a weakness of offline keyword guessing attack, besides they are based on the heavier pairing computation. We therefore devise an efficient public key encryption with keyword search (PEKS) protocol that is pairing-free and is resilient against offline keyword guessing attack for cloud storage services. Our basic construction is based on the Diffie-Hellman problem and the El Gamal encryption scheme to achieve a secure channel-free public key encryption with keyword searching (SCF-PEKS). In this design a user sends a key allowing the CSP to only identify words containing a specific keyword and return search results and learn nothing else besides.

Keywords: Cloud computing · El gamal · Keyword search · Offline keyword guessing attack

1 Introduction

Cloud computing is an advancement in computing in which dynamically scalable and often virtualized resources are provided as services over the internet [1–5]. This technology enables convenient, on-demand network access to a pool of configurable computing resource that can be deployed with great efficiency and minimal

This work was supported by the National Research Foundation of Korea Grant funded by the Korean Government (MEST) (NRF-2010-0021575).

© Institute for Computer Sciences, Social Informatics and Telecommunications Engineering 2014
T.F. Bissyandé and G. van Stam (Eds.): AFRICOMM 2013, LNICST 135, pp. 70–78, 2014.
DOI: 10.1007/978-3-319-08368-1_8

management overhead [2] such resources are networks, applications and services. So the purported cloud computing services are, software as a service (Saas), Platform as a service (Paas) and Infrastructure as a service (Iaas) all over the Internet while managed and maintained by third parties at outback locations. Central to cloud computing advancement is CSPs, whose role is to provide the abstract application services that comes with cloud computing. Specifically, the cloud-based outsourced data storage/ distribution service is most typical and promising applications. Google, Amazon and Microsoft are the well-known companies offering cloud storage services such as Google App Engine Datastore, Content Delivery Network (CDN) and CloudFront, on utility computing basis. For example Amazon simple storage service (Amazon S3) charges from $0.12 to $0.15 per gigabyte per month [3, 5]. In Iaas, a user (Alice) stores data in a cloud server of which cannot be trust entirely, as such the data is securely encrypted before storage. Even though Alice does not trust the cloud server she wishes to benefit from its services and also entrust the server with the task of informing her on incoming messages, mails containing certain keywords of interest. This provision serves Alice with much convenience as she is no longer constrained with time and space to perform her business, but can search in cloud storage account anywhere and anytime on any device. Hence Alice resorts to store encrypted data in the cloud to preserve the integrity, privacy and confidentiality of the data. Much as encryption preserves the data securely, we seek a way of retrieving a keyword searched on the encrypted data, without leaking any vital information to unwanted parties even CSP. For example, when Bob sends an email with the keyword "urgent" the mail is routed to Alice's mobile device and when the mail contains a keyword "lunch" the mail is routed to Alice's desktop for reading later [6].

To enable keyword searching over the stored encrypted data Alice creates a trapdoor for specified keywords to allow the gateway to make routing decisions, in a way, that the gateway learns nothing else about incoming mail. So the CSP is only entrusted with management of encrypted data, for the sake of preserving Alice's privacy and confidentiality in whatever sensitive transaction involved, which for example could be about, business reports, financial charts, and medical records that should be kept from exposure to unauthorized parties [7]. To ensure security and privacy while giving CSP effective data utilization of the encrypted data, cryptographic techniques have to be applied, right before outsourcing data in the cloud. For data retrieval services the technique involved is known as searchable encryption that satisfies cloud users' security needs by retaining: privacy of data, privacy of data owner and privacy of the retriever [7].

Since Song et al. proposed the first efficient keyword searching scheme on encrypted data [8], many variant searchable encryption schemes have been proposed [4, 6, 7]. In [6] Boneh et al. proposed the first PEKS built on the basic construction in [9], however Baek et al. [10] pointed out it is unrealistic and computationally demanding, due to the underlining assumption of establishing a secure channel for transporting a trapdoor. The other flaw noted with the scheme was vulnerability to, offline keyword guessing attack due to statistical analysis on cipher-text and trapdoors [8, 9]. Although Baek et al. proposed an efficient SCF-PEKS scheme to fix the problem in [10], nevertheless Jian et al. [11] found out that, offline keyword guessing attack lingers on. So the weakness of offline keyword guessing attack has been spotted with a considerable number of searchable encryption schemes [2, 11–14], and besides the schemes are based on heavy computation of pairing operation. Pairing based trapdoor has a security problem in that, it allows offline keyword guessing attack, as an attacker could choose a key to test whether the captured trapdoor includes the guessed keyword with the receiver's public key by utilizing bilinear map operation [13]. In order to improve performance Khadre [15] and Yang et al. [14] proposed pairing-free PEKS schemes, but still offline keyword guessing remains just as in the former scheme [2, 11]. So the motive of this paper is to present an efficient and secure PEKS scheme without using pairing operation that is applicable in cloud computing, while fixing the lingering problem of offline keyword guessing attack.

This paper is organized as follows: In Sect. 2 we recall preliminaries, outlining searchable encryption and the security requirements. In Sect. 3, we present an efficient public key encryption with keyword searching considering the mentioned security and privacy concerns of cloud storage services. Then in Sect. 4, we provide an analysis of the proposed protocol in regard to security requirements, computational and efficiency. Finally we conclude the paper in Sect. 5.

2   Preliminaries

We consider any cyclic group of prime order for example say a group of Z^*_q, where q is prime. The definition of the intractable problem related to the proposed protocol and El Gamal encryption scheme are given below.

Definition 2.1. The Diffie-Hellman problem (DHP)

Let be a prime number and g an integer. The DHP is the problem of computing the value $g^{ab}(\bmod\ p)$ from the known values of $g^a(\bmod\ p)$ and $g^b(\bmod\ p)$ [16].

Definition 2.2. El Gamal encryption scheme

El Gamal encryption scheme is an asymmetric encryption scheme based on DHP problem in the cyclic group with the following outlined phases: key generation, encryption and decryption [4]:

KeyGen: The algorithm picks a random p element $x \in F_q$ and computes g^x for which g is a generator of the prime order cyclic group Z^*_q. The user's public key is g^x and the corresponding private key is x.

Encryption: To encrypt a message m picks a random element $r \in F_q$, computes $c_1 = g^x$, $c_2 = m(g^x)^r$ and sets the cipher-text $c_m = (c_1, c_2)$.

Decryption: Given $c_m = (c_1, c_2)$, to recover the message, computes $c_2 . c_1^{-x} = m$.

2.1   Outline of PEKS Scheme

A non-interactive PEKS scheme consists of the following polynomial time randomized algorithms [4]:

1. *KeyGen(λ)*: Which takes a security parameters, λ_1 to generate a user's public and private key pair (A_{pub}, A_{pri}) and λ_2 to generate a CSP's public and private key pair (S_{pub}, S_{pri}).

2. *EMBEnc(A_{pub}, S_{pub}, m)*: For a user's public key A_{pub}, CSP's public key S_{pub}, and a message $m \in M$ the algorithm produces its cipher-text $c_m \in C_M$.

3. *KWEnc(A_{pub}, w)*: The algorithm takes, a user's public key A_{pub} and a keyword $w \in W$ as inputs and produces w's cipher-text $c_w \in C_W$.

4. *Tcompute(A_{pri}, w)*: Given user's private key A_{pri} and a keyword w and produces a trapdoor T_w.

5. *KWTest(A_{pub}, c_w, T_w)*: Given Alice's public key, a searchable encryption $PEKS(A_{pub}, w') = c_w$ and a trapdoor, $Tcompute(A_{pri}, w) = T_w$ as inputs, it outputs 'yes' if $w = w'$ and 'no' otherwise.

6. *PDecrypt(S_{pri}, A_{pub}, m)*: The algorithm takes CSP's private key S_{pri}, user's public key A_{pub} and a cipher-text $c_m \in C_M$ and computes an intermediate result $c_\rho \in C_\rho$.

7. *MSGRecovery(A_{pri}, c_m, c_ρ)*: The algorithm takes user's private key, A_{pri}, a cipher-text c_m, and an intermediate result c_ρ and outputs the plain-text message m.

The construction of our PEKS adopts the assumption that the DHP problem and the variant of El Gamal encryption system are intractable. There are three entities in PEKS: data sender (Bob), data receiver (Alice) and data storage server (CSP). Prior on Alice generates a trapdoor, T_{wi}, for specified keywords and present them to the CSP for future keyword searching query on a number of devices she could have: desktop, laptop, mobile device, etc. Bob encrypts an email or a message M with keywords w_1, $w_1 w_2,..., w_k$ using Alice's public key and appends the encrypted keywords: $PEKS(A_{pub}, w_1), PEKS(A_{pub}, w_2),..., PEKS(A_{pub}, w_k)$. Then Bob sends to the CSP the message: $Enc_{Apub}(m_1)||PEKS(A_{pub}, w_1),\ Enc_{Apub}(m_2)||PEKS(A_{pub}, w_2),..., Enc_{Apub}(m_k)||PEKS(A_{pub}, w_k)$. So whenever Alice wishes to search for any encrypted keyword of interest on any devices and at any time she gives the CSP the trapdoor associated with that encrypted keyword, say, "urgent". In turn the CSP has to search for the keyword and gives back a response to Alice if there is a keyword exactly corresponding to the given trapdoor, without learning anymore information besides. Unlike Boneh et al.'s construction of PEKS that requires a secure channel to protect the trapdoor during cipher-text transmission, the proposed construction adapts a SCF-PEKS, first proposed by Baek et al. [10]. Thus data sender just uses the receiver's public key and the server's public key each time he/she stores encrypted data meant for Alice in the cloud server. The design works also if Alice stores data on her own for later use in the cloud server.

2.2 Security Requirements

In order to construct a secure and privacy preserving PEKS that provides confidentiality and integrity of messages from user to the CSP the following security requirements must be satisfied:

1. *Trapdoor indistinguishability:* No adversary should get any information from any captured trapdoor.

2. *Cipher-text indistinguishability:* Since when data is encrypted for storage in the CSP, it is appended with the corresponding keyword cipher-text containing the keywords, $w_1, w_2,..., w_k$. Even if the keyword cipher-text is captured in transit no adversary can get the embedded keywords from the cipher-text. Thus an adversary will be unable to distinguish a given pair of cipher-text based on the message they encrypt.

3. *Entity anonymity:* Whenever a sender sends a message to the CSP under a receiver's public key, no adversary should deduce the identity of the authorized receiver based on keyword cipher-text.

4. *Offline keyword guessing attack protection:* Even if the trapdoor is eavesdropped during transmission or inside the CSP no adversary should expose or derive secret information from trapdoor.

3 Proposed PEKS

In this section we construct an efficient PEKS based on El Gamal encryption scheme and the DH problem, which does not require secure-channel to exchange a trapdoor.

1. *KeyGen(λ):* The key generation algorithm takes the security parameters λ_1 and λ_2 to generate public and private key pairs $(x, y = g^x)$ and $(s, Z = g^s)$ for user and the respectively.

2. *EMBEnc(y, Z, e, m):* A sender picks a random number $e \in Z^*_q$ as ephemeral private key and let $epk = g^e$ as an ephemeral public key. To encrypt the message, $m \in M$, the algorithm uses the receiver's public key, $y = g^x$, CSP's public key, $Z = g^s$ and $e \in Z^*_q$ as inputs. Then computes $C_1 = my^e$ and $C_2 = Z^e$. So the cipher-text $c_m \in C_M$ for $m \in M$ is $c_m = \{C_1, C_2\}$.

3. *KWEnc(y, w):* To encrypt m's keywords $w_1, w_2,..., w_k$ under the public key, $y = g^x$, the encryption algorithm computes $c_i = H_1(w_i||ID_A)$ and $C_{wi} = y^{ci}$ by using one-way hash function for $w_i \in \{w_1, w_2,..., w_k\}$. Then the sender conceals the keyword as $R_{wi} = C_{wi}g^e$ and sends $c_m = \{C_1, C_2, R_{wi}\}$ to CSP for storage.

4. *Tcompute(x, Z, w):* To allow retrieving the email containing only the specified keyword w_j, the algorithm computes a trapdoor $T_{wj} = (Z^{cj})^x$ under the receiver's private key and send it to the CSP.

5. *KWTest(y, c_w, T_w, s):* First CSP uses its private key to compute $C_\rho = (C_2)^{-s}g^e$ and then extracts the keyword $C_{wi} = R_{wi}g^{-e}$. To test if a given email or message in the cloud has w_j as a keyword the algorithm tests whether $(C_{wi})^s = T_{wj}$. If the algorithm outputs YES, then $w_i = w_j$ as required or else if the algorithm output NO, then $w_i \neq w_j$.

6. *PDecrypt(s, y, c_m):* As a partial decryption for a given cipher-text, $c_m = \{C_1, C_2, C_{wi}\}$, the CSP sends the simplified results, $c_m' = \{C_1, C_\rho, C_{wi}\}$, to the user.

7. *MSGRecovery(x, c_m, c_ρ):* To recover a message, m, from a cipher-text, c_m', the algorithm uses the receiver's private key and computes $(C_\rho)^x = g^{ex}$ and then $c_1.c_\rho^{-x} = m$.

Unlike [6], the proposed protocol does not need establishment of secure channel to transport the trapdoor, thus the trapdoor can be transported in public without any worry of offline keyword guessing attack. So by excluding the need for secure channel, say SSL, for trapdoor transportation, the proposed protocol improves its efficiency significantly.

4 Security and Performance Analyses

This section discusses the security analysis and the performance analysis of the proposed protocol.

4.1 Security Analysis

In this subsection, we provide the security analysis of the proposed protocol by showing how it secures against attack associated with searchable encryption.

Trapdoor security: This property prevents the attacker from deducing what the user is searching for. Since the embedded keyword of the trapdoor is in digest form, $c_i = H_1(w_i || ID_A)$ so a malicious server could not know the keyword under search from T_{wj}. The actual keyword w_j is still hidden to CSP as it is also protected by user's private key x in $T_{wi} = (Z^{cj})^x$. So due to this property, the server cannot derive a valid trapdoor, T_{wij} from two given trapdoors, T_{wi} and T_{wj} for the keywords, w_i and w_j because of the hash function and the user's private key in the construction. Thus given any two trapdoors T_{wi} and T_{wj} for the keywords, w_i and w_j a malicious server cannot distinguish which trapdoor is for which keyword with non-negligible probability.

Keyword security: This feature preserves the privacy of what keyword a user searches for in the CSP and keeps it from being exposed to the CSP or other unwanted parties. The keyword under search is not transmitted in plain but rather in a transformed in a one-way format $C_{wi} = y^{ci}$. This hides the actual query from an eavesdropper. Further to prevent statistical analysis of the search results, due to exploiting the document's frequency, by the CSP the keyword is sent in the form, $R_{wi} = C_{wi} g^e$. Since R_{wi} is dynamic depending on the random ephemeral key $e \in Z^*_q$, an eavesdropper or CSP will have no idea of the keyword under search. Therefore if given two encrypted keywords R_{wi} and C_{wj} an adversary cannot deduce the plaintext keyword w_i and w_j from them. Thus the keyword is dynamic hence protected from statistical analysis by CSP or eavesdropper.

Entity anonymity: The proposed protocol provides entity anonymity in that the cipher-text does not leak any information about the user's identity. From the transmitted cipher $c_m = \{C_1, C_2, R_{wi}\}$ from sender to CSP, no adversary can infer the correct identity of the user. In this way the proposed protocol provides user anonymity.

Off-line keyword guessing security: The proposed protocol secures against an outsider attack and a curious CSP carrying out off-line keyword guessing attack. Though the trapdoor T_{wi} for any keyword w_i is sent in public it does not leak any information about the keyword, since it is derived by user's private key. Furthermore the keyword is hidden by the one way hash function in the computation, $c_i = H_1(w_i\|ID_A)$. So to guess a keyword from a captured trapdoor, $T_{wj} = (Z^{cj})^x = g^{cjxs}$ is infeasible since it's a DHP. Thus from the trapped T_{wi} alone, the CSP cannot determine the embedded keyword w such that $w' = w_i$. Therefore this feature protects the encrypted data from a malicious CSP, however it allows processing search results without revealing the sensitive information.

4.2   Performance Analysis

The proposed protocol leverages user's computational overhead by having the CSP do partial decipherment on the encrypted keyword. Furthermore, the protocol out do most existing PEKS protocol on efficiency, for it is pairing-free. The security bases of the protocol are on the intractability of the DHP problem and El Gamal encryption, which just uses the lighter operation of exponentiation. By the fact, that pairing is the most expensive computation operation, whereas as scalar multiplication is the next while modular exponentiation is the third, then followed by operation on the finite field like modular multiplication, and the least being hash function and the XOR [17, 18], this means that the proposed protocol is more efficient than [4, 6, 10] which are based on pairing computation as shown in Table 1 below. The comparison only focuses on the operation carried out by cloud data sender or cloud data receiver with constrained computational power as we regard cloud server, CSP, to have sufficient communication capability.

So comparatively the proposed protocol is more efficient since pairing operation is at least 10 times heavier than scalar multiplication [18].

Table 1. Comparison with related protocols on computational cost.

Operation / Protocol	PA	SM	EX	HF
Li et al. in [4]	3	-	5	3
Baek et al. in [10]	2	2	1	1
Boneh et al. in [6]	1	3	1	3
Our protocol	-	3	6	1

PA: Pairing, SM: Scalar Multiplication, EX: Exponentiation, HF: Hash Function

5 Conclusion

This paper presented a pairing-free PEKS scheme which is a computationally efficient for searchable encryption scheme for Cloud computing while upholding confidentiality, integrity and privacy anytime, anywhere and on any device. The proposed scheme also addresses the noted weakness of other existing researches by withstanding offline keyword guessing attack. The design construction of the scheme is based on the intractability of the DHP problem and El Gamal encryption other than pairing operation, hence making it more efficient as compared to other schemes and is also a SCF-PEKS. Our future aspiration is integrating proxy re-encryption and multi-keyword ranked search over encrypted cloud data.

References

1. James, N.M., Daniel, E., Vasanthi, N.A.: Survey on privacy-preserving methods for storage in cloud computing. IJCA Proc. Amrita Int. Conf. Women Comput. **4**, 1–4 (2013)
2. Hsu, S.T., Yang, C.C., Hwang, M.S.: A study of public key encryption with keyword search. Int. J. Netw. Secur. **15**(2), 71–79 (2013)
3. Li, J., Wang, Q., Wang, C., Cao, N., Ren, K., Lou, W.: Enabling efficient fuzzy keyword search over encrypted data in cloud computing. IEEE Trans. Parallel Distrib. Syst. **23**(8), 1467–1479 (2012)
4. Liu, Q., Wang, G., Wu, J.: Secure and privacy preserving for keyword searching for cloud storage services. J. Netw. Comput. Appl. **35**, 927–933 (2012)
5. Agudo, I., Nuñez, D., Giammatteo, G., Rizomiliotis, P., Lambrinoudakis, C.: Cryptography goes to the cloud. In: Lee, C., Seigneur, J.-M., Park, J.J., Wagner, R.R. (eds.) STA 2011 Workshops. CCIS, vol. 187, pp. 190–197. Springer, Heidelberg (2011)
6. Boneh, D., Di Crescenzo, G., Ostrovsky, R., Persiano, G.: Public key encryption with keyword search. In: Cachin, C., Camenisch, J.L. (eds.) EUROCRYPT 2004. LNCS, vol. 3027, pp. 506–522. Springer, Heidelberg (2004)
7. Koo, D., Hur, J., Yoon, H.: Secure and efficient data retrieval over encrypted data using attribute-based encryption in cloud storage. Comput. Electron. Eng. **39**, 34–46 (2013)
8. Song, D.X., Wagner, D., Perrig, A.: Practical techniques for searches on encrypted data. In: Proceedings of the IEEE Symposium on Security and Privacy, pp. 44–55 (2000)
9. Boneh, D., Franklin, M.: Identity-based encryption from the Weil pairing. In: Kilian, J. (ed.) CRYPTO 2001. LNCS, vol. 2139, pp. 213–229. Springer, Heidelberg (2001)
10. Baek, J., Safavi-Naini, R., Susilo, W.: Public key encryption with keyword search revisited. In: Gervasi, O., Murgante, B., Laganà, A., Taniar, D., Mun, Y., Gavrilova, M.L. (eds.) ICCSA 2008, Part I. LNCS, vol. 5072, pp. 1249–1259. Springer, Heidelberg (2008)
11. Jian, W.B., Her, C.T., Gwo, J.F.: Security improvement against malicious server's attack for a dPEKS scheme. Int. J. Inf. Educ. Technol. **1**(4), 350–353 (2011)
12. Tang, Q., Chen, L.: Public-key encryption with registered keyword search. In: Martinelli, F., Preneel, B. (eds.) EuroPKI 2009. LNCS, vol. 6391, pp. 163–178. Springer, Heidelberg (2010)
13. Byun, J.W., Rhee, H.S., Park, H.-A., Lee, D.-H.: Off-line keyword guessing attacks on recent keyword search schemes over encrypted data. In: Jonker, W., Petković, M. (eds.) SDM 2006. LNCS, vol. 4165, pp. 75–83. Springer, Heidelberg (2006)

14. Yang, H.M., Xu, C.X., Zhao, H.T.: An efficient public key encryption with keyword scheme not using pairing. In: First International Conference on Instrumentation, Measurement, Computer Communication and Control, pp. 900–904 (2011)
15. Khader, D.: Public key encryption with keyword search based on k-resilient IBE. In: Gavrilova, M.L., Gervasi, O., Kumar, V., Tan, C.J.K., Taniar, D., Laganá, A., Mun, Y., Choo, H. (eds.) ICCSA 2006. LNCS, vol. 3982, pp. 298–308. Springer, Heidelberg (2006)
16. Hoffstein, J., Pipher, J., Silverman, J.H.: An Introduction to Mathematical Cryptography. Springer, New York (2008)
17. Zhu, R.W., Yang, G., Wong, D.S.: An efficient identity-based key exchange protocol with KGS forward secrecy for low-power devices. In: Deng, X., Ye, Y. (eds.) WINE 2005. LNCS, vol. 3828, pp. 500–509. Springer, Heidelberg (2005)
18. Cao, X., Kou, W., Du, X.: A pairing-free identity-based authenticated key agreement protocol with minimal message exchange. Inf. Sci. **180**(15), 2895–2903 (2010)

A Pairing Based Authentication and Key Establishment Scheme for Remote Patient Monitoring Systems

Kambombo Mtonga[1], Eun-Jun Yoon[2], and Hyunsung Kim[2(✉)]

[1] Department of IT Convergence, Kyungil University,
Gyeongsan, South Korea
[2] Department of Cyber Security, Kyungil University,
Kyungsansi, Kyungbuk 712-701, Korea
{ejyoon, kim}@kiu.ac.kr

Abstract. With the evolution of Wireless Medical Sensor Networks (WMSNs), real-time remote patient monitoring has become more feasible than ever before. Different sensors can be used e.g. at home to monitor patient's vital signs such as pulse, respiration and blood pressure. However, given the distributed nature of WMSNs for remote patient monitoring, there is a greater challenge in ensuring data security, integrity, confidentiality and access control. This is because the transmission of personal and medical information is done over insecure communication channels i.e. the Internet. At the same time, patient's physiological data are highly sensitive and remote patient monitoring systems are extremely vulnerable to many attacks. Since there is great need to access the real-time data inside WMSN nodes, proper authentication of entities (e.g. health personnel) must be ensured before allowing them access. To this end, this paper proposes a pairing based authentication and key establishment scheme for remote patient monitoring systems. The scheme is two-factor i.e. combines smartcard and password, and achieves various desirable properties such as mutual authentication, strong access control, patient identity privacy, patient un-traceability, replay attack resistance and forward secrecy.

Keywords: U-Healthcare system · Information security · Patient privacy · Bilinear pairing · Authentication and key agreement

1 Introduction

The recent technological advances in sensors, low-power integrated circuits, and wireless communications have enabled the design of low-cost, miniature, lightweight, and intelligent physiological sensor nodes. These sensor nodes capable of sensing, processing and communicating one or more vital signs, can be seamlessly integrated into wireless personal or body area networks (WPANs or WBANs) for health monitoring. Note: hereafter we refer to both WPAN and WBAN as WMSN for convenience. A WMSN contains a number of portable, miniaturized, and autonomous sensor nodes (in-body or/and on-body nodes) that monitors patients under natural physiological states without constraining their normal activities. These networks

© Institute for Computer Sciences, Social Informatics and Telecommunications Engineering 2014
T.F. Bissyandé and G. van Stam (Eds.): AFRICOMM 2013, LNICST 135, pp. 79–89, 2014.
DOI: 10.1007/978-3-319-08368-1_9

promise to revolutionize healthcare by allowing inexpensive and non-invasive continuous health monitoring with almost real-time updates of medical records via the Internet [1].

Despite the fact that wireless healthcare offers many advantages to patients being monitored, it also leaves their physiological data highly vulnerable [2]. This is because the transmission of personal and medical information is done over insecure communication channels like the Internet. Hence an adversary can easily capture the electronic medical behavior of patients and construct "patient profiles," or reveal sensitive information related to patient's medical history, leading to the violation of the patient's privacy. More importantly, the patients' vitals are very sensitive; as such they must be kept secure from unauthorized entities and common security threats [3]. Furthermore, as medical sensor nodes themselves provide services to entities (e.g. doctors, nurses, patient, and technicians) it is necessary to control who can access their information and whether they are authenticated to do so. Therefore, strong entity authentication is a core requirement to prevent illegal access to the patients' vital signs.

Attempts have been made by researchers to propose secure and privacy preserving schemes for remote health monitoring systems. In 2011 Mark et al. [4] proposed a ubiquitous healthcare framework for rural African environment. The framework was designed to assist in healthcare planning, collection and management of patient records in African developing states. However, Mark et al.'s framework is prone to password guessing attacks on the physician's side. In [5], Huang et al. proposed a secure hierarchical sensor-based healthcare monitoring architecture. They considered three real-time healthcare application scenarios i.e. in-hospital, in-home and nursing homes. Their architecture has three network tiers namely; sensor network, mobile network, and back-end network. However, Huang et al. did not consider strong entity (i.e. physician) authentication. Based on elliptic curve cryptography, Le et al. [6] proposed a mutual authentication and access control protocol which allows legitimate physicians access to their patient's data. But as noted in [7], Le et al.'s protocol is susceptible to information-leakage attacks.

Clearly there remains a gap and need for secure schemes for remote patient monitoring that can provide strong entity (i.e. physician) authentication and high level of access control. Access control to patient's vital signs is an essential part of secure remote patient monitoring systems because it protects their health data from unauthorized access by malicious parties by checking if any system user has the necessary rights to access the resources he/she requested. For example, assume a real-time scenario, and suppose a physician wants to query the patient's medical sensors for physiological information. It is vital in this case that before the medical sensors can respond to the query, the doctor/nurse should be thoroughly authenticated.

In this paper we propose a pairing based authentication and key establishment scheme for remote patient monitoring systems. In our scheme we consider an in-home patient monitoring scenario. We assume a real-time situation where a physician would like to query a specific medical sensor for real time data. Our scheme is two-factor (password and smartcard) and consists of six parties (see Fig. 1 below); namely: The registration server, the authentication server, patient, WMSN, the gateway of a patient's WMSN and physician (e.g. doctor/nurse with smartcard). In our scheme we

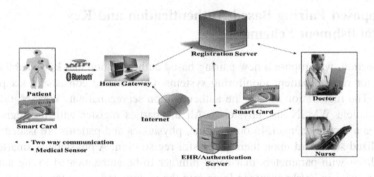

Fig. 1. Parties in our remote patient monitoring system.

require that all the parties be registered with the registration server via a secure channel and that each party (e.g. patient, doctor, nurse and surgeon) has to first prove his/her authenticity to the authentication server before he/she can access patient medical information. Furthermore, we require that any query to patient medical sensor for physiological information should first be authenticated by the gateway of the patient's WMSN.

2 Preliminaries

2.1 Bilinear Pairing

Let G_1 be an additive group of prime order q and G_2 be a multiplicative cyclic group of the same order. Let P denote a generator of G_i. Then, there exists an efficient computable bilinear map $\hat{e} : G_1 * G_1 \rightarrow G_2$ which has the following properties:

- *Bilinearity*
  Given P and Q in G_1 and $a, b \in Z_q^*$, we have $\hat{e}(aP, bQ) = \hat{e}(P, Q)^{ab}$.
- *Non-degeneracy*
$$\hat{e}(P, P) \neq 1_{G_2}.$$

- *Computability*
  There exists an efficient algorithm to compute $\hat{e}(P, Q)$ for any $P, Q \in G_1$.

2.2 Security Assumptions

- *Discrete Logarithm Problem (DLP)*
  Given $P, Q \in G_1$, find $a \in Z_q^*$ such that $Q = aP$.
- *Computational Diffie-Hellman Problem (CDH)*
  Given (P, aP, bP) for any $a, b \in Z_q^*$ and $P \in G_1$, compute abP.

3 Proposed Pairing Based Authentication and Key Establishment Scheme

In this section, we propose a new pairing based authentication and key establishment scheme for remote patient monitoring systems. Our scheme consists of six parties; namely: The registration server, the authentication server, patient, WMSN, the gateway of patient WMSN and physician. All the parties register with the registration server via a secure channel. In our scheme, physicians and patients are issued with a personalized smartcard upon their successful registration. A physician's smartcard is personalized with parameters that helps him/her to be authenticated to the authentication sever when he/she wants to login into the system and query the medical sensor for patient physiological data. While a patient's smartcard is personalized with parameters which he/she can use to register his/her home gateway to the registration server. Mutual authentication is carried out between the physician and the medical sensor via the authentication server and the gateway for the physician to access the data in the sensor node. Our scheme consist of four phases- setup phase, registration phase, mutual authentication and session key establishment phase and password change phase.

3.1 Notations

Table 1.

Table 1. Notations.

Notation	Meaning
U_i	i^{th} physician who wants to login
AS	Authentication server
PT	Patient
RS	Registration server
S_i	Medical sensor
GS	Gateway server
id_i	Identity for party i
pid_i	Pseudo-ID for party i
s	Master secret key for RS
Pub_{RS}	Public key for RS
y	Master key shared between GS and S_n
Q_i	Public key for party i
d_i	Private key for party i
$ê$	Bilinear map- $ê : \quad G_1 \times G_1 \rightarrow G_2$
$H_1(.)$	Hash function-$H_1 : \{0,1\}^* \rightarrow G_1$
$H_2(.)$	Hash function-$H_2 : \{0,1\}^* \rightarrow Z_q^*$
$\|$	Concatenation operation
PW_i	$U_i's$ password

3.2 Setup

Suppose G_1 is an additive cyclic group of prime order q, and G_2 is a multiplicative cyclic group of the same order. We assume that the CDH problem is hard in group G_1. Let P be a generator of, G_1, $\hat{e} : G_1 * G_1 \rightarrow G_2$ be a bilinear mapping and $H_1 : \{0,1\}^* \rightarrow G_1$ and $H_2 : \{0,1\}^* \rightarrow Z_q^*$ be two secure collision resistant cryptographic hash functions. The RS selects a secret key s and computes the public key as $Pub_{RS} = sP$. The RS also computes the public and private key pair (Q_{AS}, d_{AS}) for the authentication server AS, where $Q_{AS} = H_1(id_{AS})$ and $d_{AS} = sH_1(id_{AS})$. (Q_{AS}, d_{AS}) are sent to AS via a secure channel. The system public parameters are $\{G_1, G_2, \hat{e}, P, q, Pub_{Rs}, H_1(.), H_2(.)\}$. This phase is executed only once. See Fig. 2 for summery of system setup. We make the following assumption concerning our system setup.

Assumption 1: we assume that the medical sensors and GS in the same network share a master key y via any key agreement method [8]. Using this key, a medical sensor node can tell whether other nodes are in the same network or not. This key is used by the medical sensor node and the GS to authenticate each other and negotiate a session key.

3.3 Registration Phase

All parties register with the RS via a secure channel. Below we discuss the registration process of all parties.

3.3.1 Physician Registration

To register, a physician U_i (nurse or doctor) submits his/her identity id_i and password of his/her choice PW_i Note: the role of RS could also be played by the EHR server. The RS then performs following computations:

- Computes $V_i = H_1(id_i \| PW_i)$, $W_i = H_1(id_i)$ and $Reg_i = sW_i$.
- The RS then issues the physician with a smartcard personalized with $\{V_i, P, Reg_i, W_i, Q_{AS}, H_1(\cdot), H_2(\cdot)\}$, where P is generator of G_1.

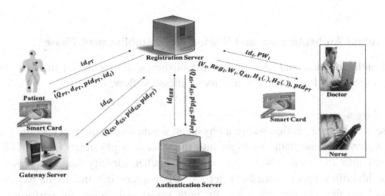

Fig. 2. System setup.

3.3.2   Patient, Medical Sensor and Home Gateway Registration

To register, a patient PT submits his/her real-ID id_{PT} to RS. The RS first validates the submitted identity. If validation is successful, then the server computes a unique pseudo-ID pid_{PT} which will be used to identify the patient in the network instead of the real-ID. This is important to ensure patient anonymity and un-traceability. We require that only RS knows the relationship between the patient's real-ID and the pseudo-ID.

The RS also computes public and private key pair (Q_{GS}, d_{ds}) for PT's GS where $Q_{GS} = H_1(pid_{GS})$ and $d_{GS} = sH_1(pid_{GS})$ respectively. Here, pid_{GS} is pseudo-ID of gateway. This is important for maintaining patient un-traceability and un-linkability.

Note: There are certain differences between monitoring in-hospital patients and patients in-home. One such difference concerns the infrastructure (computer networks, servers, etc.). In the home monitoring network, the gateway for the patient could be a desktop for example. Since we require that all registrations with RS be done via a secure channel, we make the following assumption.

Assumption 2: Upon a successful registration, the patient is issued with a smartcard. The RS personalizes the smartcard with information (e.g. $d_{GS} = sH_1(pid_{GS})$, pid_{PT}) which the patient can later use to register his/her home GS to the GS. Upon arrival at home, the patient passes over the information in the smartcard to the GS. Since some of the information is sensitive, we require that once the GS gets the parameters, it should erase the information from the memory of the smartcard to avoid security implications that may result in case the smartcard ends up in the hands of an adversary.

Once patient registration is successful, the RS issues the patient with medical sensor kit which is later strategically deployed by a qualified technician. The RS further securely passes the pseudo-ID pid_{PT} of the patient to the respective physicians and $\{pid_{PT}, pid_{GS}\}$ to the AS. This is important for authentication of communication request from physicians.

Here we assume that each patient receives one/more medical sensors depending on his/her health problems and that each sensor S_i can be independently queried to and that each is capable of communicating health data.

3.4   Mutual Authentication and Session Key Establishment Phase

Mutual authentication and session key establishment are achieved through the following stages. See Fig. 3 for a summary of message flow.

3.4.1   Login

Suppose a real time situation where a physician would like to query a specific medical sensor S_i for real time data. To login into the system, a physician U_i inserts his/her smartcard into the card reader then submits his/her identity id_i, PW_i, pid_{PT} and $S_i$which identifies specific medical sensor. Upon receiving the login request, the smartcard verifies the physician locally with pre-stored values by performing following operations:

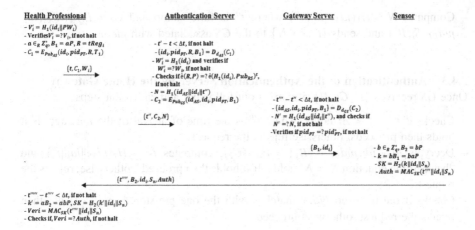

Fig. 3. Message flow for authentication and key establishment.

- Computes $V_i' = H_1(id_i\|PW_i)$ and checks if $V_i = V_i'$. If the equation is satisfied then proceeds, otherwise rejects the login request.
- Generates $a \in_R Z_q^*$. and computes $B_1 = aP$ and $R = tReg_i = tsW_i$, where t is current time stamp while $W_i = H_1(id_i)$, and encrypts $C_1 = E_{Q_{AS}}(id_i, R, pid_{PT}, S_i, B_1)$. Then the smartcard sends request $\{t, C_1, W_i\}$ to the AS. Note: for detailed analysis on the use of timestamp as nonces, please refer to [9].

3.4.2 Authentication of Physician by the Authentication Server

Once the AS receives the request $\{t, C_1, W_i\}$ it carries out the following computations to authenticate the doctor/nurse (smartcard):

- Checks if $t' - t < \Delta t$ is satisfied. Here, t' is the time of arrival of the request and Δt is tolerated transmission delay. If the check holds then proceeds, otherwise rejects the login request.
- Performs decryption on C_1 as, $\{id_i, R, pid_{PT}, S_i, B_1\} = D_{d_{AS}}(C_1)$.
- Computes $W_i' = H_1(id_i)$ and checks if $W_i = W_i'$. If it is successful proceeds, otherwise rejects the login request.
- Verifies if the following pairing holds: $\hat{e}(R, P) = \hat{e}(H_1(id_i), Pub_{RS})^t$. If the pairing holds then proceeds, otherwise rejects the login request. Note: the pairing holds, since:

$$\hat{e}(R, P) = \hat{e}(tsH_1(id_i), P) = \hat{e}(H_1(id_i), sP)^t = \hat{e}(H_1(id_i), P_{pub})^t.$$

Takes the received pid_{PT} and locates the corresponding pid_{GS}. If pid_{GS} does not exist, it means pid_{PT} is not registered patient. Hence the AS rejects the login request, otherwise proceeds.

Once the above checks are successful, the AS then authenticates the physician. The AS proceeds by carrying out the following operations:

- Computes $N = H_1(id_{AS}\|id_i\|t'')$ where t'' is time stamp and $C_2 = E_{Q_{GS}}(id_{AS}, id_i,$ $pid_{PT}, S_i, B_1)$ and sends $\{t'', C_2, N\}$ to the GS associated with pid_{PT}.

3.4.3   Authentication of the Authentication Server by the Home Gateway

Once GS receives $\{t'', C_2, N\}$, it carries out following authentication steps:

- Checks if $t''' - t'' < \Delta t$ holds, where t''' is the time of arrival of the message. If it holds then proceeds, otherwise rejects the request.
- Decrypts$\{id_{AS}, id_i, pid_{PT}, S_i, B_1\} = D_{d_{GS}}(C_2)$, computes $N' = H_1(id_{AS}\|id_i\|t'')$ and checks if the equation $N = N'$ holds. If it holds then proceeds, otherwise, rejects the request.
- Checks if the received pid_{PT} matches with the one pre-stored, pid^*_{PT}. If not then rejects the request, otherwise proceeds.

Since we assumed that the GS and the sensors share a master secret key y, the two entities $(GS\ and\ S_i)$ can now authenticate each other and establish a session key using any secure protocol. Using the established session key, theGS securely passes id_i and B_1 to S_i. Once S_i receives B_1 it then generates $b \in_R Z^*_q$ and computes $B_2 = bP$, $k = bB_1$, session key $SK = H_2(k\|id_i\|S_i)$ and $Auth = MAC_{SK}(t''''\|id_i\|S_i)$, where t'''' is time stamp. Finally S_i sends the message $\{t'''', B_2 id_i, S_i, Auth\}$ to the physician.

Once physician gets the message $\{t'''', B_2\ idi, S_i, Auth\}$ fromS_i, he/she performs the following computations:

- Checks if $t''''' - t'''' < \Delta t$ holds, where t''''' is time of arrival of the message. If it holds then proceeds, otherwise rejects.
- Computes $k' = aB_2$ followed by the session key $SK = H_2(k'\|id_i\|S_i)$. Note: $k = bB_1 = baP = abP = aB_2 = k'$.
- Computes $Veri = MAC_{SK}(t''''\|id_i\|S_i)$ and checks if $Auth = Veri$. If the equation is satisfied then the physician believes that he/she shares the same session key with S_i.

The established session key is then used in the subsequent communications between the physician and the medical sensor. Each established session key expires at the end of the session. This means that independent sessions require independent session keys. Using the information sent from S_i, the physician monitors the patient's condition and if the readings suggest any adverse health situation, medical instructions can be given and action can be taken before the situation deteriorates.

3.5   Password Change Phase

The password change phase is invoked when a physician U_i wants to change his/her password and it does not require interaction with the RS. U_i proceeds as follow:

- U_i inserts the smartcard into the card reader and enters identity id_i and his/her current password PW_i
- The smartcard checks validity of entered values by computing $V'_i = H_1(id_i\|PW_i)$ and checks if $V'_i = V_i$. If the check is successful then proceeds.

– U_i then submits his/her new password PW_i^* and the smartcard computes $V_i^* = H_1(id_i \| PW_i^*)$ and replaces V_i with V_i^*. Once this is done it implies that the password has been successfully updated.

4 Privacy and Security Analysis

Below we present privacy and security properties of our scheme and discuss how our scheme achieves these desirable properties.

- *Patient anonymity and un-traceability*
  It is important that a patients' real-ID remains unknown unless only in cases of abuse and that no any health information exchange between the patient and the health profession should be linked to a patient's real-ID. In our scheme, upon registration each patient PT receives a pseudo-ID, pid_{PT} which he/she is identified with and not the real-ID. This ensures patient identity privacy preservation since the pseudo-ID reveals nothing about the patient's real-ID. Furthermore, only RS knows the relationship between a pseudo-ID pid_{PT} and the real-ID id_{PT} of the patient. Also, there is no linkage between the pseudo-ID pid_{PT} of patient and that of his/her pid_{GS}. This means that even if the GS is compromised the patient remains un-traceable.
- *Replay attack*
  Suppose an adversary eavesdrops a physician's login request $\{t, C_1, W_i\}$ and stores this message. Then he/she could try to impersonate the physician by resending the message to AS at a later time t_{Adv}. In our scheme the time stamp t is embedded in $R = tReg_i$ Clearly even if adversary replaces t_{Adv} for t such that $t' - t_{Adv} < \Delta t$ is satisfied, where t' is the time of arrival of the request and Δt is tolerated transmission delay, but because of the DLP problem he/she cannot forge R. Hence upon verification of the pairing, the AS can detect the attack. This is because $\hat{e}(R, P) = \hat{e}(H_1(id_i), Pub_{RS})^t \neq \hat{e}(H_1(id_i), Pub_{RS})^{t_{Adv}}$. As such our scheme can successfully resist any such replay attack attempts.
- *Forward secrecy*
  This property entails that the disclosure of long term private keys of parties should not affect the secrecy of previously established session keys by corresponding honest parties. In our scheme, even if all the private keys for all the parties including the master key s for RS are compromised, the secrecy of the previously established session keys between the S_i and U_i cannot be affected. This is because the established session key $SK = H_2(kid_iS_n) = H_2(k'id_iS_i)$ is purely based on the ephemeral keys $k = baP$ and $k' = abP$ whose security is based on the hardness of the CDH problem. Hence our scheme achieves perfect forward secrecy.
- *Insider attack*
  Our scheme does not require AS to store user's passwords. This eliminates any inherent risk of passwords being stolen by insiders. Moreover, the registration and authentication of parties is done by independent servers. Such that the authentication phase does not require the registration server's long-term secret s, which is used in the registration process and unknown to AS. This makes our scheme safe against insider attack attempts.

5   Comparison

Table 2.

Table 2. Presents a comparison between our proposed scheme against work presented in [4, 5] and [6]. Note: In the table below, NA means; Not Applicable.

Schemes ↓	Mutual Authentication - U_i and S_n	Session Key Establishment	Password Guessing Attack	Strong User Authentication	Patient Id Privacy
Mark et al. [4]	NA	NA	Yes	No	No
Huang et al. [5]	NA	Yes	NA	No	No
Le et al. [6]	Yes	Yes	NA	No	No
Proposed	Yes	Yes	Yes	Yes	Yes

6   Conclusion

In this article, we have presented a pairing based authentication and key establishment scheme for remote patient monitoring systems. The pairing computation is only computed at the authentication server's side. As such the scheme is adaptable to networks with powerful authentication server. Furthermore, the patients are only pseudonymously identified, and only registration server knows the patients' corresponding real-ID. This means that in cases of apparent abuse via judicial procedure, this real-ID can be revealed.

References

1. Virone, G., Wood, A., Selavo, L., Cao, Q., Fang, L., Doan, T., He, Z., Stoleru, R., Lin, S., Stanckovic, J.A.: An advanced wireless sensor network for health monitoring. In: Proceedings Transdisciplinary Conference on Distribution Diagnosis and Home Healthcare, pp. 95–100 (2006)
2. Welch, J., Guilak, F., Baker, S. D.: A wireless ECG smart sensor for broad application in life threatening event detection. In: 26th Annual International Conference of the IEEE Engineering in Medicine and Biology Society, IEMBS'04, vol. 2, pp. 3447–3449 (2004)
3. Dimitriou, T., Loannis, K.: Security issues in biomedical wireless sensor networks. In: Proceedings of the 1st International Symposium on Applied Sciences on Biomedical and Communication Technologies, Aalborg, Denmark, pp. 25–28 (2008)
4. Mark, M., Ngwira, S.M.: Ubiquitous Health care Framework for the Rural African Environment, AFRICOM, pp. 1–6 (2011)
5. Huang, Y.M., Hsieh, M.Y., Chao, H.C., Hung, S.H., Park, J.H.: Pervasive, secure access to a hierarchical sensor-based healthcare monitoring architecture. IEEE J. Wirel. Heterogen. Netw. Selected Areas Commun. 27(4), 400–411 (2009)
6. Le, X.H., Khalid, M., Sankar, R., Lee, S.: An efficient mutual authentication and access control scheme for wireless sensor networks in healthcare. J. Netw. 6(3), 355–364 (2011)
7. Kumar, P., Lee, S.G., Lee, H.J.: E-sap: efficient-strong authentication protocol for healthcare applications using wireless medical sensor networks. Sensors 12(2), 1625–1647 (2012)

8. Lai, B., Kim, S., Verbauwhede, I.: Scalable session key construction protocol for wireless sensor networks. In: IEEE Workshop on Large Scale Real-Time and Embedded Systems (LARTES), pp. 7 (2002)
9. Neuman, B.C., Stubblebine, S.G.: A note on the use of timestamps as nonces. ACM SIGOPS Oper. Syst. Rev. **27**(2), 10–14 (1993)

Security Analysis of Some Output of RC4 Cryptosystem

Kondwani Thangalimodzi[(✉)], Gift Khangamwa, and Patrick Albert Chikumba

University of Malawi, The Polytechnic, Pvt Bag 303, Blantyre, Malawi
{thangalimodzi,giftkhangamwa,patrick_chikumba}@yahoo.com

Abstract. RC4 is one of the most widely used cryptosystem by many applications. It is used for secure communications; file encryption, Secure Sockets Layer, Wired Equivalent Protocol, potentially useful in many popular systems, it is a random bit generator. In this paper, we analyze the linear relationship in the output of RC4 over a large number of keys. In our method we test linear functions of the keystream. For each such linear function, we run the RC4 algorithm on a large randomly chosen set of keys and evaluate the corresponding output. Using statistical test we find that on some output of the RC4, the combination of output bits is not truly random.

Keywords: RC4 · Encryption · Cryptosystem · Stream cipher · Crypt-analysis · Cryptography

1 Introduction

Cryptography [1], from the Greek kryptos meaning hidden and graphein meaning to write, is the art and science of making communications unintelligible to all except the intended recipient(s). It is a tool for hiding information.

2 RC4

RC4 is the most widely used stream cipher. It is a synchronous stream cipher designed by Ron Rivest for RSA Data Security [3] (now RSA Security). It was invented in 1987. It is a variable key-size stream cipher with byte-oriented operations. The algorithm is based on the use of a random permutation. Analysis shows that the period of the cipher is overwhelmingly likely to be greater than 10^{100} [4]. Eight to sixteen machine operations are required per output byte, and the cipher can be expected to run very quickly in software. Independent analysts have scrutinized the algorithm and it is considered secure.

The source code of the Alleged RC4 was published anonymously on the Cypherpunks mailing list in 1994 [4].

© Institute for Computer Sciences, Social Informatics and Telecommunications Engineering 2014
T.F. Bissyandé and G. van Stam (Eds.): AFRICOMM 2013, LNICST 135, pp. 90–94, 2014.
DOI: 10.1007/978-3-319-08368-1_10

2.1   Use of RC4

RC4 is used for file encryption in products such as RSA SecurPC. RSA SecurPC is a software utility that encrypts disks and files on both desktop and laptop personal computers. The random key is encrypted under the users secret key, which is encrypted under a key derived from the users passphrase. This allows the users passphrase to be changed without decrypting and re-encrypting all encrypted files. Microsoft uses the RC4 stream cipher in both Word and Excel [2].

2.2   RC4 Algorithm

RC4 is a stream cipher. In theory, for a stream cipher, the n-th bit of plaintext is encrypted using the n-th bit of keystream. The RC4 algorithm generates a keystream which is XORed with the data stream. The algorithm uses a variable key from 1 to 2^n bits to initialize a 2^n-bit state table, where n is a chosen positive integer, RC4 has two parameters: key size and word size. The word size is almost always 8 bits, and if the word size is w, the key size varies from 40 bits to 2^w.

The RC4 algorithm has two parts, the key scheduling algorithm and the stream generation algorithm.

The following is the key scheduling algorithm.

```
        j=0;
        for (i=0; i < keylen; ++i) {

            j = (j + state[i] + key[i]) mod keylen;

            t = state[i];

        state[i] = state[j];

        state[j] = t;
```

The following is the stream generation algorithm.

```
        i=0, j=0;

        for (x=0; x < keystreamlen; ++x) {

            i = (i + 1) mod keylen;

            j = (j + state[i]) mod keylen;

            t = state[i];

        state[i] = state[j];

        state[j] = t;

        out[x] = state[(state[i] + state[j]) mod keylen];
```

3   Linear Cryptanalysis

Linear cryptanalysis is a known plaintext attack. This type of cryptanalysis is based on finding affine approximations to the action of a cryptosystem. It was first discovered by Mitsuru Matsui. He applied the technique to the FEAL cipher (*Matsui and Yamagishi, 1992*). Linear cryptanalysis exploits the non-linearity of the cryptosystem.

4   Our Approach

For $i \geq 0$ we denote the ith bit of the keystream by z_i. We are looking for linear functions of the variables z_i which output either 0 or 1 with probability significantly greater than 0.5 over all possible keys. We denote such a linear function [5] r.
   Then

$$r = \alpha_0 z_0 \oplus \alpha_1 z_1 \oplus \ldots \oplus \alpha_{m-1} z_{m-1} \qquad (1)$$

where each α_i is a fixed bit and m is the number of keystream bits we consider. We call $(\alpha_0, \ldots, \alpha_{m-1})$ a coefficient vector
   A keystream length is the number of n-bit words that form a keystream. Here our keystream length is 2, and $m = 2 * 6 = 12$ because there are two words of 6-bits each that form the keystream
   We run the RC4 algorithm on a large randomly chosen set of keys and evaluate the function on the corresponding output. We then keep track of how often the output is 0 or 1. For those functions that give especially unequal distributions of 0 s and 1 s, we retest those functions on larger sets of keys and then use statistics to see if the probability that the output is 1 is significantly different from 0.5. If a linear function outputs 0 s and 1 s very unequally, then we say that the coefficients in that function are good coefficients.

5   Experimental Results

RC4 essentially uses a pseudo-random number generator initialized from a secret key of up to $2^n n$-bit strings. In our experiment, we have $n = 6$. We used a program [5] which, in its first run evaluates all $2^{2.6} = 4096$ functions for a large set of keys. Those that output 0 s and 1 s most unequally are then stored for a second run. This subset of functions is then evaluated on an even larger set of keys. Then those functions are tested for the hypothesis: the function outputs 1 over all keys with probability >0.5 or <0.5, based on the data from the smaller set of keys. We consider a coefficient vector to be a binary representation of an integer and use the integer to denote the coefficient vector. For $n = 6$, the function r with coefficient vector $(\alpha_0, \ldots, \alpha_{11}) = (1, 0, 0, 0, 0, 0, 0, 0, 0, 0, 0, 1)$ would simply be denoted 2049.

5.1   Experiment

In the first run, we used $2^{13} = 8192$ keys. In the second run we took the best 255 functions (the 127 functions that output 1 least frequently and the 128 functions that output 1 most frequently) from the first run and did a second run on them with 2^{17} randomly selected keys.

In the third run, we took the best four Functions 31, 57, 14 and 23 from the second run and did a third run on them with 2^{21} randomly selected keys.

The results are presented in the table below. We present 4 pairs [5], $[r_i, oc_i]$ where r_i denotes a linear function and oc_i is the number of 1s output by that function evaluated over 2^{21} keys.

Good Coeficients:
$[[31, 1030763], [57, 1030851], [14, 1030874], [23, 1032133]]$

The null hypothesis is that $p = 0.5$. We computed the random variable measuring the proportion for a sample of keys that the Function r gives output 1 and the standard deviation for the proportion and we also computed the z - distribution. We found α, the probability of getting this output count if $p = 0.5$ is actually true. The results are shown below

$[31, 1030763]$ Proportion $= 0.491506$ Standard deviation $= 0.000345267$ $z = -24.601$ $\alpha = 0$
$[57, 1030851]$ Proportion $= 0.491548$ Standard deviation $= 0.000345267$ $z = -24.4794$ $\alpha = 0$
$[14, 1030874]$ Proportion $= 0.491559$ Standard deviation $= 0.000345267$ $z = 24.4477$ $\alpha = 0$
$[23, 1032133]$ Proportion $= 0.492159$ Standard deviation $= 0.000345267$ $z = -22.7089$ $\alpha = 0$

6 Discussion

In our experiment, the null hypothesis, for each coefficient vector is that the output is 1 with $p = 0.5$ over all keys. The alternative hypothesis, for each coefficient vector is that the output is 1 with $p < 0.5$ (respectively $p > 0.5$) over all keys if the proportion of 1s in the previous output was less than (respectively greater than) 0.5. Our significance level is $0.05/4 = 0.0125$, because we are checking four coefficients in our experiment. We computed the proportion, the standard deviation, and z. Recall that α denotes the probability that we reject the null hypothesis when it is actually true, given the z-score. Now let us test Function 3. Here α is the probability of getting a z-score less than -24.601, so $\alpha = 0$. We therefore reject the null hypothesis and we are 100 % confident in all of these cases.

We can make similar statements for Functions 57, 14 and 23.

7 Conclusion

The RC4 stream cipher provides good protection against attacks. Using statistical test we have shown in our experiment that on some output of RC4, the combination of output bits is not sufficiently random to serve its intended purpose. But the results are rather theoretical.

References

1. Konheim, A.G.: Cryptography A Primer. Wiley, New York (1981)
2. Schneier, B.: Schneier on Security. https://www.schneier.com/cgi-bin/mt/mt-search.cgi?search=RC4
3. RSA Laboratories. Crypto FAQ. 2007 RSA Security. http://www.emc.com/emc-plus/rsa-labs/standards-initiatives/rc4.htm
4. Stallings, W.: Cryptography and Network Security Principles and Practices, 3rd edn. Prentice Hall/Pearson Education Inc., Englewood Cliffs (2003)
5. Thangalimodzi, K.: Linear Cryptanalysis of RC4. Master of Science, Thesis. Mzuzu University (2008)

Sustainable ICT4D in Africa: Where Do We Go from Here?

Tegawendé F. Bissyandé[1,2]([✉]), Daouda Ahmat[3], Jonathan Ouoba[3], Gertjan van Stam[4], Jacques Klein[1], and Yves Le Traon[1]

[1] SnT, University of Luxembourg, Luxembourg, Luxembourg
{tegawende.bissyande,jacques.klein,yves.letraon}@uni.lu
[2] FasoLabs, Ouagadougou, Burkina Faso
[3] LaBRI - CNRS, University of Bordeaux, Talence, France
{adaouda,jonathan.ouoba}@labri.fr
[4] SIRDC, Harare, Zimbabwe
gertjan.vanstam@machaworks.org

Abstract. In recent years many researchers in Africa and beyond have devoted considerable resources investigating ways to harness the potential of ICT for improving users' livelihood in developing areas. Topics and domains of interest appear to be broad with recurring themes and solutions. Unfortunately there are no clear research roadmaps on what is urgent and of the state of the art solutions. In this position paper for the AFRICOMM series of conference, we propose to investigate some priorities for ICT4D in Africa. We believe that our work could motivate researchers and create a synergy around a few important challenges of ICT4D in Africa.

Keywords: ICT4D · Africa · Development · Research topics and priorities

1 Introduction

Information and Communication Technologies have shaped todays' world, and keep drawing the future by enforcing globalization and its associated challenges and opportunities for trade, cultural exchange, and innovation. In developing areas, the frontrunner initiatives to move millions of people out of poverty are recurrently said to be based on ICT. ICT for development (ICT4D) is thus the latest paradigm that occupies researchers, not only in computer sciences, but also in humanities. Unfortunately, except a few reports on experiments, there are very few studies that unequivocally show the success or ICT4D research to improve users livelihood in Africa. Furthermore, and what is more important, there are even fewer empirical studies that suggest critical fields where ICT4D would benefit the populations.

Conferences on ICT4D are now legion. At AFRICOMM, every year, researchers from Africa and beyond are proposing various techniques and approaches for ICT4D. However, as readers of papers from previous sessions of

© Institute for Computer Sciences, Social Informatics and Telecommunications Engineering 2014
T.F. Bissyandé and G. van Stam (Eds.): AFRICOMM 2013, LNICST 135, pp. 95–103, 2014.
DOI: 10.1007/978-3-319-08368-1_11

this conference, we always wonder to whom the authors make suggestions of such ideas. Indeed, often, the techniques appear to be unrealistic given the available resources and the cultural model in developing countries as well as their priorities. We thus believe that there is a need to advocate for a sustainable ICT4D research. We hope that after a solid discussion on our contributions at the conference, together with all participant researchers we will pave a new roadmap to serve African populations with ideas and solutions (1) that they care about, (2) that could really help them, and (3) that constitute a step towards overcoming the challenges of the digital divide. This position paper is also aimed at rallying young (and not so young) researchers across Africa who wish to partake in ICT4D research. Our contributions in this paper are:

1. we succinctly detail the motivation for this paper, establishing the need for questioning ICT4D research for Africa.
2. we discuss what we believe to be critical avenues of research for Africa, categorizing these topics into short, medium and long term impact-oriented research.
3. finally, we suggest research goals, by distinguishing between urban areas and rural areas in developing regions to show that unlike in developed countries, the ICT4D priorities in such areas are very much different in Africa.

The remainder of this paper is organized as follows. Section 2 provides an in-depth discussion of our motivation. Section 3 details some research avenues with their degree of priority for Africa. Section 4 discusses research topics following the context in Africa. Section 5 provides an illustrated discussion on our work and presents a proposition to implement our recommendations. We conclude in Sect. 6.

2   Motivation

The intentional use of communication to foster development is not new. As Heeks has recently described, in the mid-1950s there was already initiative for broadcasting development communication, computing/data processing for back office applications in large organization both of government and private sector in developing countries [1]. Nowadays, mobile phone has shaped its way through to become the archetypal application for ICT4D because of its affordability and because it allows to focus on the poor as producers and innovators of ICT. With the proliferation of data and bandwidth, Hilbert has suggested to now turn our eyes towards Big Data as a new paradigm for ICT4D [2].

There seems therefore to be a consensus on how ICT4D is evolving as a notion. However, in practice this evolution is not clearly witnessed in the improvement of poor people's lives. Furthermore, we note three important concerns with ICT4D research in and for Africa.

Absence of agenda. No agenda has been set on what should be done by the next decade or so to achieve any fixed goal. Even policy makers set vague objectives and then tag 'ICT' as a solution to their goals. In such a context, researchers cannot be expected to succeed in unclear endeavors. An agenda would also allow to regularly check the progress, continuously improve the means dedicated, and reassess one's ambitions. The UN ICT Task force attempts to implement such an agenda since 2005 [8]. However, it appears that they set various global and vague goals that mainly concern the government bodies and NGOs that are funded by the UN agency.

Little knowledge on needs and requirements. Second, we note that to the best of our knowledge, there are very few empirical studies that characterize the actual needs of developing countries. There are even fewer studies that discuss the requirements for ICT solutions to be proposed. Such studies however to be prerequisites in other no more important fields of research. As we discussed in previous work, the particularities of the african context should drive the design of ICT4D solutions [6].

Few return on experiences. What have researchers achieved so far to improve poor people's livelihood? Where have we failed and why? These questions persist for African developing countries because of a serious lack of documentation on failed/successful experiences. Practitioners are often afraid to report on their failures so as to maintain funding, while researchers are not keen to thoroughly validate the real adoption of their solutions, preferring to require that poor people adapt to them, rather than refining their techniques to adapt to the context.

3 Critical Research Avenues

In this section we discuss research avenues that we see as critical today. We have categorized them so as to ensure that we effectively tackle the issues that we have raised in our detailed motivation (cf. Sect. 2). First we advocate for empirical studies to shake down all beliefs about the needs of poor people and all wrong hypotheses on the context that could derail the applicability of ICT4D research.

3.1 Empirical Studies

Is broadband connectivity necessary everywhere in developing areas? Is e-Learning even an interesting topic for illiterate people in Africa? Such questions require answers for which we unfortunately do not have definite answers. ICT4D has this particularity that it employs sophisticated technologies to help people out of poverty. However, there are already a number of researchers, specially in sociology and anthropology, who conduct research on the specificities of developing areas and their inhabitants in order to provide insights that would help NGOs and government bodies to efficiently implement development plans. We believe Information Technology researchers should team up with those researchers to investigate the realities of developing areas and draw out *facts* that will direct the design of ICT solutions.

Empirical studies can also help to reduce the approximate (and often wrong) hypotheses that IT researchers make when designing their solutions. As researchers from Africa, we have personal experiences on how people regroup and stay very long close just for greeting each other. Unfortunately, we had a hard time convincing other researchers that the duration of such encounters is sufficient to establish reliable P2P connectivity to transfer sizeable data in an opportunistic scenario [6]. An empirical study on the average duration of contacts among people and their degree of recurrence would significantly help people realize the potential of opportunistic networking in Africa where it would be more suitable to our cultural context than it is in developed countries where it was first invented but remains unleverageable.

3.2   Return on Experiences

E-money, e-Learning or tele-medicine are praised everywhere as stornercones of ICT4D applications that are continuously helping the poor people. These praises however are based on very few successes which cannot be generalized. Indeed, most practitioners in many countries are aware that there are many more undocumented failures. When did those failure occur and why? Having answers to those questions will undoubtedly avoid repeated ICT4D design errors, and at the same time significantly reduce the waste of resources.

Return on experiences also participate in archiving the efforts of ICT4D for next generations of researchers. Identifying the landmarks already visited and the paths taken so far by other researchers may help in drawing new (and better) approaches.

3.3   Research Roadmaps

Use of ICT as a vehicle for sustainable economic development cannot be effective if social conditions are not first improved. Thus, it becomes imperative to first direct ICT initiatives towards such goals. To that respect, we remind the reader that ICTs, in the context of ICT4D, are constituted by tools that facilitate communication, the processing and transmission of information and the sharing of knowledge by electronic means. In this section we suggest a classification of research priorities in terms of short, medium and long term impact needs. As McNamara has stated, experience demonstrates that there is no single solution that will work in all settings [3].

Short Term Impact Research: The development of Africa is challenged by deep problems such as pandemic diseases, food and water shortage, wars, and a rapid lost of our valuable heritage. We believe that ICT4D researchers should immediately tackle issues related to these problems.

Health management. Whether it is for reducing maternal death, fighting malaria or responding to HIV spread, ICT is increasingly leveraged. Indeed, ICT initiatives have demonstrated that they can make an impact on improving dissemination public health information, on enabling remote consultation, on facilitating collaboration and cooperation among practitioners (e.g., learning best practices, and worker training), on strengthening the capabilities for monitoring threats to public health and administrative systems in health care facilities [3]. There are however no definite ICT answers to support all those needs, and ICT4D research in this area must be further pursued.

Food and Water. Once health is acquired, it cannot be sustained if food and water are lacking or are of bad quality. Around the world, initiatives to use ICT as an enabler of smart management of water and food resources are flourishing. In Africa, the room for improvement is still immense. ICT4D researchers can thus contribute to not only disseminate more efficiently information and advice, but also analyze and forecast food security issues for NGOs and government bodies.

Peace. For some time now, the United Nations Educational, Scientific and Cultural Organization has been advocating the use of ICT to promote peace. Thanks to the revolution in ICTs indeed, there is a real opportunity for "multilogue" to promote mutual understanding and peace. In Africa, there is yet to see ICT-based initiatives for peace building, although governance based on citizens' participation through ICT is increasingly advocated without real-world implementation [7].

Heritage. Finally, an urgent matter that african researchers need to look into is the preservation of the heritage. This includes the landscape, the wild life, as well as the material and immaterial legacy of African ancestors and our elders. In developed countries, national museums are taking full advantage of ICT to spark interest on their cultural heritage. In Africa, animal poaching is alarmingly threatening the Big 5 where ICT can help improve surveillance of national parks [4]. Recent events in Mali where Timbuktu's ancient manuscripts were saved in extremis remind us how fragile heritage in Africa is.

Medium Term Impact Research: To support and sustain short term impact research initiatives, ICT4D researchers should also allocate resources to investigate medium term issues.

Enhanced e-Agriculture. First, food security will not be fully ensured if e-agriculture is not better implemented. To that end, researchers need to identify opportunities for e-agriculture for illiterate populations, in accordance with the cultural models of developing areas where competition is not necessary the first incentive.

Local e-Government. Improving local participatory governance to promote stability is a noble endeavor. Since ingredients for implementing adapted ICT approaches in developing areas are now in place, ICT4D researchers could invest into proposing ICT-based schemes. These may involve online social communities, information portals, discussion forums, etc. which are implemented with the constraints of the african context, instead of being simple copies of solutions from developed countries.

Waste management. Another research avenue that needs investigation is the management of waste, specifically electronic waste. Indeed, Africa's mounting electronic waste, or e-waste, is presenting both opportunities and problems that needs to addressed. With millions of poor consumers, Africa is importing many near end-of-life electronic devices, generating a massive waste stream. How can ICT4D researchers help with solutions for analyzing, identifying and recycling these devices before they become a serious environment issue?

New Businesses of Open Source. In previous work, we have discussed how Open Source opportunities were wasted in Africa [5]. Among those opportunities are the possibilities for increasing employment of new graduate students with open-source oriented education that will help them build start ups. Indeed, ICT4D should not only focus on fixing what is broken, it should also participate in building what has never existed.

Long-Term Impact Research: ICT4D should not be short-sighted. Nor should it fail to recognize when a field is not ready for the introduction of some new paradigm. We now discuss two important research scenarios that are widely advertised and that should be (re)thought for the long run.

e-Learning. Education is and must remain a priority in Africa. Traditional class-rooms may have exhausted different possibilities for welcoming everyone in acceptable conditions. In that regard, e-Learning by using ICT to assist in the exchange of knowledge can be a solution. Unfortunately, success stories told across the web are very few, as the means to implement e-Learning are often costly in a context where even traditional school faces attendance challenges. One could advocate that new learning media would spark the interest of children. Experience in some countries have shown that such an interest is not a lasting one. The problem with E-learning thus lies within its targets. In rural areas, it serves most for advertisement (and perhaps propaganda?), while in urban areas, it can actually overcome the lack of teaching personnel in some domains.

High Connectivity. Building information highways between cities in Africa will not matter if we have not previously imagined the services that will be run with it. There is "build it and they will come" strategy that can work in areas where everything is a priority. High connectivity requires big investments that most developing african developing cannot afford to make right now. However, because of the rapid pace to which Africa is confronted to globalization, there is a need for ICT4D researchers to start devising applications and scenarios for the various connectivity needs in Africa. Thus, increasing WiFi range and using whitespace technologies will make sense if we can fully take advantage of the new bandwidth that will be delivered.

4   Mind the Context

In this section we further discuss in details why a research roadmap for ICT4D is necessary in Africa. In developed countries, almost all areas of a single countries, i.e. villages and cities, can be treated equally when offering a new ICT service or setting up a new infrastructure, even if the investments will differ. For example, when introducing the recent 4G services, operators in Europe just planned a progressive extension of the network to cover all areas. In developing countries, however, the situation would be totally, as the priorities between urban and rural areas are very much dissimilar. We exploring in the following some ICT4D priorities in each context.

4.1 Rural Areas – From Survival to Living

Rural areas are the most disadvantaged places in developing countries. People still practice subsistence farming to feed their families. However, traditional agriculture can no longer satisfy the needs of family members, and requires more information from outside world to increase productivity. Research on e-agriculture has thus become a priority for african rural areas. Another challenge for such areas is *isolation*. The lack of practicable roads and the scarce investment from network operators makes this issue persistent, although it is widely accepted that connecting rural areas with the outside world will significantly improve their livelihood, by enhancing health care, school education, farmer training, etc.

In previous work [6], we have shown how rural areas, because of the cultural model respected by inhabitants, can afford to implement ICT4D approaches based on shared technologies. Opportunistic networking is also a favorable ICT4D paradigm for bringing connectivity into such areas. Finally, ICT4D researchers should investigate the use of new free wireless technologies and the reuse/adaptation of existing open source applications.

4.2 Urban Areas – Towards Smart Cities

Urban areas in developing countries face different challenges than their rural counterparts. In African cities, infrastructure investments have already been made, and service launches (and ceases) are witnessed every day. Because the youth attempts to identify with developed countries, ICT4D researchers have a wide range of domains where solutions adapted to existing technologies and constraints are needed. We mention here research avenues and ICT paradigms that can be leveraged to incrementally improve user experience of a connected world.

Payment. Across African cities, few inhabitants have bank accounts and credit cards. Network operators have thus seen an opportunity with mobile phones and the prepaid credit system to push for mobile banking. There seems however to be a monopoly of operators to benefit from the system since payment is done through their Integrated Service Digital Network. With the democratization of Near Field Communication (NFC) on cheap smartphones, there is ample opportunity to create new scenarios of payment.

Transport. African cities are becoming crowded and the way transport systems are working is not simplifying users' life. ICT4D can improve ticketing system, enhance the dissemination of real time information about traffic, bus hours, etc.

Culture. Young Africans in cities are increasingly unaware of the cultural wealth that surrounds them and that tourists come from far away to visit. An avenue of ICT4D research could be to propose an approach for performing a collaborative census of "must-see" tourist places, and to devise plans to spark the interest of local people.

Social Networking. While online social networking is getting adepts among african populations, Internet connectivity is not fully available anytime and any-where to readily access worldwide sites. There is therefore a new to use alter-native communication vehicles such as SMS on mobile phones to create social networks that reflect our realities and capabilities.

5   Discussion

To assess the scope of the AFRICOMM conference with regards to our catego-rization, we consider all *36* papers accepted at the 2012 session of AFRICOMM and based on their titles and abstracts we count how many papers concern one of our research avenues. Table 1 summarizes our findings. It appears that *83 %* of the papers are in line with our priorities of ICT4D for Africa. Only *8 %* focus on short-term impact research, while only also *8 %* provide insights with empirical studies and returns on experience. Almost *50 %* of papers deal with problems related to our category of long term impact research. These findings reveal that there is a need to create a synergy of research to increase the value of ICT4D papers at AFRICOMM, by introducing an equilibrium among the various topics of research that can benefit african populations.

Table 1. Categories of papers presented at AFRICOMM'2012

		# of papers
Empirical studies		3
Return on experiences		0
Short term Impact	Health management	3
	Food & water	0
	Peace	0
	Heritage	0
Medium term Impact	e-Agriculture	1
	e-Governance	3
	Waste management	1
	Open Source	3
Long term Impact	e-Learning	1
	High connectivity	17
Rural areas		
Urban areas		

We propose to this end, to have a theme of research every year at AFRICOMM that will allow to focus each time on a specific topic that needs attention. We could also setup a special session (or a workshop) where all ICT4D researchers could join resources and ideas to investigate a specific challenge in Africa.

6 Conclusion

The momentum of ICT4D research has been increasing in recent years. Research conferences across the world are publishing proceedings with numerous papers proposing every day new solutions and approaches for leveraging ICT in the development of African countries. However, we note that researchers' efforts are dispersed and no clear agenda is set for delivering solutions. Furthermore, research topics are not necessarily selected based on the real needs on the ground of developing countries.

In this paper, we have discussed critical research avenues and recommended the establishment of a research theme for each edition of AFRICOMM in order to create a synergy around some challenges of ICT4D in Africa.

References

1. Heeks, R.: ICT4D 2.0: the next phase of applying ICT for international development. Computer **41**(6), 26–33 (2008)
2. Hilbert, M.: Big data for development: from information- to knowledge societies January 2013. Available at SSRN: http://ssrn.com/abstract=2205145
3. McNamara, K.: Improving health, connecting people: the role of icts in the health sector of developing countries. A framework paper, October 2007
4. Mendez, M.O., Bissyandé, T.F., Somasundar, K., Klein, J., Voos, H., Traon, Y.L.: Towards automating surveillance of national parks: the next killer App of ICT4D with UAVs? Submitted to AFRICOMM'13 (2013)
5. Ouattara/sanon, H., Ouoba, J., Bissyandé, T.F.: Open source in Africa: an opportunity wasted? -Why and how FLOSS should make sense for Africa. In 4th International IEEE EAI Conference on e-Infrastructure and e-Services for Developing Countries, Yaoundé, Cameroun, pp. 11–14, Nov. 2012 (student paper)
6. Ouoba, J., Bissyandé, T.F.: Leveraging the cultural model for opportunistic networking in Sub-Saharan Africa. In: Jonas, K., Rai, I.A., Tchuente, M. (eds.) AFRICOMM 2012. LNICST, vol. 119, pp. 163–173. Springer, Heidelberg (2013)
7. Saleh, I.: The impact of ict on peace, security & governace in africa. AoC Media Literacy Clearing House
8. UN ICT Task Force. Tools for development: Using information and communications technology to achieve the millennium development goals. Working Paper (2005)

Improving Rural Emergency Services with Cognitive Radio Networks in Sub-Saharan Africa

Dramane Ouattara[1]($\boxtimes$), Francine Krief[1], Mohamed Aymen Chalouf[2], and Tegawendé F. Bissyandé[3]

[1] LaBRI, University of Bordeaux, 351 cours de la Libération, 33405 Talence Cedex, France
{dramane.ouattara,francine.krief}@labri.fr
[2] University of Rennes 1, IRISA, IUT of Lannion, Rue Edouard Branly, 22300 Lannion, France
mohamed-aymen.chalouf@irisa.fr
[3] University of Luxembourg, Campus Limpertsberg, av. de la Faïencerie 162 A, 1511 Luxembourg, Luxembourg
tegawende.bissayande@uni.lu

Abstract. In this paper, we propose a new approach based on Cognitive Radio technology to address the challenges for ensuring connectivity in remote areas of Africa. Indeed, the current network coverage is concentrated around the cities with high density of population. Through the deployment of Cognitive Radio, emergency services in rural areas will benefit from low cost access networks. Cognitive Radio will be used to manage the selection/switching across different frequency UHF/VHF bands or TV White Spaces.

Keywords: Cognitive radio · TV white spaces · Rural areas · Remote zone connectivity

1 Introduction

The use of mobile technologies and networks in Africa is growing rapidly and services are increasingly diversified. The quality of the available networks differs from one geographical area to another. In many areas, the networks deliver a poor connectivity, while some areas have no connectivity possibility. These deficiencies are related to the operators policies and the economic benefits they should derive from their investment. However, Internet or networks access could considerably improve the inhabitants social condition in remote areas. Providing low cost Internet access anywhere through Cognitive Radio Networks (CRNs) is the main objective of this contribution. In this paper, we introduce the Cognitive Radio technology, with a more detailed description of its main modules in Sect. 2. The main advantages of this technology in African context are presented in Sect. 3 through the services that it could offer. We give an overview on the related work,

© Institute for Computer Sciences, Social Informatics and Telecommunications Engineering 2014
T.F. Bissyandé and G. van Stam (Eds.): AFRICOMM 2013, LNICST 135, pp. 104–114, 2014.
DOI: 10.1007/978-3-319-08368-1_12

referring to some work addressing the use of cognitive radio in African context in Sect. 4. The deployment plan that we propose is considered in Sect. 5, an experimentation idea and results are studied in Sect. 6. Conclusion and future work are presented in Sect. 7.

2 The Cognitive Radio Networks

2.1 Definition and Principle of Cognitive Radio Networks

Cognitive Radio [1] is a paradigm for wireless networks where a node is able to automatically modify its transmitting parameters in order to communicate efficiently, while avoiding interferences with other users, the Primary Users (PU[1]). This self-configuration and self-adaptation of parameters is based on a set of modules and several factors in the internal or the external environment of the radio such as radio frequency, user behaviour and the network state.

2.2 Cognitive Radio Modules

Figure 1 summarizes the cognitive radio modules and details of its functions are given below.

Spectrum sensing: The spectrum sensing is defined as the ability to measure, examine, learn and be aware of the parameters related to the characteristics of the radio channel. This module measures the availability of spectrum, the signal strength, the interferences and noise, scans operating environment of the radio, estimates the needs of users and applications, checks the availability of networks and nodes, learn about the local policies and other operators restrictions.

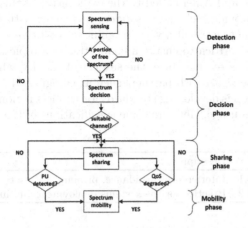

Fig. 1. Operating diagram of a cognitive radio node

---

[1] Users that have the band-use license, the TV users.

Spectrum decision: Decision-making is based on the appropriate communication channel choice, justifying the quality of service required for the data or the collected information transmission.

Spectrum sharing: Channel sharing has to comply with the requirement of synchronized access to the detected free-bands portions. This scheduling is done between the secondary[2] users on the one hand, and between these users and the primary users on the other hand.

Spectrum mobility: Spectrum mobility reflects the fact that each transceiver, must be able to change frequency band if the initial band becomes busy. Moving to a new frequency band could happen also when the initial band fails to provide the desired quality of service to service's applications.

2.3   The Standard for Cognitive Radio: IEEE 802.22

The Federal Communications Commission (FCC[3]) established the TV white spaces rules by which unlicensed devices, in our case, the cognitive radio devices, can make use of specific TV channels in the Very High Frequency (VHF) and Ultra High Frequency (UHF) bands. The table below summarises these frequency bands.

Channel	Spectrum	Bands	Channel	Spectrum	Bands
2,3,4	54–72 MHz	VHF Low	7–13	174–216 MHz	VHF High
5,6	76–88 MHz	VHF Low	14–51	470–698 MHz	UHF

The use of cognitive radio approach in rural areas in Africa is based on this principle of TV white spaces, even if the constraints and objectives are different from European and American continents. Indeed, the scarcity of spectrum resources in Europe and America led to the exploration of this new alternative. In Africa, it will provide technology services in regions with limited economic resources, often remote areas at a very insignificant cost or even free. The use of TV White Spaces in Africa to ensure a connection is a topic increasingly studied and therefore, has recently been the subject of the TV white spaces Africa Forum in Dakar (Senegal) with partners such as Google and Microsoft [2]. The 802.22 working group is developing standards for wireless regional network based on TV white spaces usage. Here are some specifications of the standard on cognitive radio[4]:

Standards	Description
IEEE 802.22.1	Interferences avoidance, primary TV users protection
IEEE 802.22.2	Practice for the systems deployment and installation

---

[2] Cognitive radio users, who do not have any band-use license, such as emergency services users in our context.

[3] http://www.fcc.gov/

[4] IEEE 802.22-2011 Standard for Wireless Regional Area Networks, July 27th 2011.

This table shows the work in progress and all the interest in the use of TV bands to provide internet services.

3 Services that Could Be Offered

Given the ability of the Cognitive Radio Networks to realize opportunistic communications, this technology could provide a set of services in rural zones, among these are:

3.1 Chronic Disease Patient Monitoring: E.g. Diabetic Patient

Chronic diseases such as diabetes are reaching an increasingly large proportion of the rural population. Patients in rural areas with appropriate monitoring, combine with timely hospital visits should save lives. In fact, diabetic patient fitted with glucose sensors connected to a smart-phone as a relay node to the internet allows to remotely inform the caregivers on abnormal high levels of sugar in the blood. This could avoid many painful movement of the patients from rural areas to the city (Hospital). The principle remains the same for other types of chronic conditions such as cardiovascular, cancer and respiratory diseases.

3.2 Hospital Services Automation: E.g. for Epidemic Disease Prevention

To accelerate treatment and diagnosis, health services in Africa should be automated. It begins with the electronic record of the patient's medical history and allows the anywhere medical records access even for people living in rural areas. The patients often helped by nurses could access, modify and control remotely their medical information or send a message on his health state to the doctors. The statistics from this automation could be helpful for early detection of health risks such as epidemics.

3.3 Emergency Alerts: E.g. Bushfire and Accident Alerts

Bushfire are often disastrous for people in rural areas and often, these people do not have the ability to call for help due to the lack of communication infrastructure. It is the same for accident occurring in very remote areas where the victims have no access networks to call the firemen. The emergency networks seem enough efficient for saving lives in similar situation with rescue arrival on time.

3.4 Internet for Children

In addition to emergency centers that could benefit from Internet, the primary schools should be connected and the children in remote villages could very soon become familiar with computers and social networks. This gives them an opening to the world, an opportunity to interact with other children, thus contributing to the reduction of social and technological gap.

3.5 Improving Government Services: E.g. Births Registration

Child births in villages are often not reported because of the distance to reach an administration office. This raises the problem of persons with no administrative paper for example in Côte d'Ivoire remote areas. The on-line registration of births through cognitive radio could significantly reduce the problem of undocumented persons. At the same time, several administrative services may be offered by the Internet access in villages.

4   Related Works

In developed countries, the growing number of wireless devices and the increased spectrum occupancy have resulted to the spectrum scarcity. Cognitive Radio is considered in Europe and USA as the new wireless communication paradigm that could address the potential spectrum exhaustion problem and should be proposed for future wireless communication devices. In the African context, this technology could mostly serve as knowledge sharing and social development tool. Cognitive Radio Networks are therefore a promising field for social networks deployment in Africa and the domain has an increasingly interest for researchers. Thus, in [3], the White space opportunity has been studied. The authors performed measurements that indicate the existence of substantial TV White Spaces available in both rural and urban areas. This work is an interesting introduction and opens up practical deployment studies which remain unexplored. Implementation of OpenBTS in rural Zambia has been studied in [4]. This work focused on providing telecommunication system such as mobile communications in rural villages. Even if this study addresses the low cost communication issue, the solution is obviously valid and valuable for the only villages with GSM networks infrastructure. However, the African countries reality proves that the majority of villages are not covered by the existing standard networks. In fact, the economic profitability in terms of return on investment is not guaranteed for telecommunications operators. The use of Cognitive Radio technology becomes therefore necessary with its bearable costs because of the existence of TV bands infrastructure in rural areas.

5   Cognitive Radio Deployment Process in Remote Areas

Depending on the isotropic radiated power, the cognitive radio base station could connect users terminals located as far as 100 km [5] as described in Fig. 2. A good base stations planning could provide a network to cover two distant areas (villages) of about 100 and greatly reduce the cost of network infrastructure. The financing by governments and the acquisition of such infrastructure and its deployment will aim to improve public services in Africa remote rural areas.

5.1   Cognitive Radio Networks Planning Scenario

Figure 2 describes the deployment scenario with a set of cities (c), villages (v) with distances estimation and the corresponding coverage plan. The cognitive radio antennas at the city allow the switching between our cognitive radio network and the existing operators networks. Also, the cognitive radio antennas set near a city, due to their sensing capability will help avoiding interferences that may be generated by the broadcasting signal of our cognitive radio networks. Relay nodes (R1) are provided to repeat the signal when the distance between two access points or base stations is greater than 100 km. Thus, it can be seen that the fundamental interest of this proposal lies in its ability to cover a large area and long distance. It should be noted that the TV band could be used only in areas lacking the standard network coverage. A proper planning and deployment will achieve a very high scope for possible internet access in the most remote locations. The cognitive radio is therefore an extension of network coverage anywhere and any-time even if its access must be controlled and limited to emergency services, public safety services or public services to avoid disorder in its usage. Based on a strong existing infrastructure such as TV bands (TV White Spaces), the solution we propose provides a stable network connection and facilitates its management and control. However, a number of challenges remain to make the effective deployment of this technology in rural areas in Africa.

5.2   Challenges

The challenges in this context concern the spectrum sensing for better detection of free TV frequencies and channel sharing. A good algorithm for free bands detection will reduce interferences and a good signalling protocol will prevent collisions.

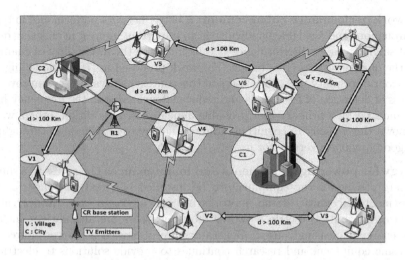

Fig. 2. Planned cognitive radio networks

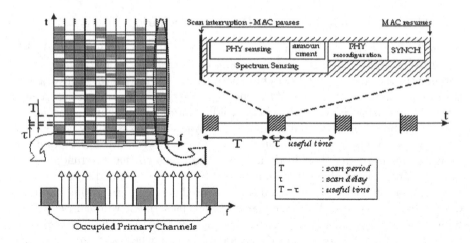

Fig. 3. Spectrum analysis for the cognitive users access [6]

Interferences avoidance with TV users: The deployment of cognitive radio networks creates a new type of opportunistic users whose major constraint remains achieving transmissions or communications without interfering with the TV users. Figure 3 shows the general principle used by the cognitive radio Medium Access Control (MAC) protocols for collisions mitigation. This figure illustrates the different steps performed by a cognitive radio node before the frequency band access. There is a sensing period (scan), a period of reconfiguration and synchronization before any transmissions on the detected free channels (useful time). Occupied primary channels denote in this case, the occupation of the frequency band by TV users and useful time are periods that can be exploited by the cognitive radio users for their transmissions.

Network performance enhancement: A better network performance in terms of throughput and available bandwidth is an important interest in ensuring quality of service to users. Performance is thus linked to the availability of channels and the quality of these free bands. The work proposed in [7] on modelling the behaviour of primary users (TV users in this context) shows how to improve the process of detection of free bands and reduce latencies due to the frequency hopping induced by a primary user probable appearance. In addition, others works [8] shown the capacity of cognitive radio technology to provide high throughput and good quality of service for users.

Energy for powering equipments and maintenance: The access to a source of energy to power the equipment to be installed is a real challenge for the deployment of cognitive radio networks in rural areas. In fact, rural areas in Africa are devoid of electric networks, however, there are alternatives such as solar energy increasingly used. Generators are also used as power source for electronic equipment and research continues to provide solutions to electricity problems in areas with limited resources (rural area) [9]. The energy problem can not therefore constitute an obstacle to the deployment of cognitive radio technology in remote areas.

Engineering and deployment: For better reduction of costs, a proper study should be conducted, that enables efficient deployment of network infrastructure. Thus, must be taken into account the best locations for cognitive radio base stations and relay nodes in order to minimize the infrastructure's cost while maximizing the network coverage area.

6   Experiments and Results

In our research work on cognitive radio networks, we perform experiments and tests on a platform acquired under the ANR[5]-LICORNE project and a platform offered by the CREW project.

6.1   The Cognitive Radio Platform LICORNE

This platform is composed of five nodes and each node is composed of a USRP-1 box, two daughter-boards for transmission/reception (Tx/Rx) operating in GSM (RX/TX 900) and in WiFi (RX/TX 2400) accompanied with the corresponding antennas. A laptop with GNU software is interconnected to the USRP box as presented in Fig. 4. This platform allowed us to do an experiment of transmission / reception on WiFi and GSM bands and to test the frequency hopping with the setup shown in Fig. 5.

To test the frequency hopping, we generate a disruptive AWGN (Adds White Gaussian Noise) signal to create interferences on the transmission channel. The signal thus generated is seen as a transmission of a primary node. This then triggers the process of frequency hopping to avoid interferences as seen in Fig. 6.

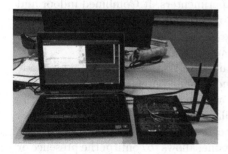   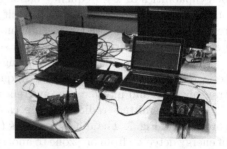

Fig. 4. A cognitive radio node   **Fig. 5.** Three nodes connected

---

[5] The French National Research Agency - ANR (Agence Nationale de la Recherche en France).

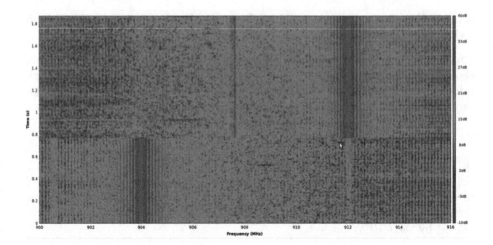

Fig. 6. Frequency hopping for interferences avoidance

This experiment in GSM and WiFi bands remains valid for mitigating interferences to TV band users with cognitive radio networks deployed in rural areas. In addition, the transmission power adaptation model proposed in [10] and tested through the LICORNE platform, represents another strategy for mitigating interferences in cognitive radio networks and therefore for TV white spaces.

6.2   The CREW Project Platform

The CREW platform [11] facilitates experimentally-driven research on spectrum sensing and sharing in licensed and unlicensed bands (TV bands). It offers testbed capabilities to TV frequency bands experimenters. It Combined indoor and outdoor installation deployed in the city of Logatec at Slovenia. The test-bed remote access portal[6] allows to show node status, choose particular cluster for performing an experiment remotely as shown in Fig. 7.

We worked on this platform during the CREW training days[7] and made tests remotely to validate the TV frequency bands potential in terms of data transmissions and interferences awareness as seen in Fig. 7.

The transmitters radio coverage calculation and visualisation is expressed through the Fig. 7. The different colors (green, blue, red) and the characteristic of energy detected from one zone to another one, allows to confirm the presence or the absence of a transmission based on the measured power. Also, this platform (CREW) allows for various tests such as the multi-hopping scenario that remains a very important aspect for transmissions reaching remote areas.

---

[6] http://www.log-a-tec.eu
[7] CREW Training Days is the day which took place on February 2013 at Brussels

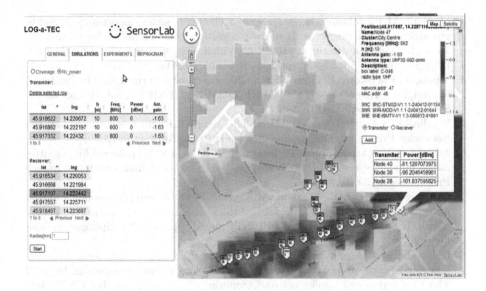

Fig. 7. Platform for remote test on the TV bands (Color figure online)

7   Conclusion

In this work, we have shown that cognitive radio is a real opportunity for network coverage in rural areas through the use of TV band. We have proposed a scenario for the deployment of this technology, noting its expansion capacity over long distances to ensure network access in remote areas. The set of services (Sect. 3) that can be offered through the cognitive radio networks demonstrates its importance in African context. This next generation network is promising to improve life of many people living in remote and often inaccessible regions in Africa. In the future, we will propose a communication architecture based on cognitive radio networks to improve health services in rural areas. Health centers to be interconnected, medical applications to develop and install, patient to be remotely monitored are some challenges for our future proposal in the context of rural areas in Africa.

Acknowledgment. This work is partially supported by the LICoRNe project, funded in part by the National Agency for Research in France ANR (Agence Nationale de la Recherche).

References

1. Palicot, J.: Cognitive radio: an enabling technology for the green radio communications concept. Leipzig, Germany, 21–24 June 2009
2. Forum website: https://sites.google.com/site/tvwsafrica2013/

3. Masonta, M.T., Johnson, D., Mzyece, M.: The white space opportunity in southern africa: measurements with meraka cognitive radio platform. In: Glitho, R., Jonas, K., Popescu-Zeletin, R., Rai, I.A., Villafiorita, A. (eds.) AFRICOMM 2011. LNICST, vol. 92, pp. 64–73. Springer, Heidelberg (2012)

4. Mpala, J., van Stam, G.: Open BTS, a GSM experiment in rural zambia. In: Jonas, K., Rai, I.A., Tchuente, M. (eds.) AFRICOMM 2012. LNICST, vol. 119, pp. 65–73. Springer, Heidelberg (2013)

5. Wyglinski, A.M., Nekovee, M., Hou, T.: Cognitive Radio Communications and Networks: Principles and Practice. Academic Press, Burlington (2009)

6. Adamis, A.V., Constantinou, P.: Intermittent DCF: a MAC protocol for cognitive radios in overlay networks. In: Wang, W. (ed.) Cognitive Radio Systems. In-tech Press, Vienna (2009)

7. Ouattara, D., Krief, F., Chalouf, M.A., Hamdi, O.: Spectrum sensing improvement in cognitive radio networks for real-time patients monitoring. In: Godara, B., Nikita, K.S. (eds.) MobiHealth. LNICST, vol. 61, pp. 179–188. Springer, Heidelberg (2013)

8. Umamaheswari, A.; Subashini, V.; Subhapriya, P., Survey on performance, reliability and future proposal of cognitive radio under wireless computing. In: 2012 Third Interenational Conference on Computing Communication (ICCCNT), July 2012

9. Gado, A., El-Zeftawy, A.: Design and economy of renewable energy sources to supply isolated loads at rural and remote areas of Egypt. In: 20th International Conference and Exhibition on Electricity Distribution, CIRED, June 2009

10. Ouattara, D., Quach, M.T., Krief, F., Chalouf, M.A., Khalife, H.: Mitigating the hospital area communication's interference using cognitive radio networks. In: IEEE International conference on E-health networking, application and services, (Healthcom), October 2013

11. http://www.crew-project.eu/

Unified Solution Towards Deployment of TV White Space in Africa

Philipp Batroff, Osianoh Glenn Aliu, Eric Schütz(✉), Mathias Kretschmer,
Christian Niephaus, and Karl Jonas

Fraunhofer FOKUS, Sankt Augustin, Germany
{philipp.batroff,osianoh.glenn.aliu,eric.schuetz,mathias.kretschmer,
Christian.Niephaus,Karl.jonas}@fokus.fraunhofer.de

Abstract. TV white spaces (TVWS), are seen as a key technology to enable the efficient use of scarce sub-GHz spectrum allowing for applications that may have a huge impact on internet penetration in rural parts of Africa. We first give an overview on TVWS, its use cases and highlight possible challenges against its uptake. Then we describe our carrier-grade wireless back-hauling solution (WiBACK) and discuss its capability for working with a geolocation database ensuring zero interference with licensed users.

Keywords: WiBACK · TVWS · White space device (WSD) · Geolocation database (GLD)

1 TV White Space

Significant efforts have been made by technology companies and development agencies to deliver cost efficient internet access to the developing areas. While the potential of improving the quality of life is higher via internet access, Africa shows the lowest penetration [1].

The challenges include deploying these technologies at a reasonable price to rural areas are among others; the huge distances to cover, a lack of infrastructure, skilled labor and low local buying power. Several technologies and concepts are addressing these points, among which is the provision of carrier grade wireless backhaul solutions. More spectrum will be required to achieve higher capacities and the global trend to make sub-GHz bands, hitherto used for TV broadcast available for wireless communication is of great interest. These bands referred to as TV White Space (TVWS), offer an interesting alternative.

There exists two main approaches towards enabling a dynamic use of the white spaces in the TV spectrum. These include the use of cognitive radios or having a geolocation database that contains information of the available white spaces. Using a database management system is the preferred option. Figure 1 gives an overview of how a TVWS based system works and summarized as

© Institute for Computer Sciences, Social Informatics and Telecommunications Engineering 2014
T.F. Bissyandé and G. van Stam (Eds.): AFRICOMM 2013, LNICST 135, pp. 115–120, 2014.
DOI: 10.1007/978-3-319-08368-1_13

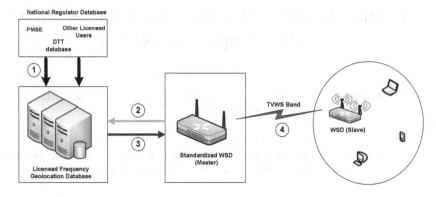

DTT: Digital Terrestrial Television
PMSE: Program Making and Special Events

Fig. 1. TV white space framework

1. The existing national regulator database of licensed users in the TV bands provides an update to the geolocation database provider.
2. A standardized WSD master[1] establishes a secure link with the geolocation database [2], queries it for the set of free channels by providing its geographical location and type of device.
3. This is used to estimate the free channels in that local area and the recommended maximum transmit power.
4. With a list of available channels and allowed transmit power the master executes a channel allocation to its associated slave devices and synchronizes with the DBMS for updates.

1.1   Applications and Current Challenges

The provision of broadband connectivity in rural areas is perhaps the most relevant use case for TVWS in underdeveloped and developing regions. It provides a cost effective solution in areas where legacy operators do not have a good business model of deploying existing wireless infrastructure. Hence, the opportunity exists to provide a carrier-grade wireless backhaul solution using this band and serve as a means for coverage extension for the last-mile mobile, DSL or satellite network. Despite the huge potential of this applications a few challenges still have to be addressed for a successful deployments.

– Standardization of WSD to aid hardware manufacturers produce radios that adhere to legal requirements of operating in the TVWS bands. Furthermore, framework for authentication and prevention of unauthorized data queries or intrusion by pseudo nodes to the database needs to be clarified [2].
– Generating an accurate TVWS database is critical as any errors would lead to severe interference both for primary and secondary users.

---

[1] Assumed placed at a fixed location such as rooftop.

- Driving locally relevant applications using the TVWS bands that will create value for local communities such as platforms for connecting agricultural centers, mobile payments, e-health, etc.
- Informing the public, incumbent licensed operators and other stakeholders on proposed plans for the broadband services in the TVWS bands as well as facilitating frameworks and schedules for testing and field trials before final deployments.
- Lack of stable power supply accounts for a major cost of telecommunication operators in Africa [3]. Solutions should incorporate a green, stable and alternate sources of power supply.

Despite the challenges highlighted, using the TVWS band for broadband applications addresses the most fundamental challenge - bridging the digital divide and can be used to provide a cost efficient carrier grade wireless backhaul solution to developing and rural areas.

1.2   Ongoing Trials and Standards

The Cambridge white space trial is one of largest field trials involving 19 sites with 2 GLDs. A summary of the technical findings can be found in [4]. This report and recommendations can help guide subsequent field trials in Africa. With South Africa expected to complete the first digital switchover in Arica by December 2013, Nigeria by January 2015 and all African countries by June 2015, various TVWS field trials have already started as the awareness of its potential begins to grow. There are planned and ongoing trials in Kenya [5], Malawi [6] and South Africa[7].

Among the various standardization activities, of particular interest are the protocols required for the communication link between the WSD and the database. Specification of this interface, communication protocols and frequency of probing the database for information. [2] specifies the protocol for accessing the GLD, use cases and requirements for the protocol. IEEE 802.22 standard specifies the air interface, MAC layer and physical layer of point to multipoint wireless regional area networks, operating in the VHF/UHF TV broadcast bands [8]. For applications in the sub-GHz band, IEEE 802.11ah WG is currently developing global wireless LAN standard [9]. IEEE 802.11af is specifically addressing modifications to the existing 802.11 physical layers and 802.11 MAC layers to meet the legal requirements for channel access and coexistence in the TV white space band [10].

2   WiBACK

A heterogeneous Wireless Back-Haul (WiBACK)[2] [11,12] architecture, which, compared to traditional fixed wireless operator back-haul networks, offers

---

[2] http://www.wiback.org

simplified deployment processes due to its flexible self-configuration and self-management characteristics. Those allow for the use of more cost-effective packet-switched equipment, such as IEEE 802.11, 802.16 or 802.22 and also support the integration with existing technologies such as DVB, 3 GPP, micro-wave or optical solutions. The scope of the WiBACK architecture is to provide or extend existing back-haul capacity which might range from single-hop long distance wireless connectivity to multi-hop connectivity with up to ten hops in urban and rural environments. Dedicated per-hop resource allocation and are used as aggregates providing resource isolation among traffic classes as well as individual *data pipes* of the same traffic class and also to detect regulatory events, such as preemptions by primary users.

3   Proposed TV White Space (TVWS) Integration with WiBACK

In this section we present the possible integration of the TVWS Framework with the existing WiBACK architecture with a focus on the management and maintenance of frequency utilization by the Topology Resource Manager (TRM). It consists of three major components: The Topology Management Function (TMF) (see [12]), Resource Management Function (RMF) (see [13]) and the Topology Database. We focus on a possible TVWS integration into the current WiBACK network, with special regard to the TVWS requirements of frequency allocation.

In [12] we have discussed in detail that our WiBACK architecture can support a Dynamic Broadcast system in parallel to Internet and data services by providing the mechanisms to dynamically manage the temporarily freed up wireless spectrum resources. As mentioned and shown in Sect. 1 and Fig. 1, the use of a *Licensed Frequency Geolocation Database* is the preferred solution to implement and deploy sub-GHz White Space. With WiBACK using a centralized management and monitoring approach, frequency changes can be triggered by the TMF. This enables the Topology Resource Manager (TRM) to react quickly and accordingly to external demands such as frequency allocation by licensed users, in this specific case other TVWS-users. Figure 2 gives an overview on the integration of the TVWS-DataBase Management System (DBMS).

To react accordingly if the TVWS-DBMS signals a change of the current channel allocation to the WiBACK network, the TMF will reconfigure the allocation to other, preferably interference-free channels in the allowed spectrum. Occupied, licensed channels can also be blacklisted by the TRM, to ensure no future collision with other licensed users for the subscription time. Based on the top level description given in this section, there exists a high level of synergy between our existing carrier grade Wireless Back-Haul (WiBACK) solution and the proposed applications of TVWS for wireless backhauling. A seamless incorporation of a geolocation database would aid our TMF to ensure resource reallocation are synchronized across the whole network with zero channel interference. Upon completion of various standardization activities, our system can be deployed on our existing testbeds in Africa.

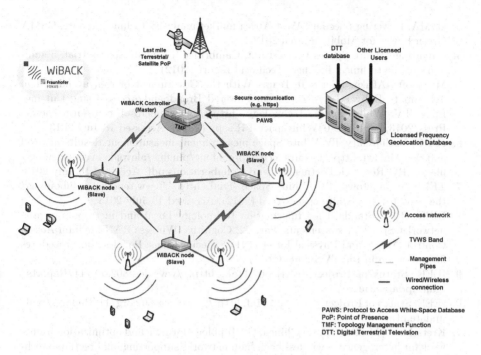

Fig. 2. WiBACK architecture for an integrated TVWS approach

4   Conclusion

The paper described challenges of TVWS and suggested some technical approaches to integrate appropriate mechanisms in the WiBACK Wireless Backhaul architecture. We are currently working on technical solutions to be ready for deployment as soon as legal frameworks allow. Most of the technical aspects have solutions that are rather straight-forward and can easily be integrated into the existing WiBACK architecture.

However it must be noted that on the physical layer spectrum is limited in the TVWS bands. If broadband backhauling shall take advantage of that spectrum, the databases need to be very accurate and the models that describes the interference areas of a long-haul (20 km) link need to be very reliable.

Acknowledgment. This work has been funded by the Federal Ministry of Education and Research of the Federal Republic of Germany (Förderkennzeichen 01 BU 1116).

References

1. ITU. The world in 2013: Ict facts and figures. Technical report (2013)
2. Mancuso, E. A., Patil, B.: RFC 6953: protocol to access white-space (PAWS) databases: use cases and requirements. Technical report, Internet Engineering Task Force (IETF), May 2013

3. GSMA. Powering telecoms: West Africa market analysis. Technical report, GSMA Green Power for Mobile, March 2013

4. Cambridge White Spaces Consortium. Cambridge TV white spaces trial, a summary of the technical findings. Technical report (2012)

5. Microsoft 4Afrika. Microsoft Teams With the Government of Kenya and Indigo Telecom to Deliver Low-Cost, Solar-Powered Broadband Access Using Cutting-Edge TV White Space Technology. https://www.microsoft.com/en-us/news/Press/2013/Feb13/02-04WhitespacesPR.aspx (2013). Accessed 18 July 2013

6. eCRG. Preliminary TV White Space measurement measurement Results in rural and city Malawi. http://ei4africa.eu/wp-content/plugins/alcyonis-event-agenda//files/eCRG_Research_Partnership_and_Collaborations.pdf. Accessed 18 July 2013

7. TENET. Capetown TV White Space Trial. http://www.tenet.ac.za/about-us/the-cape-town-tv-white-spaces-trial (2012). Accessed 18 July 2013

8. IEEE. IEEE Standard for Information technology–Local and metropolitan area networks–Specific requirements–Part 22: Cognitive Wireless RAN Medium Access Control (MAC) and Physical Layer (PHY) specifications: Policies and procedures for operation in the TV Bands (2011)

9. IEEE. Status of Project IEEE 802.11ah. http://www.ieee802.org/11/Reports/tgah_update.htm

10. IEEE. Status of Project IEEE 802.11af. http://www.ieee802.org/11/Reports/tgaf_update.htm

11. Kretschmer, M., Batroff, P., Ghinea, G.: Topology forming and optimization framework for heterogeneous wireless back-haul networks supporting unidirectional technologies. J. Comput. Commun. (COMCOM, Elsevier), Under Review

12. Kretschmer, M., Niephaus, C., Ghinea, G.: A wireless back-haul architecture supporting dynamic broadcast and white space coexistence. In: ICCCN 2012 Workshops: 6th International Workshop on Wireless Mesh and Ad Hoc Networks (WiMAN), WiMAN 2012, Munich, Germany (2012)

13. Kretschmer, M., Horstmann, T., Batroff, P., Rademacher, M., Ghinea, G.: Link calibration and property estimation in self-managed wireless back-haul networks. In: 18th Asia-Pacific Conference on Communications (APCC 2012), Ramada Plaza Jeju Hotel, Jeju Island, Korea, October 2012

Medicines Identification for African Illiterate Patients Using Near Field Communication

Mahlaku Mareli, Suvendi Rimer[✉], Babu Sean Paul,
and Khmaies Ouahada

Department of Electrical and Electronic Engineering,
University of Johannesburg, P.O. Box 524, Auckland,
Johannesburg 2006, South Africa
mmareli@hotmail.com,
{suvendic,bspaul,kouahada}@uj.ac.za

Abstract. This paper presents the application of Near Field Communication (NFC) to the healthcare sector. Although a number of papers have been written to discuss different NFC applications in the healthcare sector, none of them address the potential challenges facing illiterate patients worldwide. According to UNESCO institute for statistics, the Sub-Saharan African region has the highest percentage of illiterate people compared to other regions in the world. NFC can be used in conjunction with other technologies, especially mobile communications which provide high data speeds at cheap rates. The proposed NFC application consists of a NFC sticker placed on the medicine container, the NFC phone with an Android application that reads the sticker ID, connects to a Medicine Information Server and retrieves relevant instructions for medicine in audio form. Some of the advantages for this solution are that the NFC stickers can be recycled.

Keywords: NFC · GPRS · EDGE · 3G · Mutual inductance · Electronic health records

1 Introduction

1.1 What Is NFC

Near Field Communication (NFC) is a set of standards used to establish radio communications between NFC enabled devices by bringing them into close proximity. There are many NFC devices in the market including latest smartphones. NFC standards including ISO/IEC 14443 and FeliCa are derived from Radio Frequency Identification (RFID) .The latest ISO/IEC 18092 standards were defined in 2004 by Nokia, Phillips and Semiconductors. The NFC standards are now overseen by NFC Forum with about 60 members [1].

1.2 NFC Application

The use of Near Field Communication (NFC) has been adoption in a variety of payment systems, including bus fare, train and tickets in stadiums [2]. More implementations are expected due to its secure transaction process as a result of the short

© Institute for Computer Sciences, Social Informatics and Telecommunications Engineering 2014
T.F. Bissyandé and G. van Stam (Eds.): AFRICOMM 2013, LNICST 135, pp. 121–129, 2014.
DOI: 10.1007/978-3-319-08368-1_14

range of operation, i.e. the range is less than 10 cm. Moreover, a number of smart phones embedded with NFC technology is increasing at an exponential rate. As the prices of smart phones are also expected to drop due to high competition in smart-phone industry, many people in developing countries are likely to afford at least one NFC smart phone per family.

NFC applications in different part of the world include but not limited to the following:

- Public transport
- Mobile payment
- Loyalty program
- Commercial services
- Mobile shopping
- Access control
- Employee payment
- Event ticketing
- Home healthcare
- Field Services

1.3   UNESCO Literacy Statistics

Good healthcare systems are necessary for wellbeing of all the people including the African population which is estimated at 863 million as per 2010 UNESCO general facts about Sub-Saharan Africa [3]. Table 1 shows the statistics regarding the world distribution of adults and youth literacy. From Table 1, Sub-Sahara Africa has the lowest per cent of literate population compared to other regions of the world: 63 % of adults are literate and 72 % of youths are literate.

The mobile phone signal coverage in Africa consists of a number of technologies that complement each other. These technologies are general packet radio services (GPRS), which offers data speeds of 56–114 kbit/s. The next technology is enhanced data rates for GSM evolution (EDGE) what supports speeds of up to 296 kbit/s. The latest technology that is available in rural areas is 3G and it can support speeds of up to 56 Mbit/s. These technologies have enabled mobile devices to communicate with higher speeds and hence increased the amount of data that can be transmitted from one

Table 1. The 2010 Global distribution of adults and youths literacy in per cent.

Region	Adult	Youth
World	84	90
Arab States	75	89
Europe	98	99
Central Asia	99	100
East Asia and the Pacific	94	99
Latin and the Caribbean	91	97
South and West Asia	63	81
Sub-Sahara Africa	63	72

location to the other. The response time between the mobile devices when they exchange data has also increased due to new technologies in mobile communication.

The main purpose of this paper is to address medication identification challenges facing illiterate Africa patients using a combination of NFC and smart mobile phone technologies.

The rest of the paper is structured as follows; Sect. 2 discusses Near Field Communication theory, active and passive modes of communication and modes of operation. Section 3 discusses a literature review of NFC applications in the health-care sector, while Sect. 4 discusses the proposed NFC medication identification for illiterate African patients and finally the conclusions are made in Sect. 5.

2 Near Field Communications Theory

2.1 Basic

NFC is a short range wireless technology that operates at a distance less than 10 cm. This short range mode of operation is considered very secure and as a result trans-actions are exchanged between devices using NFC. The basic working principle for NFC is based on the induced current between two coils placed next to each other. When a coil is placed in an area covered by a changing magnetic field produced by the first coil, a changing current gets induced in the second coil. The higher the coupling coefficient (as per Eq. 1) between the two coils results in more current being induced in the second coil [4].

$$K = \frac{M}{\sqrt{(L_f * L_s)}} \tag{1}$$

where, M is mutual inductance between the two coils, and L_f and L_s are inductive values of the first and second coils respectively.

The application discussed in the previous paragraph is only true when the NFC devices operate in a passive mode. Only one device has power supply and its magnetic fields power the second device. The data communication between the devices in both directions is accomplished by using the magnetic field established between them [5–7].

2.2 NFC Active and Passive Modes of Communication

NFC employs two different coding to transfer data. If an active device transfers data at 106 kbit/s, a modified Miller coding with 100 % modulation is used. In all other cases Manchester coding is used with a modulation ratio of 10 %.

NFC devices are able to receive and transmit data at the same time. Thus, they can check for potential collisions, if the received signal frequency does not match with the transmitted signal's frequency.

Table 2 shows the relationship between coding scheme and NFC device com-munication mode.

Table 2. NFC active and passive device mode speed

Speed (kbit/s)	Active device	Passive device
424	Manchester	Manchester
212	Manchester	Manchester
106	Modified Miller	Manchester

Active Mode: in this mode both initiator and target devices provide their own power supply and create a magnetic field to transfer data between each other. Any device can be the initiator while the other will be the target. One device creates magnetic fields and the other device transfers data back to the initiator [5–7].

Passive Mode: in this mode of operation only one device (initiator) has its own power supply to power the device and creates magnetic fields for the target device (tag) as well. Upon reaching the target, the magnetic fields induce current which gets rectified and powers the target circuit. The target transfers data back to the initiator using the magnetic field channel [5–7].

2.3 NFC Standards

NFC technology utilises the 13.56 MHz frequency and is governed by ISO 18092 and EMCA 340 standards [1].

NFC Forum has defined four Tag types that are interoperable between NFC technologies and devices [8]. Table 3 shows the NFC types, corresponding standards they support and the maximum internal memory each NFC tag can accommodate.

Table 3. NFC standards and tag memory

Forum type	Standard	Memory size
Type 1	ISO/IEC 14443A	2 Kb
Type 2	ISO/IEC 14443A	2 Kb
Type 3	FeliCa	1 Mb
Type 4	ISO/IEC 14443A	32 Kb

2.4 NFC Modes of Operation

NFC can operate in one of three following modes; Card Emulator mode, Peer to Peer mode and Reader mode [9].

- **Card Emulator Mode**: in this mode mobile phone is used as a tag for external readers. This is applicable when mobile phone is used as a payment card.
- **Peer to Peer Mode**: in this mode mobile phone interact with another mobile phone for transacting.
- **Reader Mode**: in this mode mobile phone is used to read/write to external tags. This is applicable when mobile phone is used as a point of sale (POS) terminal.

3   NFC Related Work in Health Care

NFC technology has gained slow inroads in the healthcare industry. In this section, different healthcare applications based on NFC will be reviewed.

Devendran, Bhuvaneswari and Krishnan identified a need to use NFC technology in conjunction with an Electronic Medium Records (EMR) system. They proposed system can make the process of patient record keeping easier, more accurate and more efficient. Each patient is issued with a NFC tag that is read via a NFC reader connected to a computer for uploading patient information into an EMR system when the patient arrives at the hospital or clinic. The NFC data is uploaded with EMR information each time the patient leaves the hospital [10].

In addition, Devendran and Bhuvaneswari in their study of NFC and healthcare proposed a basic architecture for m-health services using NFC to facilitate the provisioning of healthcare to people using mobile phones. They highlighted that NFC and mobile phone technology can be used to allow individuals to report the following:

– Room, bed or medication identity using low cost NFC tags.
– Time, place or care giver identity by mobile phone.
– Quick filling of multiple choice forms as an option for additional information.

These applications provide real-time feedback for personal care and help improve quality assurance in the healthcare sector [11]. In their paper, the authors suggested that their proposed solution can improve quality assurance in the healthcare sector by reducing clinical errors. However, errors in most cases are human by nature rather than system oriented. That means than no technology can eliminate errors entirely if the human users are not trained to use a technological system correctly. Despite having said that, one advantage with the proposed system is that it offers systematically quick information saving and searching.

Krishna, Sreevard, Karun and Kumar are of the opinion that NFC technology can be used for real time hospital patient management. They have considered an architecture that can be used across different departments of multi specialities in hospitals. The patient's information written on the NFC tag is read by the reader when the patient enters certain doors within the hospital. This approach saves time and cost with regards to opening a new paper based file each time a patient visits different healthcare facilities [12]. This solution is considered to have positive effect when patients go to emergency departments.

Jara, Zamora and Skarmeta presented the deployment of services in medical environments that can be carried out with NFC technology also. They highlighted the following NFC services in medical environments;

– External applications to the human body; these refer to mobile phones that manage electronic health records (EHR), collecting of data from medical devices.
– Internal applications to the human body (implants); these refer to NFC devices that communicate with implant devices to collect data, setting up parameters and power supply to recharge batteries. These are possible since the NFC works at 13.56 MHz which is considered harmless to health and NFC operating frequency of 13.56 MHz is common for all countries.

Table 4. Dimensions of tags

Label	Length (mm)	Width (mm)	Area (mm^2)
Q	22	38	836
O	45	45	2025
C	65	34	2210
M	76	45	3420

Table 5. Results

Location	Depth (mm)
Below dermal fat	11
Below ribs	27 (including 11 mm of dermal fat)
With skull	15 (including 6.5 mm skin and superficial fascia

They concluded their paper by stating that in an effort to make NFC technology safe, cryptographic tags must be used to protect data stored in the NFC tags [13].

During their study regarding suitability of NFC for medical devices, Freudenthal etc. conducted a series of experiments using 15.56 MHz tags [14]. They implanted tags within human cadaver and took measurements. Table 4 shows the dimensions of the tags that were successfully read.

Their experiments furthermore determined by implant depths within which the tag information could be read accurately are shown in Table 5.

Despite the successful experiments using implanted devices, the authors noted that for distributed systems the unintended personal disclosure for private information and corruption of data integrity can occur.

Morak, Schwarz, Hayn and Schreier discussed the feasibility of using m-health and NFC based medication adherence monitoring system [15]. Their system consists of smart medication blister, a NFC phone that connects to remote tele-monitoring service which passed data to physician's phone via https protocol. Their system is depicted in Fig. 1.

Based on the obtained results, they concluded that medication adherence monitoring based on NFC enabled medication blisters and mobile phone is feasible. However, they indicated that some improvements with respect to blister and the recycling processes are required before the system can be completely adopted in the industry.

4   Proposed Solution

The previous section has covered the different healthcare applications based on NFC technology. However, none of the applications cater for illiterate patients, which can be an issue when it comes to following the correct medication regimen.

The proposed solution as depicted in Fig. 2, consists of each medicine container having an NFC sticker with data stored in it. An illiterate patient with a NFC Android smartphone can tap the NFC sticker with the phone after activating a Medicine ID

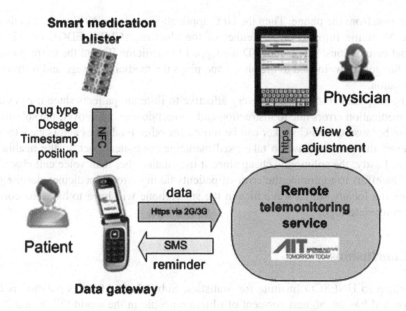

Fig. 1. Medication adherence monitoring system

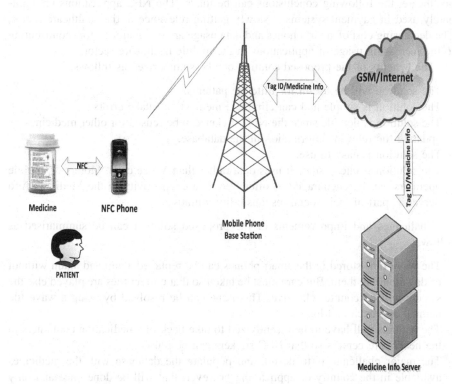

Fig. 2. Overview of NFC based solution for illiterate patients using remote audio instructions.

application from the phone. Then the NFC application reads the NFC sticker, connects to the Medicine Info Server via either of the channels (GPRS, EDGE or 3G) and Internet connections. The sticker ID is mapped to medicine ID and the corresponding wave file gets downloaded to the phone and plays the medicine dosage and instruction information.

The proposed solution can be very effective to illiterate patients since it can eliminate medication errors due to instruction and correct dosage. Moreover, the solution is flexible because the NFC sticker can be reused for other medicines and is easy to use. However, the patients have to take used medicine containers back to the healthcare centres. Lastly, the solution is cheap since it uses data rather than voice call charges.

In an effort to minimise the error of patients taking wrong medicines despite this system, the locally stored wave files in the smartphone will have to have the correct and appropriate logo.

5   Conclusions

According to UNESCO Institute for Statistics, Sub-Sahara Africa population is 863 million and has the highest per-cent of illiterate people in the world (37 % and 28 % for adults and youth, respectively). Based on the study of NFC and its application in healthcare, the following conclusions can be made. The NFC applications predominately used in payment systems is slowly getting relevance in the healthcare sector. The decreasing cost of smart phones and data usage are two major factors contributing to the increasing usage of applications in the mobile healthcare sector.

The benefits of the proposed solution can be summarized as follows;

- The solution will be useful for illiterate patients.
- The solution is simple and can eliminate medication intake errors.
- The solution is flexible since the NFC sticker can be reused for other medicines by updating the relevant information in the database.
- The solution is easy to use.
- The solution is cheap since it uses data rather than Voice calls. Moreover, mobile operators can be encouraged to offer free data connectivity to the Medicine Info Server as part of their social responsibility initiative.

Challenges and improvements of the proposed solution can be summarised as follows;

- The wave files stored in the smart phones can be replayed again and again without re-downloading them. But care must be taken so that correct files are played else the system will be counter effective. This issue can be resolved by using a wave file naming approach and logo.
- The patients will have to be incentivized to take back old medication containers to the healthcare centres so that NFC stickers can be reused.
- The major challenge is to design and populate the database with the medicines available in the country of application; however, that will be done once and only add new medicines when the need arises.

Acknowledgments. This work is based on research supported in part by the Eskom Tertiary Education Support Programme (TESP), reference number 264030.

References

1. Jung-Hyun, C., Cole, P.H., Shiho, K.: SoC Design Conference (ISOCC), International Publication, pp. 456–459 (2009)
2. Benyo, B., Vilmos, A., Kovacs, K., Kutor, L.: Intelligent Engineering Systems. 11th International Conference, pp. 277–280 (2007)
3. Adult and Youth Literacy.: Global Trends in Gender Parity. UIS Facts Sheet. UNESCO Institute for Statistics, 2 September 2012. http://unesco.org/Factsheet/Documents/ fs20-literacy-day-2013-en-v3.pdf [online 28/06/2013]
4. Agbinya, J.I., Masihpour, M.: Broadband and Biomedical Communications (IB2Com). Fifth International Conference, pp. 1–6 (2010)
5. Al-Offishat, H., Rababah, M.: Near field communication. Int. J. Comput. Sci. Netw. Secur. (IJCSNS) **12**(2), 93–99 (2012)
6. Bilginer, B., Ljunggren, P.L.: Near field communication. Master's thesis, Department of Electrical Engineering, Lund University, Sweden (2011)
7. Paus, A.: Near field communication in cell phones. White paper, Ruhr-Universität Bochum, July 2007
8. Technical Specifications: NFC Forum. http://www.nfc-forum.org/specs_list/ [online 9/06/ 2013]
9. Narada, W.: Near field communication (NFC) opportunities & standards. http://www.umts. no/files/081028%20nfc-Standards_payments%20Narada.pdf [online 20/06/2013]
10. Morak, J., Schreier, G.: MHealth based on NFC technology - preliminary results from medium scale proof of concept projects. Proceedings of the ehealth 2012. 11 May 2012; Vienna, Austria OCG (2012)
11. Vergara, M., Díaz-Hellín, P., Fontecha, J., Hervás, R., Sánchez-Barba, C., Fuentes, C., Bravo, J.: Mobile prescription: an NFC-based proposal for AAL. Near Field Communication (NFC) Second International Workshop on IEEE Conference Publications, pp. 27–32 (2010)
12. Chowdhury, B., Khosla, R.: Computer and information science. 6th IEEE/ACIS International Conference Publication, pp. 363–368 (2007)
13. Jara, A.J., Zamora, M.A., Miguel, A., Skarmeta, A.F.G.: Secure use of NFC in medical environments. RFID Systems and Technologies (RFID SysTech), 2009 5th European Workshop on VDE Conference Publications, pp. 1–8 (2009)
14. Freudenthal, E., Herrera, D., Kautz, F., Natividad, C., Ogrey, A., Sipla, J., Sosa, A., Betancourt, C., Estevez, L.: Suitability of NFC for medical device communication and power delivery. Engineering in Medicine and Biology Workshop, 2007 IEEE Dallas Conference Publication, pp. 51–54 (2007)
15. Morak, J., Schwarz, M., Hay, D., Schreier, G.: Engineering in Medicine and Biology Society (EMBC), Annual International Conference of the IEEE Publication, pp. 272–275 (2012)

Spatial Analysis of Location of Mother's Choice for Delivery: A Case of Blantyre and Mwanza Districts in Malawi

Priscilla Maliwichi[(✉)] and Patrick Albert Chikumba

Department of Computing and Information Technology,
University of Malawi-The Polytechnic, Private Bag 303, Blantyre 3, Malawi
pmaliwichi@yahoo.co.uk, patrick_chikumba@yahoo.com

Abstract. As all pregnancies involve some risks to mother or infant, it is important to prevent, detect and manage complications. The provision of antenatal care can give a chance to detect existing conditions of pregnant women that can cause complications during child birth. Location where women live affects their health, nutrition and decision to choose where they will deliver their babies. This research has focused on mapping and analysing the locations where mothers choose to deliver their babies. It has been found apart from distance and lack of transport to a health facility availability of health facilities and maternal services can affect the choice of where to deliver. There are some demographic and cultural factors that affect mothers when making their decisions such as their education background, number of children that they have and age of the mothers.

Keywords: TBA · Pregnant women · GIS · Mapping · Spatial analysis · Baby delivery · SBA

1 Introduction

Location where women live affects their health, nutrition, and decision to choose where they will deliver their babies [20]. Urban residences are associated with a higher percentage of pregnancies assisted by a skilled attendant than those in rural areas [20]. Pregnant women can plan to deliver at home, traditional birth attendant (TBA) or government/private health facility. But sometimes due to other circumstances such as social, cultural, economical factors and poor infrastructure of road network, women can deliver their babies in locations which they have not planned. Distance to a health facility can be an obstacle to access the facility [20].

Malawi Government expects all women to deliver their babies at health facilities. Developing countries, including Malawi, are trying to meet MDG 5 and 6 which are to improve the maternal and infant mortality rates. The target is reduction of maternal mortality by three-fourths between 1990 and 2015 [49]. Safe motherhood projects are being introduced to improve maternal health care. Gruenberg [26] points out that complication during pregnancy and delivery often arises unexpectedly.

The maternal mortality rate in Malawi is at 810 per 100,000 live births and one of the highest in the world [53]. It is estimated that each year about 600,000 women die

© Institute for Computer Sciences, Social Informatics and Telecommunications Engineering 2014
T.F. Bissyandé and G. van Stam (Eds.): AFRICOMM 2013, LNICST 135, pp. 130–139, 2014.
DOI: 10.1007/978-3-319-08368-1_15

as a result of pregnancy and childbirth and almost 99 % of these deaths occur in developing countries [57]. Skilled attendant at childbirth is crucial for decreasing maternal and neonatal mortality [30].

Ronsmans et al. [46] suggest five major direct causes of maternal mortality such as hemorrhage, sepsis, hypertensive disorders, prolonged labour and unsafe abortion. These could be prevented with proper medical monitoring, information and services. Improved nutrition and the reduction of harmful practices such as female genital mutilation may also reduce the risk. Unsafe abortion can be prevented with access to family planning information and services.

In order to prevent maternal mortality, it is very important that all pregnant women have access to quality prenatal and postnatal care as well as good care at the time of delivery. Assuring access requires proper organization of health care services and the introduction of programs in family planning as well as education and preventive programs during pregnancy, delivery and post-natal period. Differences in access arise for several reasons such as distance to health centres and lack of women's empowerment to make independent decisions regarding their reproductive health [9].

The advancement in ICT has made it possible to use Information System (IS), such as Geographic Information System (GIS), to analyse data and help in decision making. GIS is a powerful set of tools for collecting, storing, retrieving, transforming and displaying spatial data from the real world for a particular set of purposes [8]. The GIS acts as a spatial database containing attribute information in which specific data themes can be integrated and explored cumulatively in order to derive new information on a particular question. GIS is commonly used to make decisions that involve locations [25].

This research aims at finding factors that influence women when making decision of where they want to deliver. It focuses on their socio-economical status, the distance to the health facility, the mode of transport used to travel to health facility and their place of residence. Poor availability and accessibility to a health facility is a problem which this research is addressing. GIS has been used to map and analyse the availability and accessibility of the required services for safe motherhood.

The data has been analysed using point processes and discrete variation inferential models. According to [7], point processes are defined as a set of irregularly distributed points in a terrain, whose location was generated by a stochastic mechanism. The inferential models of discrete variation concern the distribution of events whose localization is associated to areas delimited by polygons. This case occurs much frequently when dealing with phenomena aggregated by population, mortality and income. In this case, there is no exact locality of the events, but value aggregated by area. The objective is to model the pattern of spatial occurrence of the geographic phenomenon under study.

2   Geographic Information System and Maternal Healthcare

According to [46], maternal mortality is one of the great neglected problems of health care in developing countries. Maternal mortality rates in developing countries are as much as 100 times higher than those in industrialized countries. The causes include obstructed labour and ruptured uterus, postpartum haemorrhage, eclampsia, post-partum infection, and complications of illegal abortion. Most obstetric complications occur around the time of delivery and cannot be predicted [17]. Therefore it is important that all pregnant women have access to a skilled birth attendant. The net-works of maternity care facilities, trained personnel, and means of transport are necessary to provide needed emergency maternity care services.

Inaccessibility of essential health information is only part of the problem [50]. Even when a woman reaches a health facility, there are a number of obstacles receiving adequate and appropriate care. These are a result of failures in the health services delivery system: the lack of minimal life-saving equipment at the first referral level; the lack of equipment, personnel, and know-how even in referral hospitals; and worst of all, faulty patient management. Prevention of maternal deaths requires fun-damental changes not only in resource allocation, but in the structures of health services delivery. According to [23], creating a functioning health system is the most obvious means of providing this type of environment. In a functioning district health system the availability, accessibility, use, and quality of essential obstetric care are expected to be high and maternal mortality is expected to be low. Some developing countries, such as China, Sri Lanka, and Malaysia, have reduced maternal mortality dramatically after improving the coverage and quality of their health services [23].

Places where people live affect their health, nutrition, and access to health care services [35]. Researchers can link Demographic and Health Survey (DHS) data with routine health data, health facility locations, land use, local infrastructure, and envi-ronmental conditions by using GIS [35]. The geography of health care comprises the analysis of spatial organization (number sizes, types, and locations) of health services, how and why spatial organization changes over time, how people gain access to health services, and the impacts on health and well-being [15].

New forms of health care delivery are emerging and the persistently high costs of health care are raising concerns about quality, effectiveness, and access [34]. GIS and related spatial analytic techniques provide a set of tools for describing and under-standing the changing spatial organization of health care, for examining its relation-ship to health outcomes and access, and for exploring how health care delivery can be improved. Although GIS has been used for several decades to examine health care systems, the scope of GIS contributions has grown rapidly in recent years [34].

Geographic variation in population provides the foundation for analysis and planning of health services [34]. People are not spread evenly across the Earth's surface, and populations differ along many dimensions that affect their need for health care, their ability to travel to obtain health care, and the types of services they are willing and able to utilize [34]. Increasingly, GIS is being used to map and explore geographical variation in need for health services and to develop innovative indicators of health care need.

GIS has an important role in assessing health care needs for small areas by facilitating the spatial linking of diverse health, social, and environmental data sets. Although the layering capabilities of GIS have been used for many years, researchers are now making use of the analytic capabilities to relate data sets that rely on non-consistent areal units and to generate meaningful service areas [32]. As digital information on morbidity, demographics, and utilization becomes more widely available, health needs data will be incorporated in GIS-based decision support tools that allow communities and decision-makers to examine questions of health care needs, access, and availability [34].

Access describes people's ability to use health services when and where they are needed [1]. Health care decisions are strongly influenced by the type and quality of services available in the local area and the distance, time, cost, and ease of traveling to reach those services [24, 27, 42]. For medical conditions that require regular contact with service providers, travel time and distance can create barriers to effective service use [15, 27]. GIS is being used to create better measures of geographical access and to analyze geographical inequalities in access as well as those patterned along social and economic lines.

One of the advantages of GIS is that it can combine spatial information on roads, transportation and population to create much accurate measures of geographical separation. To assess travel along transportation networks, many studies have used GIS to calculate network distances [3, 15, 54] and travel times based on road type and quality [27, 45]. A given area typically contains a mix of people who rely on different transportation modes and thus have varying levels of geographical access [33]. Health care providers differ greatly in the range, type, and quality of services offered. Most people are willing to travel farther to obtain specialized or higher-quality care, so there is a trade-off between distance and facility size/quality [34].

Health care analysts have been involved with questions of location, for example deciding where to locate new service resources, which existing facilities to close, and how best to improve service locations. Location-allocation models, and related optimization methods, provide tools for addressing these types of questions [37]. Relying on spatial data commonly available in GIS, location-allocation models are increasingly being implemented in a GIS environment.

Today it is common to use GIS in calculating network travel times from demand areas to potential health facility sites [5, 10, 54]. It is also straightforward to incorporate differences in mobility and transportation access among population groups, but few published location-allocation studies appear to have done this. Using tools readily available in GIS, analysts can better represent geographical context in identifying optimal health care locations, and they can visualize and explore model results [48, 58].

3 Methodology

This research used both quantitative and qualitative research methods. This is so because there are a number of quantitative data. Interpretivism research paradigm was used for all qualitative data. In this research, experiences of women during antenatal, delivery and postnatal were collected using interviews and observations.

The study population was from Mwanza and Blantyre districts of Malawi. Mwanza has a population of 92,974 and Blantyre has a population of 1,001,984 [39].

Both probability and non-probability sampling were used. Probability sampling was used when interviewing mothers. Snowball sampling of non-probability sampling was used when interviewing members of staff at a health facility and TBAs.

The sample size was 70 for both in Mwanza and Blantyre districts. Observation was used at health facilities when dealing with maternal cases.

GPS system was used to collect the coordinates of the locations where mothers choose to deliver babies, as well as the locations where they actually delivered their babies. Maps were generated using Quantum GIS 1.6.0.

4 Mapping and Analysing Locations Mothers Choice of Delivery

In Mwanza and Blantyre, women have wide choice of where to deliver based on various factors that influence their choices. They can deliver at home, TBA and health facilities. In some cases, if they delay, women can deliver on road on the way to the health facility as the case in Mwanza (see Fig. 1).

One woman in Mwanza delivered at home because when labour started, she was waiting for her mother in-law and sister in-law to come to take her to the hospital. This shows that cultural factors affect women in making decision of even starting off from home to the hospital. Women in some cultures may avoid facility delivery due to cultural requirements of seclusion in the household during this time of "pollution" [17, 36].

A TBA in Blantyre commented that, sometimes a health centre calls her to assist in delivery. If this woman delivers again certainly she is going to use the TBA because she feels that using TBA's is the same as using the hospital.

TBAs are usually deemed affordable for poor families since their payment is negotiable in terms of amount and timing and can be in kind [2]. TBA assisted deliveries are common in T/A Makata and Kapeni since the nearest hospital offering basic obstetric care is Mlambe mission hospital and is not free. However, Thaddeus and Maine [52] finds out that the financial cost of receiving care is often not a major determinant of the decision to seek care.

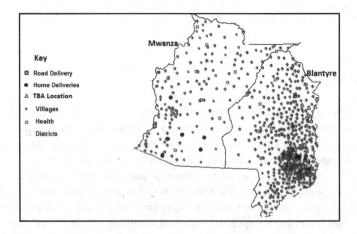

Fig. 1. Mapping locations of mother's choices of delivery

The type and severity of complications that lead to a change in place of delivery depend on the perception of what is abnormal and what is amenable to medical treatment [52]. People who consider "normal deliveries" or minor problems as not justifying cost, time and travel to a facility may attempt to overcome those barriers if there is a danger to life, even if the cost is much higher.

Bad roads make the women not to reach the health facility in time. For example in Thambani, the health centre has an ambulance which goes to Mwanza district hospital every day to deliver all maternal emergencies and other patients who need to be admitted. This is so because Thambani is very far and it is not appropriate to be calling for ambulance from the district hospital when there is an emergency. When taking emergencies to Mwanza district hospital sometimes babies are born on the way due to the condition of the road.

Mode of transport is also another factor that affects women on the place of delivery. Using the finding from T/A Chapananga, there is no mode of transport from Chapananga to Tulonkhondo. As a result people either have to walk to Tulonkhondo health centre or deliver at home. It is argued that there is a clear relationship between antenatal follow up for delivery care and the distance to the nearest health centre due to lack of convenient transport and the bad road conditions and concluded that rural women access to maternal care services is relatively low as they have to travel long distance to the nearest health facility which has a negative impact on the maintaining consistency in their health seeking behaviour.

Thaddeus and Maine [52] suggests that patients who make a timely decision to seek care can still experience delay, because the accessibility of health services is an acute problem in the developing world. In rural areas, a woman with an obstetric emergency may find the closet facility equipped only for basic treatments and education, and she may have no way to reach a regional centre where resources exist.

Perceived quality of care, which only partly overlaps with medical quality of care, is thought to be an important influence on health care-seeking. Assessment of quality of services "largely depends on [people's] own experiences with the health system and those of people they know" [52]. Most women from villages in Mwanza are delivering their babies at home or at far health centre because there is no nurse at the closest maternity centre. Although some elements such as waiting times can be measured objectively, the perception of whether these are a problem and affect quality is more subjective (ibid). When using far health centre, these women stay for long time at the hospital until they deliver. Elements of satisfaction cover satisfaction with the outcome, the interventions and with the service received – including staff friendliness, availability of supplies and waiting times [52].

At some health facilities, all nurses are male nurses and they are the ones who carry out all ANC and delivery services. In many cases, the medical 'culture' may clash with the woman's. For example, when family members are not allowed to be present, supine birthing position is imposed or privacy not respected; this may lead to perceptions of poor quality [52].

From the findings, antenatal care, basic obstetric care and emergency obstetric care are important services that need to be found at a health facility. But it has been found that though some health facilities can conduct emergency obstetric care, due to lack of equipments and resources, the needed treatment cannot be provided to mothers. Looking at a case that happened at Mwanza district hospital which offers emergency obstetric care, a woman died just because the hospital did not have vitamin K to give a woman who had severe bleeding after delivery. In this case, the hospital did not have blood to give to this woman to buy time until the woman can be referred to QECH where they refer more complicated cases.

Arriving at the facility may not lead to the immediate commencement of treatment. In this research, lack of personnel, equipment, shortage of supplies and type of services offered at the health facilities delay the patients in receiving adequate and appropriate care. This supports Thaddeus and Maine [52] findings that reveal that shortages of qualified staff, essential drugs and supplies, coupled with administrative delays and clinical mismanagement, become documentable contributors to maternal deaths.

The birth order also influences women on where to deliver. In this research, 66 % of later birth occurs outside the health facility. The study also found that young girls from Thambani area are having children at a very young age. The first birth is known to be more difficult and the woman has no previous experience of delivery. Normally, health workers may recommend a facility delivery for primipara. Often a high value is placed on the first pregnancy and in some settings the woman's natal family helps her get the best care possible [38]. This is the reason why all first pregnancies are referred to the main hospital, like Mwanza district hospital and Mlambe Mission Hospital. By contrast, women of higher parity, can draw on their maternity experiences and may not feel the need to receive professional care if previous deliveries were uncomplicated [43]. Very high-order births, however, are more risky. Like at Thambani health centre, all order women and women delivering their fourth born are referred to Mwanza District Hospital.

Mother's education is another factor. About 94 % of women interviewed had no formal education. This shows that there is high illiteracy rate among rural women and this affects the decision on where to deliver. There are multiple potential pathways that could explain why maternal education is consistently and strongly associated with all types of health behaviour [4]. These include increased knowledge of the benefits of preventive health care and awareness of health services. Education also reflects a woman's childhood background, including familiarity with health services and certain beliefs and norms, and some recommend this should be controlled for [14, 38, 44].

5   Conclusion

In conclusion, all levels of assistance that a woman receives during the birth of her child also are important for both the mother and the child. Women's health issues in general and women health care need in particular are foremost among the public health priorities of the countries around the world. In this regard, the Malawi government has started safe motherhood projects whose mission is to encourage health facility based deliveries. Women deliver now their babies at the hospital. For people who still have home deliveries they go to the health centre and claim that the baby was born on the way to the hospital, just for the hospital to record in their health passport so that they should not be charged a goat.

References

1. Aday, L.A., Andersen, R.M.: Equity of access to medical care: a conceptual and empirical overview. Med. Care **19**(12), 4–27 (1981)
2. Amooti-Kaguna, B., Nuwaha, F.: Factors influencing choice of delivery sites in Rakai district of Uganda. Soc. Sci. Med. **50**(2), 203–213 (2000)
3. Bamford, E.J., et al.: Accessibility to general practitioners in rural South Australia. Med. J. Aust. **171**(11–12), 614–616 (1999)
4. Bell, J., Curtis, S.L., Alayón, S.: Trends in delivery care in six countries. Calverton, MD: ORC Macro: 62 (2003)
5. Branas, C.C., MacKenzie, E.J., ReVelle, C.S.: A trauma resource allocation model for ambulances and hospitals. Health Serv. Res. **35**(2), 489 (2000)
6. Burgard, S.: Race and pregnancy-related care in Brazil and South Africa. Soc. Sci. Med. **59**(6), 1127–1146 (2004)
7. Câmara, G., et al.: Spatial analysis and GIS: a primer (2000). www.dpi.inpe.br/gilberto/tutorials/spatial_analysis/spatial_analysis_primer.pdf
8. Chang, K.: Introduction to Geographic Information Systems, pp. 15–27. McGraw-Hill Publishing Company, New York (2002)
9. Cook, C.A.L., et al.: Access barriers and the use of prenatal care by low-income, inner-city women. Soc. Work-albany N.Y. **44**, 129–141 (1999)
10. Cromley, E., Wei, X.: Locating facilities for EMS response to motor vehicle collisions. In: Proc. Health GIS Conf., 2001 (2002)
11. D'Ambruoso, L., Abbey, M., Hussein, J.: Please understand when I cry out in pain: women's accounts of maternity services during labour and delivery in Ghana. BMC Public Health **5**(1), 140 (2005)
12. Derekenaris, G., et al.: Integrating GIS, GPS and GSM technologies for the effective management of ambulances. Comput. Environ. Urban Syst. **25**(3), 267–278 (2001)
13. Duong, D.V., Binns, C.W., Lee, A.H.: Utilization of delivery services at the primary health care level in rural Vietnam. Soc. Sci. Med. **59**(12), 2585–2595 (2004)
14. Elo, I.T.: Utilization of maternal health-care services in Peru: the role of women's education. Health Transit. Rev. **2**(1), 49–69 (1992)
15. Fortney, J., et al.: The impact of geographic accessibility on the intensity and quality of depression treatment. Med. Care **37**(9), 884 (1999)
16. Furuta, M., Salway, S.: Women's position within the household as a determinant of maternal health care use in Nepal. Int. Fam. Planning Perspec. **32**(1), 17–27 (2006)
17. Gabrysch, S., Campbell, O.: Still too far to walk: literature review of the determinants of delivery service use. BMC Pregnancy Childbirth **9**(1), 34 (2009)
18. Gage, A.J.: Barriers to the utilization of maternal health care in rural Mali. Soc. Sci. Med. **65**(8), 1666–1682 (2007)
19. Gage, A.J., Calixte, M.G.: Effects of the physical accessibility of maternal health services on their use in rural Haiti. Popul. Stud. **60**(3), 271–288 (2006)
20. Geubbels, E.: Epidemiology of maternal mortality in Malawi. Malawi Med. J. **18**(4), 208 (2007)
21. Gibson, A., et al.: Geographies of need and the new NHS: methodological issues in the definition and measurement of the health needs of local populations. Health Place **8**(1), 47–60 (2002)
22. Glei, D.A., Goldman, N., Rodríguez, G.: Utilization of care during pregnancy in rural Guatemala: does obstetrical need matter? Soc. Sci. Med. **57**(12), 2447–2463 (2003)

23. Goodburn, E., Campbell, O.: Reducing maternal mortality in the developing world: sector-wide approaches may be the key. Br. Med. J. **322**(7291), 917 (2001)
24. Goodman, D.C., et al.: The distance to community medical care and the likelihood of hospitalization: is closer always better? Am. J. Public Health **87**(7), 1144 (1997)
25. Gorr, W., Johnson, M., Roehrig, S.: Spatial decision support system for home-delivered services. J. Geogr. Syst. **3**(2), 181–197 (2001)
26. Gruenberg, B.U.: Birth Emergency Skills Training: Manual for Out-of-Hospital Midwives. Birth Guru Publications, Duncannon (2008)
27. Haynes, R., Gale, S., Mugford, M., Davies, P.: Cataract surgery in a community hospital outreach clinic: patients' costs and satisfaction. Soc. Sci. Med. **53**(12), 1631–1640 (2001)
28. Hounton, S., et al.: Methods for evaluating effectiveness and cost-effectiveness of a skilled care initiative in rural Burkina Faso. Trop. Med. Int. Health **13**, 14–24 (2008)
29. Khan, M.M., et al.: A cost-minimization approach to planning the geographical distribution of health facilities. Health Policy Plan. **16**(3), 264 (2001)
30. Lawn, J.E., et al.: 4 million neonatal deaths: when? where? why? Lancet **365**(9462), 891–900 (2005)
31. Love, D., Lindquist, P.: The geographical accessibility of hospitals to the aged: a geographic information systems analysis within Illinois. Health Serv. Res. **29**(6), 629 (1995)
32. Lovett, A., Haynes, R., Bentham, G.: Improving health needs assessment using patient register information in a GIS. GIS Health **6**, 191 (1998)
33. Martin, D., et al.: Increasing the sophistication of access measurement in a rural healthcare study. Health Place **8**(1), 3–13 (2002)
34. McLafferty, S.L.: GIS and health care. Annu. Rev. Public Health **24**(1), 25–42 (2003)
35. MEASURE DHS: Mapping for improved health (2009). www.measuredhs.com/What-We-Do/.../GIS_DHS_Brochure.pdf. Accessed on 1 October 2011
36. Mesko, N., et al.: Care for perinatal illness in rural Nepal: a descriptive study with cross-sectional and qualitative components. BMC Int. Health Hum. Rights **3**(1), 3 (2003)
37. Moller-Jensen, L., Kofie, R.Y.: Exploiting available data sources: location/allocation modelling for health service planning in rural Ghana. Geogr. Tidsskr. Dan. J. Geogr. **101**, 145–154 (2001)
38. Navaneetham, K., Dharmalingam, A.: Utilization of maternal health care services in Southern India. Soc. Sci. Med. **55**(10), 1849–1869 (2002)
39. NSO: The National Statistical Office of Malawi (2008). http://www.nso.malawi.net/. Accessed 6 September 2010
40. Olson, D.L.: Introduction to Information Systems Project Management. Irwin, Illinois (2004)
41. Patton, M.Q.: Qualitative Evaluation and Research Methods, 2nd edn., 532 p. Sage, Newbury Park (1990)
42. Phillips Jr., R.L., et al.: Using geographic information systems to understand health care access. Arch. Fam. Med. **9**(10), 971 (2000)
43. Potter, J.E.: Use of maternal health services in rural Mexico. Salud pública de México **30**(3), 387 (1985)
44. Raghupathy, S.: Education and the use of maternal health care in Thailand 1. Soc. Sci. Med. **43**(4), 459–471 (1996)
45. Ramsbottom-Lucier, M., et al.: Hills, ridges, mountains, and roads: geographical factors and access to care in rural Kentucky. J. Rural Health **12**(5), 386–394 (1996)
46. Ronsmans, C., Graham, W.J., et al.: Maternal mortality: who, when, where, and why. Lancet **368**(9542), 1189–1200 (2006)

47. Rubin, A., Babbie, E.R.: Essential Research Methods For Social Work. Brooks/Cole Pub. Co., Salt Lake City (2009)
48. Rushton, G., West, M.: Women with localized breast cancer selecting mastectomy treatment, Iowa, 1991–1996. Public Health Rep. **114**(4), 370–371 (1999). (Washington, DC: 1974)
49. Sachs, J., McArthur, J.: The Millennium Project: a plan for meeting the millennium development goals. Lancet **365**(9456), 347–353 (2005)
50. Sundari, T.K.: The untold story: how the health care systems in developing countries contribute to maternal mortality. Int. J. Health Serv. Plann. Adm. Eval. **22**(3), 513 (1992)
51. Tanser, F., et al.: New approaches to spatially analyse primary health care usage patterns in rural South Africa. Trop. Med. Int. Health **6**(10), 826–838 (2001)
52. Thaddeus, S., Maine, D.: Too far to walk: maternal mortality in context. Soc. Sci. Med. **38**(8), 1091–1110 (1994)
53. UNICEF: UNICEF - Malawi – Statistics (2010). http://www.unicef.org/infobycountry/malawi_statistics.html Accessed 3 September 2010
54. Walsh, S.J., Page, P.H., Gesler, W.M.: Normative models and healthcare planning: network-based simulations within a geographic information system environment. Health Serv. Res. **32**(2), 243 (1997)
55. Wennberg, J.E., Fisher, E.S., Skinner, J.S.: Geography and the debate over Medicare reform. Health Affairs-Millwood va Then Bethesda Ma **21**(2), 10–10 (2002)
56. WHO: World Health Statistics (1997). http://www.who.int/whosis/whostat/EN_WHS10_Full.pdf
57. WHO: Second Generation, WHO Country Cooperation Strategy, 2008-2013, Malawi - AFRO Library Cataloguing-in-Publication Data (2009) http://www.who.int/countryfocus/cooperation_strategy/ccs_mwi_en.pdf
58. Wong, D.W.S., Meyer, J.W.: A spatial decision support system approach to evaluate the efficiency of a meals-on-wheels program. Professional Geogr. **45**(3), 332–341 (1993)

Diabetes Advisor – A Medical Expert System for Diabetes Management

Audrey Mbogho[1]([✉]), Joel Dave[2], and Kulani Makhubele[1]

[1] Department of Computer Science, University of Cape Town,
Cape Town, South Africa
audrey.mbogho@uct.ac.za, kulani.makhubele@absacapital.com
[2] Division of Endocrinology and Diabetic Medicine, University of Cape Town,
Cape Town, South Africa
joel.dave@uct.ac.za

Abstract. Access to medical services in rural communities, especially in the developing world, is extremely limited. Medical expert systems can play a significant role in alleviating this problem by providing decision support in the giving of advice on diagnosis, treatment and disease management. This study built a prototype for diabetes, a chronic illness affecting millions across the globe. Preliminary evaluation suggests that such a system could be useful for expanding medical services in rural communities and as an educational tool for unskilled medical staff.

Keywords: Expert systems · Diabetes · Decision support

1 Introduction

Diabetes is a serious, life-threatening, chronic disease affecting over 300 million people [1]. It is estimated that this figure will reach 366 million by 2030 [2] with 81 % of these diabetics being in developing countries, where medical care remains severely limited.

Fortunately, diabetes can be managed very effectively through healthy lifestyle choices, primarily diet and exercise. Furthermore, people who are at high risk can avoid developing the disease also through diet and exercise. This paper reports on a prototype expert system for the provision of medical advice on diabetes which can be used at home or at a rural clinic.

2 Expert Systems

An expert system is a computer program that emulates the decision making ability of a human expert [3]. The expert system developed in this project, Diabetes Advisor (DA), is designed to give advice to patients with diabetes. DA can also be used to educate people without diabetes in order to raise awareness about the disease and to enable people to assess their own risk and take appropriate action.

© Institute for Computer Sciences, Social Informatics and Telecommunications Engineering 2014
T.F. Bissyandé and G. van Stam (Eds.): AFRICOMM 2013, LNICST 135, pp. 140–144, 2014.
DOI: 10.1007/978-3-319-08368-1_16

In addition, DA can be used as an educational tool by unqualified medical staff to learn more about diabetes and become better prepared to attend to patients safely and effectively.

Expert systems can provide *decision support* or can be used as *decision makers* [4]. In the decision support role, expert systems assist the clinician. This can reduce the cost of healthcare for the patient because the clinician can consult with the expert system in the same visit instead of referring the patient to a specialist. In rural communities, an expert system can provide decision support or can be the decision maker if medical staff are unqualified or completely absent. In the decision making role, expert systems would be used in place of the clinician. While this might be seen as risky, the risk from getting no medical attention at all is greater than that posed by getting it from a computer.

2.1 Expert Systems for Diabetes

In [5], Hernando *et al.* described DIABNET, an expert system whose purpose was to assist clinicians in treating patients with gestational diabetes. As this form of diabetes tends to be temporary, patients do not have enough time with the disease to learn how to manage it, and frequent visits with clinicians are necessary. DIABNET aimed to reduce the frequency of such visits by giving recommendations on insulin dose adjustment and meal planning. In addition, DIABNET could monitor patient data continuously and alert clinicians when unusual readings appeared, allowing clinicians to attend to patients remotely. Rudi *et al.* proposed a similar expert system [6] for giving diabetes management advice as well as storing clinical data and enabling doctors to remotely monitor patients. In [7], Garcia *et al.* described ESDIABETES, an expert system for helping patients monitor and control their blood glucose level. These systems suggest that diabetes management is particularly amenable to expert system intervention.

3 Development of DA

DA is a medical expert system prototype for medical advice provision on diabetes built using the JESS expert system shell [8]. DA is designed as a menu based interactive system and the language is simplified so that novice users can easily understand it. It gives advice at various points in the course of the consultation to avoid giving a large amount of advice at the end of the consultation as this could overwhelm and confuse the user. People might not have the patience to read so much information at once. The system gives some information for each symptom to the user during the consultation process and thus helps the user to gain more understanding of diabetes. This is an advantage over consulting a human because doctors do not normally have time to explain their reasoning to each patient. The final output of a DA session is a summary of the main recommendations that a patient will need to take note of and may tell the patient to visit a clinic or to see a doctor.

3.1   Knowledge Engineering

Acquiring high quality knowledge and validating it can be extremely time-consuming. Converting it into a form suitable for a computer program (knowledge representation) adds another layer of complexity. In this project, knowledge acquisition occurred through meetings with the diabetes expert in which notes were written by hand and conversations were audio-recorded. This knowledge was converted to IF-THEN rules as required by JESS.

3.2   System Development Methodology

An iterative system development approach was used. After the first meeting with the diabetes expert, the first prototype was designed. This prototype gave advice on exercise plans, eating plans and monitoring sugar level. The system first asked the patient about the symptoms or warning signs they were experiencing. A second meeting with the expert revealed certain flaws and what improvements were needed, as follows: the system was not able to consider all aspects relevant for decision making; advice was only provided at the end of the consultation; the system was not giving enough advice to patients; the language used was not simple enough for people with poor literacy; the system asked for unnecessary information that was never used in formulating advice; the system assumed only people with diabetes would use the system (this assumption was removed in the final system). The expert also provided magazines, leaflets and other documents to aid in the implementation of the improvements identified in the first prototype. A second prototype was designed incorporating the suggestions made. Below are some of the questions the system asks the user.

Do you experience increased thirst? (y/n)
Have you experienced unexplained weight loss? (y/n)
How often do you eat fruits and vegetables? (0–9)
How many meals do you eat per day? (0–9)
Do you smoke? (y/n)
Do you consume alcohol? (y/n)
Do you monitor your blood sugar level? (y/n)
Do you experience unexplained weakness and exhaustion? (y/n)

The final system had a simple text-based user interface which provided entry into the following use cases.

1. Receive diabetes advice
2. Learn more about diabetes

The next section gives two scenarios of the system in use.

3.3   Use Case for Diabetes Advice

Patient A, who has diabetes, provides information to DA. This information is represented as facts within DA. These facts, then, cause the appropriate rules to fire, and these rules in turn generate output for the user which is tailored to her needs. Different output would be generated for someone without diabetes.

Patient A is a 20 year old woman, who has been living with diabetes for 2 years. She does not know enough about diabetes management and has been taking insulin to treat her diabetes. DA responds with various recommendations as the interaction proceeds. Some of the recommendations given to patient A are shown in the listing below. (Intervening prompts by the system are not shown.)

Advice for Patient A: Now that you have diabetes, you must make sure that you manage your diabetes properly. Please remember to take your medication as your doctor tells you. Remember that you must not use the same place for injection every time because your medication can stop working. It is good that you have a healthy eating plan. Remember to eat your meals in small portions. 3 meals a day with snacks in between your meals is advisable. High fibre food: Eat 2–3 portions of this type per meal.

3.4   Use Case for Diabetes Information

If the user selected to learn more about diabetes, the system displays a menu of eight topics covering what diabetes is, its different forms, its causes, symptoms, treatment, prevention, medication and complications. We consider this to be an equally, if not more, important feature of the system because getting people educated about the disease can help them keep it at bay.

4   Evaluation

The diabetes expert used in developing the system checked the knowledge and behaviour of the first prototype and gave feedback, including suggestions for improvement. It was also important, as recommended in [5], to use other evaluators who had not taken part in the development of DA. Therefore four medical students nearing completion of their degree were used as additional domain experts. They were asked to interact with the final prototype and to give feedback via a questionnaire. The questionnaire contained desirable properties in such a system, and the respondents were required to use a Likert scale to rank how strongly these were present in DA. The feedback was largely positive; respondents' median response was Agree to 7 of the 9 statements below and Strongly Agree to Statements 7 and 8; these were the two highest ranks, the others being Neutral, Disagree, Strongly Disagree and Not Applicable. This indicated that the system was useful and met its intended goals.

1. A person with no computer skills can be able to use this system.
2. The clinics or hospitals can use this system to learn more about the required expertise.
3. This system can free physicians from boring routine tasks.
4. This system can be very useful to physicians or nurses in rural areas.
5. This system does look at all branches needed to be considered by a physician while giving advice.

6. Even though I am a medical student I can rely on this system for advice instead of going to a specialised doctor.
7. I would recommend this system to my diabetic patient if necessary.
8. The advice provided by the system is correct and useful.
9. The advice provided by the system can be understood by people with poor literacy.

5   Conclusion and Future Work

In this study, a prototype expert system for the provision of advice on diabetes was constructed. It was evaluated and found to be useful. As this was only a preliminary phase of a planned larger study, the evaluation was not very extensive. A larger number of domain experts are needed to more fully evaluate the system and to confirm the positive results seen here. Secondly, field testing is critical before actual deployment. That is, the system needs to be tested with a random sample of actual rural patients so that its efficacy in its intended environment can be confirmed.

Another important improvement that is needed is in the user interface. The DA prototype has a basic textual interface, which falls short in terms of usability. A graphical user interface or a speech-based interface would be more desirable, and this is included in the plan for future work. In addition, a system like this one could be made accessible to more people if deployed as a Web application. This is also a planned extension to the work in the near future.

References

1. International Diabetes Federation. http://www.idf.org
2. World Health Organisation. Diabetes Program. http://www.who.int/diabetes
3. Jackson, P.: Introduction to Expert Systems. Addison Wesley, Harlow (1999)
4. Metaxiotis, K., Samouilidis, E.: Expert systems in medicine: academic illusion or real power? Inf. Manag. Comp. Sec. **8**(2), 75–79 (2000)
5. Hernando, M., Gómez, E., Corcoy, R., del Pozo, F.: Evaluation of DIABNET, a decision support system for therapy planning in gestational diabetes. Comp. Meth. Prog. Biomed. **65**, 235–248 (2000)
6. Rudi, R., Celler, B.: Design and implementation of expert-telemedicine system for diabetes management at home. In: International Conference on Biomedical and Pharmaceutical Engineering, pp. 595–599. Research Publishing Services (2006)
7. Garcia, M., Gandhi, M., Singh, T., Duarte, L., Shen, R., Dantu, M., Ponder, S., Ramirez, H.: Esdiabetes (An Expert System in Diabetes). In: Meinke, J. (ed.) J. Comp. Small Coll. **16**(3), 166–175 (2001)
8. Friedman-Hill, E.: Jess in Action: Java Rule-Based Systems. Manning Publications, Greenwich (2003)

Assessing Spatial Distribution of Maternal Health Related Resources in Health Facilities in Malawi: Case of Skilled Birth Attendants in Zomba District

Chipiliro Awali$^{(\boxtimes)}$ and Patrick Albert Chikumba

Department of Computing and Information Technology,
University of Malawi-The Polytechnic, Private Bag 303, Blantyre 3, Malawi
awali.chipi@gmail.com, patrick_chikumba@yahoo.com

Abstract. Primary care with proper resources is recognized as the most important form of healthcare and if properly distributed it is most effective in preventing avoidable maternal deaths on a large scale. Since a place where pregnant women go for delivery is very important, the distribution of maternal health related resources in health facilities is one of guides to achieving the goal of "health for all" and hence reducing maternal mortality. This study therefore, focuses on the assessment of distribution of maternal health related resources in health facilities at district level in Malawi using GIS. Eight health facilities in Zomba were involved. The qualitative research method was used to analyze findings of the research. Interviews and questionnaires were used for data collection. The study has revealed that there are disparities in the distribution of maternal health related resources in various health facilities.

Keywords: Disparity · Equity · GIS · GPS · Spatial · Distribution · Maternal health related resources · Skilled birth attendants

1 Introduction

Malawi is one of the countries in the Sub-Saharan Africa where the deaths of women due to pregnancy or pregnancy related causes are high [40]. Maternal mortality ratio (MMR) in Malawi is one of the highest in this region. According to the annual Millennium Development Goals (MDG) Report MMR decreased from 1,120 per 100,000 live births in 2000 to 807 per 100,000 births in 2006 [40], whereas the current maternal mortality ratio for Malawi is still high at 675 deaths per 100,000 live births and the 95 % confidence interval for the 2010 maternal mortality ratio ranges from 570 to 780 deaths per 100,000 live births [23]. It is projected that by 2015, MMR will be at 338 per 100,000 live births, which is greater than the MDG target of 155 per 100,000 live births [22, 28, 38].

This high MMR is due to various factors which include poor availability and accessibility to proper medical care and hence poor deliveries in cases of complications [1]. Some of the maternal deaths that lead to high MMR have been identified as hemorrhage, Sepsis, Pregnancy-induced hypertension, obstructed labor and abortion complications [2, 13, 24].

© Institute for Computer Sciences, Social Informatics and Telecommunications Engineering 2014
T.F. Bissyandé and G. van Stam (Eds.): AFRICOMM 2013, LNICST 135, pp. 145–152, 2014.
DOI: 10.1007/978-3-319-08368-1_17

All these causes are said to be avoidable if attended by Skilled Birth Attendants (SBAs) such as midwives/nurses and with proper care [1, 19, 41]. If a system is in place to recognize problems promptly and to transport a woman to a healthcare facility where she can receive appropriate and timely treatment by SBAs, then the majority of maternal mortalities could be avoided [18, 26].

District Health Office (DHO) is responsible for distribution of health resources to public health facilities. However, Zomba DHO indicates that there is no specific criterion that is used in the distribution of resources and that most of the times they depend on health facility-in-charge to request for some. This could contribute to having some health facilities with little needs to have more resources than those with greater needs.

Disparities in turn have an impact on the maternal mortalities. For instance, the percentages of maternal deaths for rural are higher than those for urban areas [3]. In Malawi however, disparities in geographic distribution of health professionals persist though not readily available up-to-date information exists. Previous reports have shown that this is to be problematic [4, 25]. For the MoH, the figures can be compared at district level by population density, but this does not show the disparity within districts where facilities may be a long way from the district headquarters [4].

This study, therefore, was to fill in this gap by using Geographical Information System (GIS) to assess the spatial distribution of resources to various health facilities. The main focus was on the distribution of maternal health related resources including SBAs. GIS was chosen as an analysis tool in assessing the spatial distribution of the maternal health related resources because this problem of disparities is spatial in nature and can be understood properly with geographical means.

2 Maternal Health and GIS

One of studies was carried out in London where GIS was used as a key element of both the service mapping and gap identification parts. The particular focus was to look at capacity, stability and funding and particularly to identify gaps in relation to service provision, unmet need, and accessibility [11].

Tanser [36] used GIS technology to equitably distribute fieldworker workload in a large rural South African health survey. Fuzzy accessibility model was used within a GIS to adjust for the heterogeneities and a multiple regression analysis was performed on the average fuzzy variables to predict the number of homesteads mapped per fieldworker per day, and then equitably distributed workload among the Demographic Surveillance System (DSS) fieldworkers.

In Kenya however, GIS was used to highlight the disparities in physical access to health care services [30]. Euclidean distances between centroid of each sub-location and the nearest public health facility were computed. It was found that 82 % of the populations lived within 5 km of a public health facility. Twelve percent of the populations were living at a distance of between 5–10 km to the nearest health facility and 6 % lived at a distance of more than 10 km to a health facility.

GIS usage is not limited to studies of accessibility to primary health facilities, but it has also potentials for assessing how primary health centre and resources have been distributed to different population groups in a country. For example, a study carried out in Nepal [35] examined the factors explaining the utilization of maternal and child health services. A prominent relationship was found between the overall structural quality of the nearest health centre and the service uptake was evident.

Maps of health infrastructure were used in eastern Indonesia to inform the allocation of resources by the district health departments. For instance, in the district of Timor Tengah Selatan, maps of midwives were used in the planning of staff allocations. Maps of clinic facilities were used to plan the upgrading of clinics to provide Basic Emergency Obstetric Care (BEmOC) [10].

In Mozambique GIS was used as a Service Availability Mapping (SAM) tool to perform analysis of data related to the "Second Delay" level of the "Three Phases of Delay" conceptual framework proposed where the spatial data including administrative boundaries, location of health facilities, rural hospital and referral facility for the four districts in cases of emergency, distance between one health facility to another, and between one health facility and it's referral [31]. The use of GIS tool allowed the easy visualization and consistent monitoring of service availability within and between districts.

GIS has been used in a number of ways in Malawi. For example, (a) the use of GIS in the Drug Logistic MIS at the district level in Malawi [5]; (b) GIS was applied in the monitoring and management of HIV/AIDS [29]; (c) investigating access to reproductive health services [17]; and (d) GIS was used in the monitoring of tuberculosis (TB) programme performance at the district level [5].

3 Methodology

According to the nature of this study, purposive sampling was used to select only health facilities that provide maternity services. Eight health facilities were selected out 26. Sixty-nine the health personnel were involved including 7 person-in-charges. Semi-structured interviews and self-administered questionnaires were used to collect data at the district health office and at various health facilities visited.

Spatial data was collected in the form of shape files from the Faculty of Built Environment at The Malawi Polytechnic, Department of Geography at Chancellor College and National Statistical Office (NSO). On the other hand, attribute data was collected from Zomba DHO and the health facilities visited.

4 Distribution of Skilled Birth Attendants (SBAs)

Data in Table 1 was drawn from different maps generated by the GIS prototype. Catchment populations, villages, bearing age women, pregnant women and deliveries at each health facility were mapped in order to compare with the spatial distribution of skilled birth attendants. By 2011, in Zomba health district, there were eight health facilities (health centres) which provide maternal health services.

Taking into consideration the population of women of child bearing age, it has been shown that the catchment area of Namikango is the one having the highest

Table 1. Estimated catchment population, villages, bearing age women, pregnant women and deliveries in Zomba health district by 2011

Facility	Catchment population	Villages	Bearing age women	Pregnant women	Deliveries
Bimbi	22774–26222	49–57	5239–6031	1–1067	63–162
Chamba	22774–26222	49–57	5239–6031	1140–1311	1–62
Domasi	1–22773	58–61	1–5238	1068–1139	255–356
Makwapala	32723–37336	62–90	7527–8587	1842–2375	255–356
Matawale	32723–37336	1–48	7527–8587	1637–1841	163–254
Matiya	31190–32722	91–96	7175–7526	1312–1636	357–431
Namikango	37337–51721	97–137	8588–11933	1312–1636	163–254
Pirimiti	26223–31189	62–90	6032–7174	1312–1636	432–589

population of women of child bearing age and that of Domasi has the least. So by applying the concepts of vertical equity, Namikango health facility is supposed to have a greater number of SBAs, and Domasi health facility should have the least number of SBAs (Fig 1).

However, the findings have shown that Pirimiti is the one having the largest number of SBAs, despite having a smaller population size for women of child bearing age and Chamba health centre with the least number of SBAs. As such, if the population for women of child bearing age is used as the criterion, then it can be concluded that there are disparities in the distribution of SBAs in the health facilities.

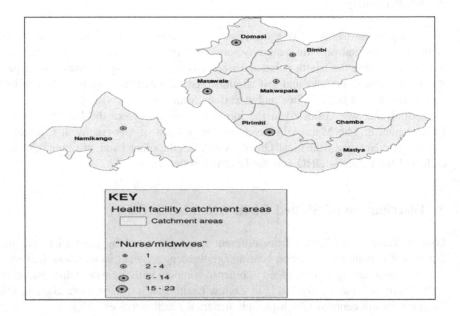

Fig. 1. Spatial distribution of nurses/midwives in Zomba health district by 2011

Pregnant women are the ones that are supposed to visit health facilities frequently to receive the maternal health services. These services require skilled personnel who have been well trained to provide such services [1, 7, 14, 16, 18, 19, 26].

The findings have revealed that Makwapala health facility is the one with the largest population of pregnant women and Bimbi health facility having the least population. So using the population of pregnant women as the criterion for the distribution of SBAs whilst at the same time applying the concept of vertical equity, it implies that Makwapala health facility should have a greater number of SBAs and Bimbi should have the least number of SBAs because it serves a smaller population of 'pregnant women'.

It has been observed that Pirimiti is the one with the large number of SBAs and Bimbi has the least number of SBAs. This suggests that there are some disparities in the distribution of SBAs in the health facilities as far as the population of pregnant women they serve and the concepts of vertical equity are concerned.

If a health facility has few SBAs but serves a large population of pregnant women, then both the SBAs and the clients (pregnant women) are affected in one way or the other. For instance, the SBAs may have too much workload thereby failing to assist all the clients timely. As a result, the women may be discouraged and decide not to visit the health facility again. Most of the women in the rural areas walk longer distances to get to the nearest health facilities. So when the time to give birth comes, the women may just opt to deliver at home/TBAs and this may lead to avoidable maternal deaths [32, 33].

Taking into account the number of deliveries at a health facility, the findings have revealed that Pirimiti health facility is the one that has the largest number of deliveries while Chamba health facility has the least number of deliveries. In this case, if the number of deliveries at health facility is chosen as the criterion for distributing health personnel (SBAs) and by taking vertical equity into consideration, Pirimiti health facility deserves to have the largest. As for Chamba health facility, it has the least number of SBAs which, somehow, corresponds to the number of deliveries.

This seems to suggest that there are some disparities in the distribution of SBAs as deliveries are concerned. It would be better that if the distribution of SBAs is based on the average deliveries at a health facility. It is recommended that all deliveries should take place at a health facility, and be managed by well trained personnel (SBAs) [1, 7, 14, 16, 18, 19, 26] who can detect complications and be able to refer the case to the appropriate facility where the complications can be properly handled.

On the other hand, it is surprising to note that the health facilities that do not have large population of pregnant women (i.e., Pirimiti and Matiya) are the ones those having larger number of deliveries than the health facilities that have higher population of pregnant women (e.g., Makwapala and Matawale).

One possible reason, for example, could be that Pirimiti and Matiya health facilities are under CHAM whose services are mostly described to be much better than in health facilities that belong to the government [12]. So, may be because of that, women wish and ready to deliver at these health facilities despite other obstacles such as distance, since they are assured that they will receive quality attention and services.

However, if so, what about Namikango health facility which is also under CHAM. Another possible reason could be that women in the other catchments areas prefer to deliver at home/TBAs due to some obstacles such as long distances. Sometimes, women do not appreciate the services offered in their respective health facilities, as such they choose to deliver at home/TBAs or at another health facility.

5 Conclusion

This study has shown that the disparities are present in the way maternal health related resources have been distributed to various health facilities in Zomba district. District Health Office (DHO) needs to have specific criteria for distributing maternal health related resources (such SBAs) to health facilities. Based on the criterion established, GIS can be used in the process of distribution of the maternal health related resources to the health facilities through monitoring and management since health facilities that need more resources could be easily identified by the use of GIS application. This is so because equity is an important criterion in evaluating health system performance, and developing a framework for equitable and effective resource allocation for health depends upon knowledge of service providers and their location in relation to the population they serve or should serve [30].

References

1. Ali, M.: Make Every Mother Count: Maternal mortality in Malawi, India and United Kingdom. Degree Thesis in Public Health Science. School of Health, Care and Social Welfare (2009)
2. Bisika, T.: The effectiveness of the TBA programme in reducing maternal mortality and morbidity in Malawi. East Afr. J. Pub. Health 5(2), 103–110 (2008)
3. Bradley, S., McAuliffe, E.: Mid-level providers in emergency obstetric and newborn health care: factors affecting their performance and retention within the Malawian health system. Hum. Resour. Health 7(14) (2009). http://www.human-resources-health.com/content/7/1/14. Accessed 22 October 2011
4. Carlson, C., et al.: Malawi Health SWAp Mid Term Review. Norwegian Agency for Development Cooperation. Oslo, Norway (2008)
5. Chikumba, P.A.: Application of the Geographic Information System (GIS) in the Drug Logistics Management Information System (LMIS) at the district level in Malawi: Opportunities and Challenges. Master Thesis. University of Oslo, Norway (2009)
6. Coeytaux, F., Bingham, D., Strauss, N.: Maternal Mortality in the United States: A Human Rights Failure, CSDH, 2010. A Conceptual Framework for Action on the Social Determinants of Health, Commission on Social Determinants of Health (2011)
7. Diderichsen, F.: Resource Allocation for Health Equity: Issues and Methods September 2004, Washington, DC 20433: The International Bank for Reconstruction and Development/The World Bank 1818 H Street, NW (2004)
8. Elgazzar, H.A.: Raising Returns: The Distribution of Health Financing and Outcome in Yemen, Washington DC (2011). http://siteresources.worldbank.org/HEALTHNUTRITION ANDPOPULATION/Resources/281627-1095698140167/RaisingReturnsTheDistribution ofHealthFinancingandOutcomesinYemen.pdf. Accessed 3 October 2011

9. Fauveau, V., Sherratt, D.R., de Bernis, L.: Human resources for maternal health: multipurpose or specialists? Hum. Resour. Health, **6**(1), 21 (2008). http://www.human-resources-health.com/content/6/1/21/abstract. Accessed 25 July 2012

10. Fisher, R.P., Myers, B.A.: Free and simple GIS as appropriate for health mapping in a low resource setting: a case study in eastern Indonesia. Int. J. Health Geogr., **10**(1), 15 (2011). http://www.ij-healthgeographics.com/content/10/1/15. Accessed 13 July 2012

11. Foley, R., Platzer, H.: A Good Place to Talk: Mapping Mental Health Advocacy Services in London using a GIS (2002). http://www.google.com/#hl=en&output=search&sclient= psyab&q=A+Good+Place+to+Talk:+Mapping+Mental+Health+Advocacy+Services+in++ London+using+a+GIS&psj=1&oq=&aq=&aqi=&aql=&gs_sm=&gs_upl=&bav=on.2,or.r_gc. r_pw.r_qf.,cf.osb&fp=ed30f6c244bfee50&biw=1366&bih=656. Accessed 21 February 2012

12. Galimoto, M.S.: Integration of Health Information Systems. Master Thesis. University of Oslo, Norway (2007)

13. Geubbels, E.: Epidemiology of maternal mortality in Malawi. Malawi Med. J. **18**(4), 206–225 (2006)

14. Graham, W.J., Bell, J.S., Bullough, C.H.: Can skilled attendance at delivery reduce maternal mortality in developing countries? Stud. Health Serv. Organ. Policy **17**(1), 97–130 (2001)

15. Graves, A.: A model for assessment of potential geographical accessibility: a case for GIS. Online J. Rural Nurs. Health Care **9**(1), 46–55 (2009)

16. Guagliardo, M.F.: Spatial Accessibility of Primary Care: Concepts, Methods and Challenges. Int. J. Health Geographics **3**, 3 (2004)

17. Heard, N.J., Larsen, U., Hozumi, D.: Investigating access to reproductive health services using GIS: proximity to services and the use of modern contraceptives in Malawi. Afr. J. Reprod. Health, **8**(2), 164–179 (2004). http://www.ncbi.nlm.nih.gov/pubmed/15623130. Accessed 28 December 2011

18. Jahn, A., De Brouwere, V.: Referral in pregnancy and childbirth_: concepts and strategies. Stud Health Serv. Organ. Policy **17**(1), 229–246 (2001)

19. Johnson, L.S.: The right to maternal health care: developing international human rights law to prevent maternal mortality. Univ. Botswana Law J. **1**(1), 40–80 (2010)

20. Lazaro, D., Namasasu, J.: Ministry Of Health and UNFPA: Needs Assessment of Obstetric Fistula in Malawi (2005)

21. Liese, B.: The State of the Health Workforce in Sub-Saharan Africa: Evidence of Crisis and Analysis of Contributing Factors. The World Bank/Georgetown University, Washington, DC (2004)

22. Lunan, B., Clements, Z., Mahony, S.: 2011–2012 Maternal Health in Malawi: Members' Report, Scotland Partnerships Malawi (2011)

23. Malawi National Statistical Office and ICF Macro: 2010 Malawi Demographic and Health Survey: Key Findings. NSO and ICF Macro, Calverton, Maryland, USA (2011)

24. Malawi National Statistical Office and ORC Macro: 2000 Malawi Demographic and Health Survey. NSO and ORC Macro, Calverton, Maryland, USA (2001)

25. Martineau, T., et al.: Factors affecting retention of different groups of rural health workers in Malawi and Eastern Cape Province. WHO Alliance for Health Policy and Systems Research: Liverpool School of Tropical Medicine, South Africa, Geneva (2006)

26. Maternity World Wide: Causes of Maternal Mortality (2011). http://www. maternityworldwide.org/pages/causes-of-maternal-mortality.html. Accessed 12 May 2011

27. Milind, D.M.: Socio-economic inequality and its effect on healthcare delivery in India: inequality and healthcare. Electron. J. Sociol. (2004). http://www.sociology.org/content/ vol8.1/deogaonkar.html

28. Ministry of Development Planning and Cooperation: 2009 Malawi Millennium Development Goals Report, Lilongwe, Malawi (2009)
29. Msiska, B.C.: Challenges and Opportunities in Using GIS for Monitoring and Management of HIV/AIDS: A Case Study from Malawi. Master Thesis. University of Oslo, Norway (2009)
30. Noor, A., et al.: Creating spatially defined databases for equitable health service planning in low-income countries: the example of Kenya. Acta Trop. **91**(3), 239–251 (2004)
31. Saugene, Z.B.: Achieving the Health Millennium Developing Goals using GIS Knowledge Networks: the case of Maternal Health in Mozambique (2011)
32. Shaikh, B.T., Hatcher, J.: Health seeking behaviour and health service utilization in Pakistan: challenging the policy makers. J. Publ. Health **27**, 49–54 (2004)
33. Shaikh, B.T., Hatcher, J.: Health seeking behaviourand health services utilization trends in national health survey of pakistan: what needs to be done? J. Pak. Med. Assoc. **57**(8), 411–413 (2007). http://www.jpma.org.pk/full_article_text.php?article_id=1184. Accessed 15 April 2012
34. Tanser, F. et al.: New approaches to spatially analyse primary health care usage patterns in rural South Africa. Trop. Med. Int. Health **6**(10), 826–838 (2001). http://doi.wiley.com/10.1046/j.1365-3156.2001.00794.x. Accessed 8 February 2012
35. Tanser, F., Gijsbertsen, B., Herbst, K.: Modelling and understanding primary health care accessibility and utilization in rural South Africa: an exploration using a geographical information system. Soc. Sci. Med. (1982), **63**(3), 691–705 (2006). http://www.ncbi.nlm.nih.gov/pubmed/16574290. Accessed 23 April 2012
36. Tanser, F.C., Le Sueur, D.: The application of geographical information systems to important public health problems in Africa. Int. J. Health Geographics **1**(4), 4–12 (2002)
37. UNICEF: Progress for Children – Maternal mortality, UNICEF (2007). http://www.unicef.org/progressforchildren/2007n6/index_41814.htm. Accessed 6 July 2011
38. United Nations: Country Assessment Report 2010: Malawi, Lilongwe, Malawi: United Nations (2010). http://www.unmalawi.org
39. White, S.: Malawi: Country Gender Profile (2007)
40. WHO: Malawi Country Office: 2009 Annual Report, World Health Organization (2009)
41. WHO: Maternal Mortality: Fact Sheet, World Health Organization (2008)
42. Zwarenstein, M., Krige, D., Wolff, B.: The use of a geographical information system for hospital catchment area research in Natal/KwaZulu. S. Afr. Med. J. (Suid-Afrikaanse Tydskrif Vir Geneeskunde) **80**(10), 497–500 (1991). http://www.ncbi.nlm.nih.gov/pubmed/1948466. Accessed 9 February 2012

Reporting in the Health Systems:
Case Study of Ghana

Ivy de-Souza[✉]

Accra, Ghana
lution2@yahoo.com

Abstract. In this paper, we analyse the current reporting systems or regimes as performed in Ghana's health system. Reporting not only allows detection of disease outbreaks, it also contributes greatly to enable good management of the health system nationally and internationally, because objective data is required to enable planning, follow-up and management towards improvement. Based on the results, considering the availability of current ICT tools, we hope to propose improvements to the model.

Keywords: Ghana health system · E-health · Data management · Reporting

1 Introduction

The World Health Organization (WHO) report 'The World Health Report 2000, Heath system: improving performance' emphasises on health reporting systems in order to give a clear overview of the world health statistics [1]. In Ghana, various health system levels exist [2]. For long, reporting was paper-based. This is cumbersome, expensive and requires a heavy work-load.

The current reporting system uses computer software. It is called the District Health Information System (DHIMS2) [3]. Ghana's health system is structured in a hierarchic way; All health facilities submit their health activities reports to a higher level. The National office then summarizes the data into regions. DHIMS2 is not available at the sub-district level [4].

The core capacity of validating and analysing DHIMS data lies with the Ghana Health Services (GHS) [5].

2 Materials and Methods

This research performed data collection using questionnaires. The questionnaires were specifically aimed at obtaining performance, efficiency and quality data on the reporting system in place. The study divided the country into three zones and questionnaires were distributed to four groups in the health sector.

The Heads of Department and Data Managers were interviewed at each health institute. The data collection officer at the Ministry of Health was interviewed and an officer responsible for data collection at the world level (WHO) was also contacted.

© Institute for Computer Sciences, Social Informatics and Telecommunications Engineering 2014
T.F. Bissyandé and G. van Stam (Eds.): AFRICOMM 2013, LNICST 135, pp. 153–156, 2014.
DOI: 10.1007/978-3-319-08368-1_18

Questionnaires

The purpose of the study is to obtain quantitative and qualitative information on the current reporting practice. Therefore the questionnaires contain questions about:

- time spend in filling in and processing the monthly health care statistics
- quantity of reported data
- quality of reported data
- usefulness evaluation by the participants in the reporting system
- feedback.

The questionnaires were planned to be distributed to a representative sample of health care institutions: health centers, sub-district hospitals, district hospitals, regional hospitals, referral hospitals, Ministry of Health and finally WHO. We also try to involve both rural and urban representatives of the above, where possible, this leads to a total of 40 questionnaires that will be processed for the complete study.

3   Preliminary Results

Out of the 32 questionnaires currently distributed to 16 hospitals (1 to the data manager and 1 to the head of department), 28 were returned. Four more questionnaires are yet to be collected. 26 questionnaires were returned by the health facilities, with respondents:

- 13 heads of department
- 13 data managers
- 1 respondent from the Ministry of Health
- 1 respondent from the World Health Organization (WHO).

Sources of Information

See Table 1.

Human Resources for Reporting

The mean time spent on the reporting is 4 man-days with a standard deviation of 1.5 man-days.

18 respondents judged the required workload as "too much", 6 "just enough" and 2 had no opinion.

Table 1. Sources and tools for reporting per type of institution.

	Sources used					
	Register	Spreadsheet	Paper tables	Patient dossier	Immunization cards	EMR
Private	3/3	2/3	1/3	1/3	1/3	2/3
Subdistrict	5/5	4/5				
District	3/3	2/3	1/3	1/3	1/3	1/3
Regional	2/2	1/2		1/2	2/2	2/2

If we extrapolate this over the whole Health Care System in Ghana (276 hospitals) we come to an estimated total work load (per month) of about 60 full-time equivalents.

Feedback Obtained

Out of 26 respondents, 24 reported they obtained feedback, only 2 did not.

4 Discussion

So far, only 32 filled-in forms were collected, so we can only draw preliminary conclusions.

4.1 Head of Department (HoD)

The register is the most common tool used for data reported combined with either one or other tools. Out of 13 responses obtained, only two facilities experienced stock out of immunization cards in the last six months.

4.2 Data Manager

Community health workers are involved mostly in data collected for reporting at the public or government health facilities but the administrative staffs do the bulk of reporting work at the private facilities. Average time spent filling in reports is 4 days in a month with a standard deviation of one and half days. Some data managers are not comfortable with the deadline dates and need 2–5 extra days to ensure accurate reporting. Data verification mechanisms are in place at some facilities (how many?).

4.3 Both Head of Department (HoD) and Data Managers

Out of the 26 responses obtained, 24 receive feedback to their reports and only 2 do not receive feedback. All sub-districts receive regular feedback, some districts do not receive any feedback and the regional hospitals receive feedback once a year. Some of the private facilities receive feedback and others do not. Upon receiving feedbacks, necessary correction is made and important issues raised are noted. Some of the health facilities also just filed the feedbacks for further actions. From the responses obtained it is clear that the workload associated with reporting is demanding and time consuming especially at the sub-district and district levels.

4.4 Ministry of Health (MoH)

The Ministry of Health analyses all monthly data submitted by health facilities using statistical means. Feedbacks are given to respective agencies. The feedbacks are sent in form of report which is both electronic and hard-copy. The feedbacks are sent quarterly and yearly on performance indicators. Codes, passwords and authorized users are security systems used to protect the data. Districts league table and reward systems and sanctions at facility levels are measures taken by the ministry towards late reporting by health institutions. The Ministry also reports to international bodies such as WHO and GLOBAL FUND.

4.5 World Health Organization (WHO)

Reporting to WHO is not regular. It is generally weak, less quality and less reliability. There no good system, most data are not classified according to ICD.

Although the internal reporting system seems to work, according to our respondents, Ghana their cause of death information is still reported to WHO with long delays. An interview with a WHO official revealed that the country level reporting towards WHO is far from ideal.

Some reports on immunization are received by WHO and UNICEF but sometimes with 5 months delay. There are also some reports on MDGs to WHO and UNICEF on population. To obtain relevant information, WHO itself has to employ people to do the job. WHO reports the acquired estimates via Global Health Observatory (GHO). Data verification by WHO is done via registers [6].

5 Preliminary Conclusions

This study (so far) identified that even though Ghana has a Health Information management System (HIMS) in place; it is not fully used in the whole country. Other HIMS are used in some facilities. Some private facilities report to the ministry of health and others do not.

The work-load associated with reporting is huge. Based on our data, the total work-load represents an estimated 4 man-days on average per institution with a standard deviation of 1.5 days.

Only about half the institutions apply data verification and most of the centres get feedback after their reports are sent in.

Acknowledgments. I am grateful to my promoter Professor Marc Nyssen whose guidance, patience, assistance and constructive ideas have resulted in the achievement of this paper. Thanks to all who collaborated and responded by carefully filling in their questionnaires.

References

1. WHO's report: the world health report 2000 health systems: improving performance Geneva: World Health Organization (2000)
2. Durairaj, V., D'Almeida, S., Kirigia, J.: Ghana's approach to social health protection (2010)
3. Ghana Health Service. Ghana Health Service 2011. Annual report (2012)
4. Ghana Health Service. 2009 GHS Annual report. Ghana Health Service (2009)
5. Ministry of Health Ghana. Independent Review Health Sector Programme of Work 2010 (2011)
6. Ties, B.: World Health Organization, Geneva (2013)

Real-Time Communication over Wireless Sensor Network – A Prototype for Disaster Areas

Sarantorn Bisalbutra[1(✉)] and Elisa Jimeno[2(✉)]

[1] Ericsson Research, Nomadic Lab, Kirkkonummi, Finland
sarantorn.bisalbutra@ericsson.com
[2] VTT Technical Research Centre of Finland, Espoo, Finland
elisa.jimeno@vtt.fi

Abstract. Disasters introduce challenges in providing affordable and reliable communications. Before temporary GSM base stations are in place, rescue teams have to deploy and cope with VHF radios as well as high-cost satellite connections without packet-based local connectivity between the members. The above issues became one of our motivations to develop a low cost and low energy consumption wireless sensor network based on the IEEE 802.15.4 standard, in order to provide fast and easy to deploy infrastructure. In this paper, we describe a design and current implementation of a wireless sensor network prototype. We also propose a design of a gateway. It interconnects the wireless sensor network and an IP-based wireless backhaul, enabling voice and data communication, e.g., between headquarters, command posts and field rescuers, in real-time. Finally, we show initial results and an evaluation of our system, which lead to the plan for future improvements.

Keywords: WSN · Voice over sensor · WiFi-to-WSN gateway · WSN prototype for disaster areas · Multi-hop WSN

1 Introduction

Natural disasters, such as tsunamis, earthquakes, and landslides usually cause severe damage to communication infrastructure. Telephone and Internet lines immediately collapse and the remaining network quickly overloads. These hazards render the underlying infrastructure unusable during rescue operations. Cost and capacity of communication equipment are other obstacles. On-site personnel generally rely on high-cost and low capacity medium like VHF radios, GSM and satellite phones. In most cases, small organizations cannot afford such equipment.

After the crisis, lifesaving is crucial. Rescue operations require coordination between public organizations, relief workers, and victims. Fast communication establishment thus becomes essential for a successful rescue strategy.

In addition to providing broadband Internet connectivity to emerging areas, the Converged Infrastructure for Emerging Regions (CIER) project [1] also aims to develop an efficient, robust, reliable and affordable heterogeneous wireless network to overcome the above challenges. Currently, the CIER project is developing two types

© Institute for Computer Sciences, Social Informatics and Telecommunications Engineering 2014
T.F. Bissyandé and G. van Stam (Eds.): AFRICOMM 2013, LNICST 135, pp. 157–166, 2014.
DOI: 10.1007/978-3-319-08368-1_19

of wireless networks, the so-called, Wireless Backhaul (WiBACK) [2] and Wireless Sensor Network (WSN). The Wireless Backhaul bridges fixed infrastructure and different wireless access technologies. It uses the IEEE 802.21 standard [3] and Multi-Protocol Label Switching [4] to manage handovers and data forwarding.

This paper presents the Wireless Sensor Network based on IEEE 802.15.4 [5]. The target is to provide a wireless personal area network (WPAN) between on-site rescue workers. The system will be easy to deploy, allowing them to exchange information as fast as possible. In addition, we propose a design of a gateway between the WSN and the backhaul. It provides connections to other sites and enables them to exchange information with the workers in real-time. Our system, as a result, tries to assure availability, mobility, and reliability in the communication.

2 Background

In this section, we explain the theoretical background of the CIER wireless networks. Because the wireless technologies are high in cost but low in bandwidth, we consider them as a complement of the wired infrastructure. They offer better features when the wired deployment is difficult or time-consuming.

2.1 CIER Wireless Backhaul

The Wireless Backhaul (WiBACK) is a wireless mesh network. It consists of nodes connected via heterogeneous radio interfaces. The backhaul bridges the gap between a fixed backbone and access networks, offering self-management, autonomous operation and carrier-grade service provisioning.

The WiBACK solution composes of two main components: control plane and data plane. The control plane utilizes outcomes of the CARrier grade wireless MEsh Network (CARMEN) project [6] and IEEE 802.21 [3] for cross layer management and media handovers. The Interface Management Function (IMF) is the core of the control plane. It is an interface between different media access technologies and management functions, where channel switching, handovers, etc. are controlled.

The WiBACK network guarantees quality of service and fast packet delivery by utilizing Multi-Protocol Label Switching (MPLS) in the data plane. Instead of relying on IP routing, an ingress router inserts a 4 bytes label between the packet's data link and networking headers. This label carries forwarding information, QoS prioritization, and time to live. Intermediate routers forward the packet according to mappings between the label and outgoing interfaces. Finally, the MPLS label is removed when the packet reaches an egress router.

MPLS is lightweight and protocol independent. It indicates a bi-directional link as a pair of unidirectional paths and allows the backhaul to carry packets of various types and sizes including IPv4 and IPv6.

2.2 IEEE 802.15.4-Based Wireless Technologies and Related Works

The IEEE 802.15.4 standard defines physical layer and media access control for low-cost, low-power and low-rate Wireless Personal Area Network (WPAN). We selected XBee radio developed by Digi International [7] for this research. The radio provides wireless connectivity between devices and supports up to 65,000 nodes with point-to-point, point-to-multipoint, and mesh configurations.

The 802.15.4 standard specifies three operating frequencies: 868 MHz, 915 MHz and 2.4 GHz. Our radio communicates over the 2.4 GHz, ISM band. There are 16 channels with 5 MHz channel spacing available inside this range. In theory, the maximum bit rate of XBee radio is 250 Kbps over-the-air and at the serial interface.

XBee supports network layer protocols like ZigBee [8], and Digimesh [9]. In addition, there are standardized approaches, e.g., 6LoWPAN [10], available for the implementation. In densely connected networks, these protocols allow users to create mesh topologies instead of the usual end-to-end connection. They offer network resiliency through self-healing and self-discovery.

Despite reducing interference with Direct Sequence Spread Spectrum (DSSS), the ZigBee and Digimesh protocols are quite different. ZigBee classifies wireless nodes into three categories: coordinators, routers, and end devices. The coordinators initiate and maintain information of the network topology. The routers extend the range of connection by relaying data. Finally, end devices are the nodes that communicate to either the coordinators or the routers without relaying any packets. In ZigBee, the coordinators and routers are not allowed to sleep. They consume more energy and can become points of failure. The nodes in Digimesh, on the contrary, are all equals. The protocol allows them to sleep and forward packets at anytime. Regarding the addresses, a network address in ZigBee occupies 16 bits of the payload, while routing in Digimesh is based on MAC addresses only.

Even though XBee radios are commonly used to convey sensor and control data, some research shows interests in utilizing them for voice communications. They address challenges, evaluate the performance, and suggested some improvements to IEEE 802.15.4 wireless networks. The authors of [11] present a voice over sensor solution for rescuing coal miners in emergency situations. They build the sensor network on top of the Firefly platform [12]. Also, they handle multihops data transfer and voice delivery by using a TDMA-based Nano-RK real-time operating system [13] and RT-Link protocol [14]. Researchers in [15] and [16] study voice communications over ZigBee, where mobile devices communicate with a coordinator in a star topology. They suggest suitable configurations for the voice communications and propose the usage of WiFi routers to extend the range of ZigBee.

3 Prototype

In this work, we concentrate on design and implementation of the Wireless Sensor Network and the gateway for real-time communication. Figure 1 depicts the network overview of our prototype. We plan to deploy the Wireless Sensor Network during an early stage of the crisis, especially in areas without energy supply and wired infrastructure. The field rescuers will be equipped with Sensor Clients. These clients allow them to communicate among themselves and the headquarters, represented by a WiBACK Client. Our gateway accesses the WiBACK network through WiFi and converts the IEEE 802.15.4-based traffic to the IEEE 802.11-based, and vice versa. Alice and Bob will represent WiBACK and Sensor Clients in the following sections.

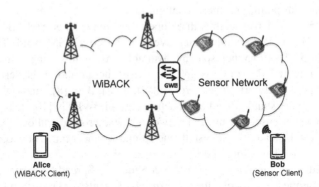

Fig. 1. Network overview of the prototype

3.1 Wireless Sensor Network

Our Wireless Sensor Network is utilizing the IEEE 802.15.4 standard. The rationale behind this choice is affordability. Moreover, in comparison to mobile ad hoc network (MANET), the WSN offers more static infrastructure, resulting the network to be easier to configure, control, and maintain. As the WSN will only be deployed for a few days before temporary base stations are in place, we assume that the battery is sufficient. We consider quality of voice and data communication as the main priority in this research. Figure 2 demonstrates the topology of our WSN prototype. We expand the range of our network by implementing forwarding mechanism in the wireless nodes, which we will explain in the following sections.

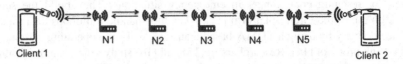

Fig. 2. The topology of Wireless Sensor Network

Hardware. The wireless nodes are equipped with XBee-Pro radios [17]. They are built on top of Arduino Fio boards with 2 KB SRAM, 1 KB EEPROM, and 8-bit microprocessors [18]. Each node relies on a rechargeable lithium battery. Theoretically, the achievable range of the XBee-Pro is up to 90 m indoor and 1.6 km outdoor. The radio transmit power is 63 mW with −100 dBm sensitivity.

Software Configuration. Our radios operate in the API mode over channel C, a 2.45 GHz frequency. We disabled acknowledgement since voice communication is in real-time and does not get any benefit from packet retransmission. Moreover, we deactivate XBee beacon-enabled mode because the beacon frame degrades our network capacity. Also, time synchronization in beacon frame does not allow voice packets to be transmitted according to voice codec specifications [15].

Packet Forwarding. Our wireless nodes communicate to the next hop using 16-bit link layer addressing. We indicate types of XBee frame, e.g., received/transmitted, 16-bits/64-bits addresses, and AT commands according to the specification in [17].

We adopt the basics of 6LoWPAN and header compression defined in RFC 4944 [10] for networking layer. We encapsulate mesh header in Fig. 3 to the API frame. This header occupies 12 bytes of the payload. V and F fields in the header are set to 1, stating that we are using 16-bit addressing in both the originator and the receiver. The HC1 flag indicates that networking addresses of the source and destination are acquired from the source and destination address fields. Bits 5–6 and 7 point to the following HC2 flag and UDP compression, respectively. Inside the HC2 flag, bits 0 and 1 tell that the UDP source and destination ports are compressed into 4 bits with respect to a reference number. To derive the actual port, our applications add the compressed values to the reference port 61616.

0				7	15		23	31		39
1	0	V	F	Hops Left	Source Address			Destination Address		
HC1 Dispatch 0100 0010					HC1 Flag 1111 1011		HC2 Flag 1110 0000	Hops Limit 0100 0000		Src and Dst Ports 0010 0010
Checksum						12 Bytes Application Header …		Payload …		

Fig. 3. The format of 6LoWPAN header in this prototype

During the early stage of this work, we decided to use static routing. It gives us a clear insight of the forwarding path and allows us to evaluate the effects of hops and distance on the quality of service. The relay nodes have preconfigured routing tables. They forward the packets by inspecting destination addresses in the 6LoWPAN header, acquire next hop ID from the routing table, and finally forward the packets to the next hop using link layer address.

3.2 Enabling Voice and Data Communications – The User Terminals

WiBACK and Sensor Clients are user terminals in this prototype. They are Android applications developed within the CIER project to support voice and data communications. The functionalities of these applications are basically the same except that they communicate over different technologies. The WiBACK Client connects to the wireless backhaul using a built-in WiFi adapter. It sends and receives packets through an IP socket. The Sensor Client, on the other hand, controls an XBee radio by using Universal Asynchronous Receiver/Transmitter (UART) and an IOIO board as depicted in Fig. 4.

Both clients support half- and full-duplex voice communication. Talk and Listen buttons in Fig. 5 allow the users to send and receive voice packets. The applications present statistics on the graph. They also summarize number of received and dropped

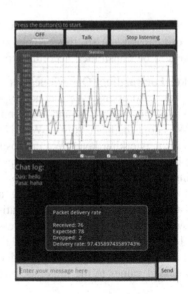

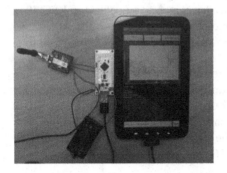

Fig. 4. Hardware configuration of the sensor client

Fig. 5. User interface of the WiBACK and Sensor Clients

frames as well as delivery rate in the pop up window. Users can also send and receive text messages in the box below. The text messaging is one form of data communication. It demonstrates that our prototype has an ability to transfer any type of information, including sensor and control data.

We use 16-bit Pulse Code Modulation [19] with 8 kHz sampling frequency to convert voice signal to digital pulses. We utilize the Speex codec [20], a speech encoding over low latency networks, to compress the packets. The codec provides packet-loss concealment and noise suppression to our communication.

3.3   Interconnection Between the Wireless Sensor Network and the Backhaul

We connect the CIER wireless networks through a gateway. The gateway has one interface to the Backhaul and the other to the WSN. We assume that the WiBACK and Sensor devices are in the same subnetwork, with 16-bit mask, and communicate with IPv4. This is because the WSN is using 16-bit address to support larger payloads. It allows us to encode only the last two octets of the IP address in the 6LoWPAN header.

In addition to converting the traffic, the gateway handles some challenges due to limitations of the low-rate Wireless Sensor Network [21]. These limitations include the maximum payload size and data rate. The IEEE 802.15.4 limits the payload to 102 bytes, which is significantly small compared to the maximum transfer unit in the WiBACK network. Moreover, the WiBACK data rate is much higher than what is achievable in the WSN.

Gateway Initialization. When the gateway is started, it automatically retrieves and configures an IP address of the WiBACK interface. Then, the gateway initiates an XBee connection with the next-hop towards the WSN.

Packet Transfer. Figure 6 summarizes packet transfer between the CIER wireless networks. The communication from Alice to Bob requires several configurations on the WiBACK Client. The user needs to configure addresses of the gateway, and Bob's device. The WiBACK Client uses this information to create a 6LoWPAN header. After this, it encapsulates voice or data packet and sends the packet over UDP protocol. In the 6LoWPAN header, source address field is the last two octets of the WiBACK device's IP address. The destination is Bob's 16-bit link layer address. We allocated port 61618 to the communications in this prototype. Once the packet reaches the gateway, the gateway re-encapsulates this packet with an XBee header. To deal with the limitation of the Wireless Sensor Network, we design the gateway to control outgoing traffic by checking payload size and limiting the sending interval to 100 ms.

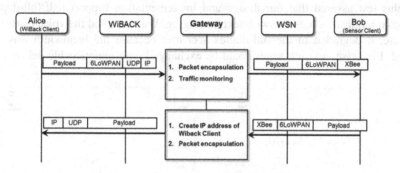

Fig. 6. Diagram of the packet transfer

The communication from Bob to Alice is slightly different. The Sensor Client does not need to know the gateway address. If the destination is outside the WSN, forwarding nodes will automatically route the packet to our gateway. When the gateway receives packets from Bob, it does not need to concern itself with the WiBACK capacity. Our gateway reads destination address and port from the 6LoWPAN header, creates IP address of the WiBACK Client and directly sends it over UDP. The first two octets of the IP address comes from the information we obtained in the initialization phase. The last two octets are the first and the second bytes of destination address field in the 6LoWPAN.

Current Implementation. We currently have two versions of the gateway. The first one is an android application written in Java. It connects to the backhaul through the WiFi and controls XBee radio over a USB cable similar to the Sensor Client. The second version is a C++ program implemented on a Linux system. In addition to operating on a stand-alone device, this program can be integrated to the CIER WiBACK node or bullet radio [22]. In this version, we utilize the libxbee [23] over a serial-to-USB adapter to control the XBee module, while the android application needs to construct the API header from scratch.

The gateway composes of three modules. *WiBACK_Messenger* and *XBee_Messenger* threads are interfaces to the WiBACK and the Wireless Sensor networks. They continuously listen to incoming packets from one side and dispatch the payload to the other. The *WiBACK_Messenger* is responsible for creating an IP address from the 6LoWPAN and deliver it to the WiBACK Client over the socket API. The *XBee_Messenger*, on the other hand, takes care of WiBACK-to-WSN traffic. It monitors and adjusts the traffic according to the design we have described. The last module is *Utilities*. It supports both WiBACK and XBee threads to create and parse 6LoWPAN and API headers in our implementation.

3.4 Initial Results

Functional testing was carried out to observe the behavior and accuracy of our prototype. First we analyzed the communication between two Sensor clients. Then, we moved on to the communication between the Sensor and WiBACK clients. The results from this test assured that our design and implementation support half/full-duplex voice communication together with text messaging. We evaluated the voice quality as moderate. It degraded in the full-duplex scenario, because the bandwidth was distributed. Likewise, text messages could be exchanged with unnoticeable delay.

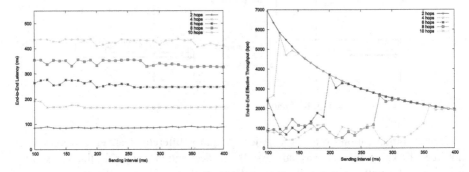

Fig. 7. Correlation between latency and number of hops

Fig. 8. Correlation between throughput and number of hops

In addition to the functional testing, we evaluated performance of our Wireless Sensor Network by performing tests on different setups. We studied influences of hop count, distance between the sensor nodes, baud rate, transmission delay, transmission power, capacity of the Arduino board and sending interval. The tests were conducted indoor with a line of sight between the wireless nodes. Figures 7 and 8 show some of the results we have. In these measurements, we continuously injected 120 bytes packets from an Android phone and collected data at the destination. Even though we could achieve a longer range with multi-hops transfer, the quality of transmission degraded and the end-to-end delay increased. Furthermore, the graph in Fig. 8 shows that with more hops, the network is less tolerant to congestion. We expected high throughput during small sending intervals, but the graphs start to improve when the transmission was less frequent.

Hardware performance is another aspect we would like to explore. We measured the time an Arduino board spent on each task. At 115200 bps, the board took 13 ms to transmit a 120-byte packet. In the echoing test, we configured node 5 to reflect the same packet back after different number of delays. The tests showed that network throughput slightly improved when the destination buffered the packet and echoed it back after 5 ms delay. Finally, the comparison between ACK disabled and enabled mode convinced us that the decision to omit acknowledgment is optimal since the throughput from the non-ACK mode was higher.

4 Conclusion and Future Work

In this paper, we proposed a design for a wireless sensor network and a gateway to the CIER wireless backhaul. The system was designed to be fast and easy to deploy in order to establish a prompt, efficient, and well-organized rescue procedure. We also presented the gateway mechanism to handle network constraint and traffic monitoring. This was a first step towards development of a self-configured and self-provisioned system. The prototype implementation and its initial results showed that the design is practical and feasible to be developed further. The evaluation gave us a clearer insight and helped guiding the system improvements to a reasonable direction.

Future Work. Our goal in the future is not only to develop the wireless sensor network, but also to build up more advanced functionalities to the system according to existing problems and requirements.

The plan is to further improve functionalities such as a support for Session Initiation Protocol (SIP) [24] at the gateway and a Device Directory. We intend to use a SIP application on the WiBACK device. The SIP support allows different organizations and the field rescuers to seamlessly exchange information using any SIP applications. The directory service stores identities of devices, including IP addresses and also their capability such as support for voice, data, location tracking, etc.

Moreover, we will investigate suitable routing protocols for the Wireless Sensor Network and evaluate them on the basis of the voice quality and energy efficiency. Another improvement is the hardware configuration. As an alternative to the IOIO board, we will investigate possibilities to integrate WiFi radio to the WSN. It enables wireless connectivity to the sensor device without any hardware modification. Finally, we will conduct outdoor testing to examine network range and radio propagation.

Acknowledgments. The work reported in this paper was partly supported by the Finnish Funding Agency for Technology and Innovation (Tekes) in the framework of the EUREKA/ Celtic project Converged Infrastructure for Emerging Regions (CIER). The authors would like to thank Daoyuan Li for his collaboration in the prototype implementation and testing, especially the WiBACK and Sensor applications. We also would like to show our appreciation to Juha Zidbeck, Patrik Salmela, and Sami Ruponen for their comments and support.

References

1. CIER project information. http://www.celtic-initiative.org/Projects/Celtic-projects/Call7/CIER/cier-default.asp
2. Niephaus, C., Petrov, D.: Management of Heterogeneity in Wireless Backhauls. CIER Celtic Project: Deliverable-D3.2.1, October 2012
3. IEEE Standard for Local and Metropolitan Area Networks- Part 21, Media Independent Handover, January 2009
4. Ghein, L.D.: MPLS Fundamentals: A Comprehensive Introduction to MPLS Theory and Practice. Cisco Press, Indianapolis (2007)
5. IEEE 802.15.4, IEEE 802.15 WPAN Low Rate Alternative PHY Task Group 4a (TG4a)
6. Banchs, A., et al.: Carmen: delivering carrier grade services over wireless mesh networks. In: IEEE 19th International Symposium on Personal, Indoor, and Mobile Radio Communications PIMRC 2008, September 2008
7. Digi XBee. Digi International XBee Technology. http://www.digi.com/xbee/
8. ZigBee Alliance.: ZigBee Specification. ZigBee Alliance, 053474r17 edn., January 2008
9. XBee/XBee-PRO Digimesh^{TM} 2.4 RF Modules. Digi International, 90000991_B (2011)
10. Montenegro, G., et al.: Transmission of IPv6 Packets over IEEE 802.15.4 Networks. RFC 4944, September 2009
11. Mangharam R., et al.: Voice over sensor networks. 27th IEEE Real-Time Systems Symposium (RTSS), Rio de Janeiro, Brazil, December 2006
12. Rowe, A., et al.: FireFly: A Time Synchronized Real-Time Sensor Networking Platform. Wireless Ad Hoc Networking: Personal-Area, Local-Area, and the Sensory-Area Networks, CRC Press Book Chapter, Boca Raton, November 2006
13. Eswaran, A., et al.: Nano-RK: an energy-aware resource-centric RTOS for sensor networks. IEEE Real-Time System Symposium (2005)
14. Rowe, A., et al.: RT-link: a time-synchronized link protocol for energy-constrained multi-hop wireless networks. The Third IEEE SECON, September 2006
15. Song, H.Y., et al.: Implementation and analysis of IEEE 802.15.4 MAC for voice communications. The 4th Joint Workshop Between HYU and BUPT (2011)
16. Yoon, H.C., et al.: Efficient voice communications over wireless sensor network. The 4th Joint Workshop Between HYU and BUPT (2011)
17. XBee/XBee-PRO RF Modules. Digi International, 90000982_B (2009)
18. Arduino Fio Website. http://arduino.cc/en/Main/ArduinoBoardFio
19. Black, H.S., Edson, J.O.: Pulse code modulation. Trans. Am. Inst. Electr. Eng. **66**(1), 895–899 (1947)
20. Valin, J.M.: Speex: a free codec for free speech. In: Australian National Linux Conference (2006)
21. Sakhawat, H., et al.: Interconnection between 802.15.4 devices and IPv6: implications and existing approaches. Int. J. Comput. Sci. Issues (IJCSI) **7**, 19–31 (2010)
22. Mannweiler, C., Sihvonen, M.: Architecture and Hardware Specification. CIER Celtic Project Deliverable-D.2.3.1, 8 October 2012
23. Libxbee. A C/C++ library to aid the use of Digi XBee radios in API mode. http://code.google.com/p/libxbee/
24. Rosenberg, J., et al.: SIP: Session Initiation Protocol. RFC 3261, June 2002

Wireless Sensor Networks and Advanced Metering Infrastructure Deployment in Smart Grid

Omowunmi M. Longe$^{(\boxtimes)}$, Khmaies Ouahada, Hendrick C. Ferreira, and Suvendi Rimer

Department of Electrical and Electronics Engineering Science,
University of Johannesburg, Johannesburg, South Africa
{omowunmil,kouahada,hcferreira,suvendic}@uj.ac.za

Abstract. The increasing demand for has necessitated the introduction of information and communication technologies (ICT) in the development of the smart grid. Advanced Metering Infrastructure (AMI) and Wireless Sensor Networks (WSNs) are contributing technologies. In this paper, a review on AMI and WSN in the smart grid is carried out. Also, the introduction of WSNs with AMI in the in-home energy management system of the smart grid is also presented with challenges faced in the deployment of WSNs for the smart grid. The low power and low-cost nature of WSN has presented itself as a technology that can be used with AMI and smart home appliances in achieving home energy management within the great goal of the smart grid.

Keywords: Wireless sensor network · Advanced Metering Infrastructure · Smart Grid

1 Introduction

The rapid global growth in science and technology has greatly increased the number of gadgets and cities to be electrically powered, but the present power generation cannot meet this growing demand for electrical energy; hence, the need to introduce information and communication technologies to the present power grid to give birth to a smart grid. The smart grid is expected to provide energy efficiency, reliability, security and economic savings. To achieve this paradigm every stage of the power system namely: generation, transmission, distribution and consumption would have information and communication technologies incorporated into it. Four major steps have been pointed out as necessary for the actualization of a smart grid, but the foremost is Advanced Metering Infrastructure (AMI) [1]; while others are Advanced Distribution Operations (ADO), Advanced Transmission Operations (ATO) and Advanced Asset Management (AAM). The smart grid will include the use of smart appliances, switches and plugs at consumer premises. In South Africa, the industry specification for AMI is set as NRS049. This specification was prepared on behalf of the Electricity Suppliers Liaison Committee (ESLC) and approved for use by supply authorities. The first iteration of NRS049 was published in 2008 by the South African

© Institute for Computer Sciences, Social Informatics and Telecommunications Engineering 2014
T.F. Bissyandé and G. van Stam (Eds.): AFRICOMM 2013, LNICST 135, pp. 167–171, 2014.
DOI: 10.1007/978-3-319-08368-1_20

Bureau of Standards (SABS). Eskom, the national electricity utility provider intends implementing the AMI solution for its qualifying customers in a phased approach [2].

2 Advanced Metering Infrastructure

AMI is defined as the communications hardware and software; associated system and data management software that create a network between advanced meters and utility business systems and which allows collection and distribution of information to customers and other parties such as competitive retail providers, in addition to providing it to the utility itself [3]. The meter data is received by the AMI host system and sent to the Meter Data Management System (MDMS) that manages data storage and analyses data to provide the information in useful form to the utility. AMI enables two-way communications between utility and the meter. Communication media for AMI are wired, wireless and cellular.

2.1 Benefits of AMI

The benefits of AMI can be categorized basically into two namely: system operational benefits and customer service benefits.

System Operational Benefits. These include eradication of personnel for meter reading and monthly bills dispatch, elimination of errors in reading and missing meter readings, increased consistency in billing periods, theft reduction, provision of detailed data to inform energy advisors actions, better troubleshooting can be done by grid operations engineers, reduced fuel and maintenance cost on meter reading and maintenance, less labour cost to service providers, improved cash flow budgeting and management, provision of monitoring tool for demand and line losses etc.

Customer Service Benefits. These include energy savings and a lowered bill, accurate bill as consumer, payment of electricity bill at convenience, no arbitrary high bill to the consumers etc.

2.2 Components of AMI System

An AMI system is comprised of a number of technologies and applications that have been integrated to perform as one:

- Smart meters
- Wide-area communications infrastructure
- Home (local) area networks (HANs)
- Meter Data Management Systems (MDMS)
- Operational Gateways

Smart Meters. These are solid state programmable devices that perform many more functions, including time-based pricing, consumption data for consumer and utility, net metering, loss of power (and restoration) notification, remote turn on or turn off operations, load limiting or demand response purposes, energy prepayment, power quality monitoring, tamper and energy theft detection and communications with other intelligent devices in the home [1, 4]. The AMI communications infrastructure supports continuous interaction between the utility, the consumer and the controllable electrical load.

Home Area Networks (HAN). HAN interfaces with a consumer portal to link smart meters to controllable electrical devices. Its energy management functions may include in-home displays so the consumer always knows what energy is being used and what it is costing, responsiveness to price signals based on consumer-entered preferences, set limits for utility or local control actions to a consumer specified band, control of loads without continuing consumer involvement and consumer over-ride capability, security monitoring [4, 5].

Meter Data Management System (MDMS). MDMS is a database with analytical tools that enable interaction with other information systems such as Consumer Information System (CIS), billing systems, utility website, Outage Management System (OMS), Enterprise Resource Planning (ERP), power quality management, load forecasting systems, Mobile Workforce Management (MWM), Geographic Information System (GIS) and Transformer Load Management (TLM) [4, 6]. One of the primary functions of an MDMS is to perform validation, editing and estimation (VEE) on the AMI data to ensure that despite disruptions in the communications network or at customer premises, the data flowing to the systems described above is complete and accurate.

Operational Gateways. AMI interfaces with many system-side applications to support Advanced Distribution Operations (ADO), Distribution Management System with advanced sensors, Advanced Outage Management for real-time outage information from AMI meters, Distributed Energy Resources (DER) Operations (using Watt and VAR data from AMI meters), Distribution automation (including Volt/VAR optimization and fault location, isolation, sectionalization and restoration (FLISR)), Distribution GIS and also application of AMI communications infrastructure for microgrid operations (AC and DC), Hi-speed information processing, Advanced protection and control and Advanced grid components for distribution [4].

AMI has many challenges which include interoperability, non-standard protocols and multiple open protocols such as DLMS/COSEM, ANSI C12, Modbus, IEC 1107, legacy meters with limited communication functionalities, data security and integrity, handling of huge volume of data and real-time data update, commercial losses due to theft and tampering of smart meters [6, 7].

3   Wireless Sensor Network Enabling AMI Communications

WSN technology addresses two-way communication efficiently by providing low-cost and low-power wireless communications. With the invention of low-cost, low-power radio sensors, wireless communication is one of the most cost efficient ways to collect utility meter data.

The contribution of WSNs brings significant advantages over traditional communication technologies including rapid deployment, low cost, flexibility, and

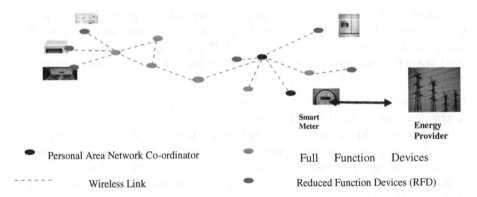

Fig. 1. A Typical WSN Topology in a HAN

aggregated intelligence through parallel processing. The recent advances of WSNs have made it feasible to realize low-cost embedded electric utility monitoring and diagnostic systems [8–10]. In these systems, wireless multifunctional sensor nodes are installed on the critical equipment of the smart grid and monitor the parameters critical to equipment condition. Such information enables the smart-grid system to respond to the changing conditions in a more proactive and timely manner. In this regard, WSNs play a vital role in creating a highly reliable and self-healing smart electric power grid that rapidly responds to online events with appropriate actions. However, the realization of these currently designed and envisioned applications directly depend on efficient and reliable communication capabilities of the deployed WSNs. A typical WSN topology in a HAN is shown in Fig. 1.

4   Challenges of WSNs in Smart Grid

In WSN-based smart grid applications, a good link quality metric is essential for a reliable and energy-efficient system operation. Some of the challenges faced in WSNs deployment in the Smart Grid are described below [9, 10].

Harsh Environmental Conditions. Sensors may also be subject to radio frequency interference, highly caustic or corrosive environments, high humidity levels, vibrations, dirt and dust, or other conditions that challenge performance [8]. These may lead to malfunctioning of sensor nodes.

Reliability and Latency Requirements. The wide variety of applications envisaged on WSNs for smart grid will have different quality-of-service (QoS) requirements and specifications in terms of reliability, latency, network throughput, etc while it is important to receive the data at the controller node in a timely manner.

Packet Errors and Variable Link Capacity. In WSNs, the bandwidth of each wireless link depends on the interference level perceived at the receiver and wireless links exhibit widely varying characteristics over time and space due to obstructions and noisy environment in electric power systems.

Resource Constraints. The design and implementation of WSNs are constrained by three types of resources namely: energy, memory and processing. Therefore, communication protocols for WSNs are mainly tailored to provide high energy efficiency.

5 Conclusion

The impact that AMI and WSNs would have in smart grid cannot be over-emphasized as energy management has grown beyond generation, transmission and distribution, but has moved right into the consumer premises, be it an individual home or commercial and industrial premises. AMI and WSNs are therefore very promising technologies for the success of the smart grid even as their introduction would bring benefits to both utility and energy consumers including energy efficiency, saving, reliability and security.

Acknowledgment.   This work is based on research supported in part by the Eskom Tertiary Education Support Programme (TESP), reference number 264030.

References

1. Yan, Y., Qian, Y., Sharif, H., Tipper, D.: A survey on smart grid communication infrastructures: motivations, requirements and challenges. IEEE Commun. Surv. Tutorials **15**(1), 5–20 (2013)
2. Eskom, Frequently asked questions – Advanced Metering Infrastructure (AMI) (2011)
3. SmartGrid/AEIC AMI Interoperability Standard Guidelines for ANSI C12.19/IEEE 1377/ MC12.19 End Device Communications and Supporting Enterprise Devices, Networks and Related Accessories, Version 2.0, 19 November 2010
4. Fang, X., Misra, S., Xue, G., Yang, D.: Smart grid – the new and improved power grid: a survey. IEEE Commun. Surv. Tutorials **14**(4), 944–980 (2012)
5. National Energy Technology Laboratory (NETL): Advanced Metering Infrastructure, U.S. Department of Energy Office of Electricity Delivery and Energy Reliability, NETL Modern Grid Strategy Powering our 21st-Century Economy (2008)
6. Seal, B.K.: Challenges and benefits of AMI development in the USA, Electric Power Research Institute (EPRI). In: APEC Workshop on Addressing Challenges in AMI Deployment and Smart Grids in APEC (2011)
7. Rodriguez, R.H.L., Cespedes, G.R.H.: Challenges of advanced metering infrastructure implementation in Colombia. In: IEEE PES Conference on Innovative Smart Grid Technologies (ISGT), Latin America (2011)
8. Gungor, V.C., Hancke, G.P.: Industrial wireless sensor networks: challenges, design principles, and technical approaches. IEEE Trans. Ind. Electron. **56**(10), 4258–4265 (2009)
9. Gungor, V.C., Bin, L., Hancke, G.P.: Opportunities and challenges of wireless sensor networks in smart grid. IEEE Trans. Ind. Electron. **57**(10), 3557–3564 (2010)
10. Tuna, G., Gungor, V.C., Gulez, K.: Wireless sensor networks for smart grid applications: a case study on link reliability and node lifetime evaluations in power distribution systems. Int. J. Distrib. Sens. Netw. **2013**, 11 (2013)

Mobile Sink Wireless Underground Sensor Communication Monitor

Cedrick S. Nomatungulula, K.G. Ngandu, Suvendi Rimer[(⊠)],
Babu Sean Paul, Omowunmi M. Longe, and Khmaies Ouahada

Department of Electrical & Electronic Engineering,
University of Johannesburg, Johannesburg, South Africa
{cedrick.noma,gilbertngandu}@gmail.com,
wunmigrace@yahoo.com,
{bspaul,suvendic,kouahada}@uj.ac.za

Abstract. Mine disasters claim thousands of human lives and cause millions of property loss every year. The safety of the mine worker is of paramount importance in any underground environment. Advances in the development of Wireless Sensor Networks (WSNs) for monitoring infrastructure health, and environmental conditions provide end users with the benefit of low-cost installation, maintenance and scalability. This paper will investigate the challenges around a development of a real-time mine monitoring system using wireless sensor nodes to prevent mine disasters such as gas explosions or mine collapses. We propose a mobile, real-time gateway that will be able to process data collected from static wireless sensor nodes monitoring underground infrastructure, to prevent underground disasters.

Keywords: Wireless sensor network · Mobile sensor network · Underground mobile processing · Underground mobile sink communication monitor

1 Introduction

Drill and blast mining operations conducted on underground mines can cause explosions and tunnel collapses resulting in loss of life of mine workers, extensive property damage and reduced productivity. To improve the safety of the mine worker and minimize damage to mine infrastructure it is important to monitor the underground environment in real-time and collect data about the current state of the system. The disadvantages of using wired networks include costs (both labor and capital), inflexibility in adapting to changing environmental conditions and the requirement for a readily available power source. Wireless sensor networks (WSNs)are cheaper both in terms of labor installation and capital costs, more flexible and easily adaptable to changing environmental conditions and easily and rapidly deployable in environments where there is no or limited power and communication structures. Wireless communication systems in underground mines and tunnels are influenced by harsh environmental conditions, tunnel length and width, and the layout of the tunnel walls and ceilings [4]. Radio frequency (RF) waves in underground systems do not propagate well in due to the bounding effects of the tunnel infrastructure [5] and experience high

© Institute for Computer Sciences, Social Informatics and Telecommunications Engineering 2014
T.F. Bissyandé and G. van Stam (Eds.): AFRICOMM 2013, LNICST 135, pp. 172–177, 2014.
DOI: 10.1007/978-3-319-08368-1_21

attenuation of the transmitted signal power [2]. These problems present serious difficulties in using WSNs for tunnel infrastructure monitoring. This paper proposes a mobile real-time wireless gateway node, which will collect data from static infrastructure wireless nodes. The mobile node communicates with static nodes strategically placed within the underground tunnel and processes the received data in real-time to determine the current strength of the surrounding infrastructure and air quality. Each mobile node will be equipped with a trigger event that broadcasts data. Any surrounding level 1 static nodes that receives a high priority message will re-broadcast the message until it is received by all level 1 nodes which will alert workers of the potential danger in that environment.

The rest of the paper is structured as follows. In Sect. 2, related work in the use of wireless sensor nodes to monitor underground systems is reviewed. Section 3 provides a brief summary of the algorithm description. In Sect. 4, the experimental setup is described. In Sect. 5, the results of the experiments are analyzed and Sect. 6 provides a conclusion and discusses future work.

2 Related Work

Li and Liu designed a system to rapidly detect structure variations caused by underground collapses [3]. Mohanty proposed miner tracking and detection of hazardous conditions in underground mines, using stationary wireless sensor nodes placed at selected locations throughout the mine so that each node could communicate with gateway node(s) (called "sink") using one or more hops [6]. Bandyopadhyay et al. propose a Wireless Information and Safety System for Underground Mines based on RFID for tracking miners and moveable equipment in an underground environment [2]. Akyildiz et al. [1] describe signal propagation techniques for wireless underground communication networks. The channel model and signal propagation characteristics for electromagnetic (EM) waves and magnetic induction (MI) techniques in the soil transmission medium is described and the effects of various interference, noise and signal attenuation factors are discussed. A multimode channel model characterizing the wireless channel in a tunnel or a room-and-pillar in underground mines and road/subway tunnels is discussed [1].

3 System Overview

Figure 1 shows the structure implemented for monitoring hazardous conditions. The mobile processing gateway node (MP), at the lower level of the hierarchy (level 3), scans the environment to locate which static node is in communication range and stores the address in an array. After storing the addresses, the MP requests data from each stored static node address at the time in order to avoid collision messages at the MP. The static nodes, in the middle of the hierarchy (level 2), collect the data then send it to the MP, which stores the values in a second array in order to compare it to the threshold value set and to keep records. The threshold is considered as the highest level value status information of the environment. Three environmental states

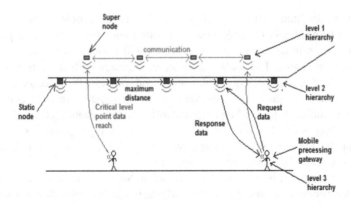

Fig. 1. Structure implementation

condition will be displayed, namely: normal, warning, and dangerous condition. The case of warning condition will be displayed when the threshold level is passed before reaching the critical point value. This condition is taken in order to make aware workers that the sensors are detecting unwanted change in the environment. When dangerous condition is detected, the mobile processing gateway node will broadcast the message to the high hierarchy or level 1 node (super node) which will send it to all super nodes then activate the alarm system. The super node (high hierarchy) communicates with each other and also scan all static nodes to check if they still functioning. When a super node cannot detect a static node, in case of battery failure or node malfunctioning, an alert message will be sent to workers informing which specific place of the node is malfunctioning.

4   Experimental Setup

An experimental setup was conducted in a passageway at the University of Johannesburg as a representation of an underground tunnel. South African underground mines have stringent safety requirements and an actual mine tunnel in which to conduct the experiment could not be found. A node is placed on a belt at shoulder level and tested on different human heights. Static nodes are placed on the center of the ceiling the maximum communication range distance apart. The maximum range distance is divided in sectors. For each sector, a pedestrian walks toward the static wireless node from the maximum point sector and from the static wireless node to the maximum point sector. For each pattern, time is recorded. The process continues while communication between the two nodes exists. Each pattern has time and distance variables that determine the relationship among pedestrian mobility and communication. Different speed behavior is tested for specified distance in order to determine the effect of pedestrian mobility on communication reliability. At specified distance point X, an angle of communication can be determined by assuming that the communication between two nodes is in straight line condition.

5   Results and Discussion

The maximum communication range between two wireless nodes in the passage way for good reliability is 30.5 m. The size of the message used in the experiment is 8 and 16 bits long. A communication reliability threshold was set at 98 % to test the propose algorithm structure.

A. Using 8 bit message with mobile node at height Mh = 1.44 m above ground.

Figure 2 shows the correlation between the pedestrian velocities and the communication reliability. It was noticed that for different pedestrian velocity, the reliability of the communication was mostly good while the mobile wireless node is in the communication range but the faster the pedestrian, the communication reliability decreases. Figure 3 shows the reliability of communication was inversely proportional to the angle, the bigger the angle means that the mobile wireless node is closer to the static node the better the communication.

B. Using 16 bit message with mobile node at height Mh = 1.44 m above ground.

Figure 4 shows the correlation between pedestrian velocities and the communication reliability. Figure 5 shows the correlation between angle and the communication reliability. The result shows that most of the data collected was above that threshold.

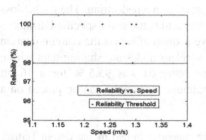

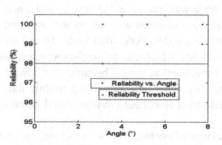

Fig. 2. Reliability vs. speed, 8-bit Mh = 1.44 m

Fig. 3. Reliability vs. angle, 8-bit Mh = 1.44 m

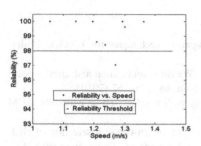

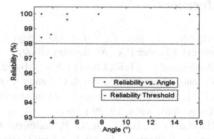

Fig. 4. Reliability vs. speed, *16-bit Mh* = *1.44 m*

Fig. 5. Reliability vs. angle, *16-bit Mh = 1.44 m*

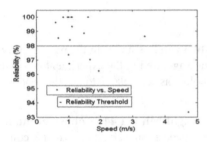   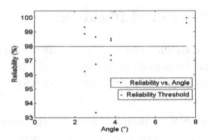

Fig. 6. Reliability vs. speed, *16-bit Mh =*   **Fig. 7.** Reliability vs. angle, *16-bit Mh = 1.47 m*
1.47 m

C. Using 16 bits message with mobile node at height Mh = 1.47 m above ground.

Figure 6 shows the signal strength drops to 93.5 % for high speed and is 100 % for slow speeds. It was also noticed that at a distance between nodes greater than 15 m the average signal strength is 98 %. Figure 7 shows the correlation between angle and the communication reliability.

6   Conclusion

The effect of pedestrian mobility on communication reliability in a WSN is analyzed. A node was placed on the ceiling and a node gateway on a pedestrian. The packet loss rate was measured with different movement speeds and patterns for specified distances between nodes. Pedestrian mobility and do have a small effect on the communication reliability which can be neglected when both wireless nodes are sharing data within communication range because the lowest rate obtained was 93.5 % for a 16 bit message. This indicates that a mobile data communicator (sink) can be placed on a pedestrian to collect environmental behavior.

Acknowledgments. This work is based on research supported in part by the Eskom Tertiary Education Support Program (TESP), reference number 264030.

References

1. Akyildiz, I.F., Sun, Z., Vuran, M.C.: Signal Propagation Techniques for Wireless Underground. Elsevier B.V, Amsterdam (2009)
2. Bandyopadhyay, L.K., Chaulya, S.K., Mishra, P.K.: Wireless information and safety system for underground mines. Wirel. Commun. Undergr. Min. **68**, 175–262 (2010)
3. Li, M., Liu, Y.: Underground coal mine monitoring with wireless sensor networks. ACM Trans. Sens. Netw. **10**, 29 (2009)
4. Hancke, G. P., Hancke Jr, G. P.: Industrial wireless sensor networks: a selection of challenging applications. In: 6th European Conference on Antennas and Propagation (EUCAP), pp. 64–68 (2012)

5. Sun, Z., Akyildiz, I.F.: Channel modeling and analysis for wireless networks in underground mines and road tunnels. IEEE Trans. Commun. **58**(6), 1758–1768 (2010)
6. Mohanty, P. K.: Application of Wireless Sensor Network Technology for Miner Tracking and Monitoring Hazardous Conditions in Underground Mines. Ohio

Consumer Adoption of Mobile Payment Systems in Malawi: Case of Airtel Malawi ZAP in Blantyre City

Menard Nyirenda[1] and Patrick Albert Chikumba[2(✉)]

[1] Malawi Revenue Authority, Private Bag 247, Blantyre, Malawi
mdnyirenda@mra.mw
[2] Department of Computing and Information Technology,
University of Malawi-The Polytechnic, Private Bag 303, Blantyre 3, Malawi
patrick_chikumba@yahoo.com

Abstract. Mobile payment enables consumers to purchase goods and services as well as transfer money using a mobile phone. This qualitative study aimed at investigating the factors that are affecting consumers in using mobile payment in Malawi using Zap [mobile payment system] as an example. Snowball sampling technique was used to identify study participants in Blantyre District. Inductive and deductive qualitative data analyses were carried out based on the transcriptions of interviews. Study findings show that relative advantage, complexity, compatibility, cost, trust and security, network externalities and situational factors affect use of mobile payment systems. In addition, personal characteristics and use of mass media play a role in the adoption of mobile payment systems. The findings reinforce the existing theory of Diffusion of Innovation and adoption of mobile payment systems. The study recommends improvement in the network stability, extension of the service to banks and utility service providers, and recruitment of more mobile payment agents across the country.

Keywords: Adoption · Innovation · Mobile payments · Mobile phone · Zap

1 Introduction

Making payments for goods and services is an everyday activity for most households worldwide. Payment is the transfer of value via a financial asset from one person to another, usually in return for some good or service received in a transaction [10]. According to [1] any payment where a mobile device is used to initiate, authorize and confirm an exchange of financial value in return for goods and services is referred to as a mobile payment. Mobile devices may include mobile phones, PDAs, tablets and any other device that connect to mobile telecommunication network and make it possible for payments to be made [21]. In so doing, mobile phones bring together services that cross existing boundaries.

According to ITU [17], there were 2.43 million mobile cellular subscribers in Malawi as of 2009 for the two mobile operators, namely Telekom Networks Malawi (TNM) and Zain Malawi. Zain Malawi was formerly known as Celtel Malawi Limited. Zain Malawi changed to Airtel Malawi in 2010.

© Institute for Computer Sciences, Social Informatics and Telecommunications Engineering 2014
T.F. Bissyandé and G. van Stam (Eds.): AFRICOMM 2013, LNICST 135, pp. 178–187, 2014.
DOI: 10.1007/978-3-319-08368-1_22

Airtel Malawi and TNM offer their customers downloadable materials for purchase using their phones which include ring tones, caller tunes and music. Airtel Malawi and TNM customers can also purchase mobile phone units using "Zachangu" [local language which literally means 'quick'] service offered by agents. This is another form of mobile payment, an alternative way of purchasing prepaid airtime instead of buying scratch cards or using an auto teller machine. Airtel Malawi was the first mobile company to introduce phone-to-phone airtime credit transfer service in 2005 [43] which are dubbed "Me2U" ['me to you'].

Khanje [22] and Mashni [28] indicate that Zain Africa [now being called Airtel Africa] introduced a mobile payment service called "Zap" in Kenya, Uganda, Tanzania, Siera Leone and Niger. Notably, Zap was introduced in countries where M-PESA was already successfully implemented, namely Kenya and Tanzania.

Airtel Malawi introduced Zap mobile payment service in 2010 in Malawi as a full commercial pilot [22, 44]. Zap enabled customers to withdraw cash or pay for goods and services, school fees and utility bills, including electricity and water; receive/send money from/to friends and family; send and receive money to their bank accounts; top-up airtime and manage their bank accounts [22, 28, 43].

Several banks in Malawi, namely: Inde Bank, First Merchant Bank (FMB), National Bank of Malawi (NBM) and Opportunity International Bank of Malawi (OIBM) have mobile banking services [9, 16, 31, 37].

It seems to be an overlap between mobile banking and mobile payments in the sense that within mobile banking there are payment transactions. However, according to [37], the main difference is that mobile banking uses a 'bank-led' model while mobile payment usually uses a 'telco-led' model. In 'telco-led' model a telecommunication company runs payment services while in 'bank-led' model, it is a bank that offers banking services in partnership with a telecommunication company.

In the telco-led model, regulations bar telecommunication companies from offering savings or loan products, so their programs typically focus on helping people to move money quickly and securely (ibid) unlike the bank-led model where the money is subjected to bank interest calculations. From these two approaches on how mobile payment service is implemented, this research focused on mobile payment services run by mobile network operators.

Mobile payment is an alternative way of making payments for goods and services as well as an alternative means of money transfer among people who are not carrying out business transactions. The question that this research intended to answer was: What factors affect consumers in adopting mobile payment systems in Malawi?

2 Mobile Payments

There are different ways in which consumers make payments for goods and services in their day to day living. Among the numerous methods of making payments are cash, credit card, Electronic Funds Transfer, cheque and direct debit [10]. In addition, technological development has allowed more efficient and secure payment systems through the Internet. Electronic payment technologies include magnetic stripe card, smartcard, contactless card and mobile handset.

Preference of payment instruments varies from country to country. Jonker [19] found that people in Netherlands mostly use cash in comparison with debit cards, e-pulse and credit cards. In USA, Stavins [39] noted that retail payment transactions made with electronic payment instruments still constitute only a small fraction of all payments. A recent study by [15] indicates that USA has historically relied on cheques; Europe had a well-established nationwide electronic payment system before USA; and Japan currently uses cash more than twice as much as Europe and over six times as much as USA. Stavins [39] argues that, in USA, differences in cost among payment instruments typically are not evident to consumers, who are charged the same amount regardless of how they pay.

ECB [8, 20] defines mobile payments as a subgroup of e-payments, where mobile phones or other wireless communication devices are used to access accounts for payment services. Mobile payments are typically made remotely via SMS, WAP billing, Mobile Web, Direct-to-subscribers' bill and direct to credit cards [23].

Different countries have had different experiences regarding mobile payments. In 2007, Kenya's largest mobile network operator (Safaricom) launched M-PESA [14]. "Pesa" is the Swahili word for cash and "M" is for the mobile.

Most people preferred sending the money with friends or family members. Use of courier companies and post office money orders was also popular. However, there was a massive reduction in the use of delivery by hand, post office orders and courier companies, following the introduction of M-PESA which people now prefer most [2]. Furthermore, Kenyan farmers, who insure their crops against drought or other weather problems to Union Insurance and Provincial Insurance (UAP), receive their insurance claims via M-PESA [29].

A mobile payment model similar to M-PESA was introduced in Tanzania but has not been as successful as it has been in Kenya [2]. In South Africa, WIZZIT (a mobile banking service), allows a bank holder to move money from one bank account to another using a mobile phone that is linked to the bank account.

Mallat [26] identified the following current and potential mobile payment applications for Finland: vending, ticketing, purchase of mobile content services, peer to peer fund transfers, payments on the Internet, and payments of goods and services in shops, restaurants and corner stores. In Finland, Helsinki City Transport offers a mobile subway and tram ticket—an example of a successful mobile payment service [27]. In addition, mobile devices can be utilized in a variety of payments, such as payments for digital content, concert or flight tickets, parking fees, and bus, tram, train and taxi fares [23].

In Europe and North America with few exceptions such as Austria, Spain and Scandinavian countries the developments of mobile payments have not been successful. However, mobile payment services in Asia have been fairly successful especially in South Korea and Japan [4].

In Philippines, the uptake of mobile payment systems has been particularly strong, where three million customers use systems offered by mobile operators Smart and Globe [7]. The main difference between successful implementations of mobile payment services in the Asia Pacific region and failure in Europe and North America is primarily attributed to the 'payment culture' of the consumers that are country-specific

[4]. In agreement, consumers from different cultures may differ considerably in perceptions, beliefs, selection, and use of m-commerce [12, 24].

3 Methodology

This study adopted the qualitative research method since the research was about exploring and understanding perceptions and experiences of consumers in using mobile payment systems. According to [30], the qualitative research methods were developed in the Social Sciences to enable researchers to study social and cultural phenomena.

The case study research strategy was used to describe what mobile payments are and how people are utilizing them. Based on the argument by [36] that a case study can be a worthwhile way of exploring existing theory, this study intended to explore theories on factors that influence adoption of mobile payments for instance Rogers' Innovation Diffusion theory.

The study used Zap mobile payment system for Airtel Malawi as a case study because it was the only mobile payment system being managed by a mobile network operator by that time as such it does not require a consumer to have a bank account. As such Zap seemed to have the potential of being widely used by people in both rural and urban areas.

Data for the study was collected in the months of February and March in 2011. It was collected using semi-structured interviews, document analysis and participatory observations. Data was solicited from customers of Airtel Malawi in Blantyre District who registered and used Zap mobile payment system.

The study also gathered information from documents that were obtained from institutions that offer money transfer services. The documents included sending and receive forms; and deposit and withdraw slips for banks. Other documents were obtained from the mobile network operators and contained information on the services they offer together with the charges. In addition, information about what Zap can do and where Zap dealers are located was extracted from newspaper articles.

The researcher participated in the research by registering to Zap services in August 2010. The reason was to acquire hands-on experience and understanding on the usage of Zap mobile payment system before gathering data from research participants.

4 Factors Affecting Use of Mobile Payment (ZAP)

Zap was a new innovation for money transfer as well as making payments. The ordinary ways of money transfer include: using bank accounts, money transfer services, and through hand delivery. As for payment, the ordinary methods include: cash, debit card and cheque.

Participants compared Zap with other ordinary methods of money transfer and payment methods which they have used. Previous researches [3, 18, 26] found independence of time and place as relative advantage of mobile payments. This means that the consumers are able to transact at any time and any place where there is network coverage for service providers. Ubiquitous is a general characteristic of mobile payments and the study found other ways in which a mobile payment method can be compared with ordinary means of money transfer and payment.

A Zap customer can transact at any time of the day and anywhere as long as there is a network for Airtel and the electronic money is in the mobile phone. In so doing, participants are saved from travelling distances when making payments for goods which are in electronic form such as airtime as well as paying for services that are administered remotely.

However, the service of loading electronic money into the Zap account requires Zap agents who are available at certain times of the day and at certain places. Whenever a Zap customer has money in the account, a transaction can be initiated and completed instantly on the spot. For a transaction such as purchasing airtime, it can be initiated and completed instantly as long as the network is functional.

The study found that the mobile payment system can provide safety to a consumer when used at an awkward time in a crime prone environment which other previous research on mobile payments did not reveal this relative advantage of mobile payment over traditional method of payment using cash. The customer does not need to travel when using mobile payment system. This is applicable to all transactions that are associated with goods in electronic format or a service that is provided remotely. For instance to buy airtime using Zap, a consumer has to specify the mobile phone number and amount of money regardless of time and place.

A mobile payment system enables a consumer to avoid carrying a lot of cash which is prone to theft and difficult to recover. High crime rate in Kenya, and Nairobi in particular created a greater demand for a safe way of sending money compared to Tanzania where the risk of robbery is lower [2]. However, when a mobile phone which has electronic money is stolen the thief cannot access the money in the Zap account because it is protected by a password. In addition, the consumer is given the equivalent electronic money into a new SIM card.

According to [25], complexity and problems with usability have contributed to low adoption of a variety of payment systems including smart cards and mobile banking. None of the participants complained on how the procedures are followed when carrying a Zap transaction. This might be because the participants attained basic education qualification. However, it was learnt from the participants that Zap was mostly meant for people living in the rural areas to receive money from relatives staying in urban areas. Some participants noted that most people in rural areas are illiterate and this might hinder fast adoption of mobile payment system.

Once the receiver has the money in Zap account, the electronic money has to be transferred from the recipient's Zap account to the Zap account of the agent in order to get cash. In sending the money, there are several steps which require the sender to choose the Zap transaction type and then specify the recipient mobile number or nickname, the amount being transferred and the password to authorize the transaction. It requires a consumer to be familiar with reading instructions and pressing appropriate buttons on the mobile phone.

Limitations of usability of mobile payment systems as indicated by [26, 32, 38] were not evident in the study. However, the limitations might affect people in the rural areas on learning how to use the mobile payment system.

More than half of participants had a background of information technology and most of them had used an auto-teller machine which has similar features with mobile payment system. Zap uses technology which is menu driven like that of an ATM. Therefore, it was easy for them to learn and start using Zap.

This concurs with how [35] defined compatibility as a degree to which an innovation is perceived as consistent with individual values, beliefs, past experiences and needs. Past experiences of using an ATM has assisted participants on how to operate Zap. However, the participants did not use the innovation much on money transfer which is an indicator that the innovation is not addressing their needs.

Consumers are not willing to use mobile commerce when transaction costs are high [5, 42]. It was found that commissions are charged when a Zap customer is exchanging cash with electronic money from a Zap agent and when a Zap customer is sending electronic money to another Zap account holder. When purchasing goods in shop using a mobile payment system, there is an additional charge on top of the item price. These findings agree with previous research findings that cost is a factor that affects consumers to use or not use mobile payments. Most of the participants were aware of costs associated with Zap and they felt that the costs were high.

Participants felt that a large amount of money is safer in the mobile phone than cash. The participants felt confident that even if the mobile phone that has a Zap account is stolen, the thief cannot use the money in the phone due to the authentication mechanism. Similarly, [7] suggest that mobile banking systems might reduce loss of money to petty theft. All the services on Zap require a password just before carrying out the last step in a transaction. The importance of authentication in mobile payment system was evident in this study and concurs with [26, 34].

Other participants expressed concern that money in the Zap account is not safe since some time they had experienced a loss on mobile phone credit. They expressed fear that the same can happen with their money in the Zap account. Another fear was that unauthorized people, who were called 'hackers', would access the electronic money in the phone as they do with money in the bank account.

Additionally, most participants expressed concern on the instability of the network while transacting using Zap. Some participants received a 'no network coverage' message from the mobile network operator when they were about to complete the Zap transaction even though there was network coverage in that place. Participants showed lack of trust in the mobile phone network due to its instability when sending SMS as well as in using the Zap services. These network problems deny participants to use the service when they need it. Tsiakis and Sthephanides [40] indicate service availability is a security requirement of any electronic payment system. The service should be continuously and uninterruptedly provided.

This network unreliability might result into lack of trust in the Zap service which deals with financial transactions. Despite that participants expressed that a Zap transaction is faster than a bank transaction, this is only true when the mobile network is functioning properly. The network problems affected some participants to reconsider using Zap until there is an improvement in the network as indicated by one participant.

A perceived risk which is not evident in previous research of mobile payments is that mobile payments can lead a consumer to financial mismanagement since the electronic money is easy and tempting to use. Participants stated that it is easy to purchase items such as airtime using money in the mobile phone than cash since the transaction can take place anywhere and anytime.

There are few Zap agents within Blantyre who are operational. The network of Zap agents is essential as it provides the interface between Zap consumers and the mobile network operator. Some of Zap agents were shop owners. As such consumers would buy goods using Zap money from these shops. Apart from the shops efforts are being made to extend Zap services to bank services. Commercial banks have consumers who are also subscribers of Airtel Malawi and some consumers might find Zap services convenient for managing their bank accounts.

Furthermore, Airtel Malawi has been negotiating with water and electricity utility providers to use Zap for bill payments. This is also another way of expanding the network for mobile payment consumers and merchants. Most households in urban areas use water and electricity meaning that the customer base is big and Zap can take this advantage. Zap is only functional within the Airtel mobile network and only among Airtel subscribers. This limits number of customers using Zap.

There were several factors that depended on the context in which mobile payments are used. These include: Zap services availability and mobile network coverage. Zap service availability encompasses availability of Zap agents and availability of cash and electronic money with the Zap agent.

Some participants compared the availability of Zap agents with availability of banking and post offices in terms of times of operation. Most banks are opened from 8:00am to 3:00pm while post offices are opened from 8:00am to 4:30pm. On the other hand, most shop owners who might be also Zap agents open their shops earlier than 8:00am and close later than 4:30pm. Consequently, a Zap customer can still transact after the banks and post offices are closed. In addition, the banks and post offices are closed from Saturday afternoon until Monday morning while a Zap agent remains open during the weekend as well. In some cases a Zap agent can be there but without resources such as cash and electronic money.

Zap agents can only be found where there is network coverage. Some participants pointed out that some remotest areas are not covered by Airtel mobile network. These are the places where Zap would be most helpful because there are no banks and post offices. It is most likely that where there is no mobile network coverage there are no Zap agents. Therefore, Zap will not work in that area even if a person registers to Zap.

According to [33], there are five steps involved in the decision process of an innovation. These stages are: knowledge, persuasion, decision, implementation, and confirmation. The innovation diffusion model by [35] illustrates that the decision process of an innovation is influenced by communication sources.

It was found that Zap was advertised through the radio, television, flyers, posters, newspapers and a minibus that was dedicated for Zap registration. Some of the participants explained that the adverts prompted them to register for the service. It was also mentioned that the time Zap was being introduced; there were many adverts.

Some posters were meant to direct Zap customers where Zap agents are located in case they want to transact. And some participants made complaints about the unavailability of these posters which makes identification of Zap agents difficult. Some participants complained that Zap adverts are no longer being heard on audio-visual media and not seen in print media. A consumer sounded confused as he complained about disappearance of Zap advertisements.

The study found that the media played a role in the innovation decision process and therefore concurs with the model of innovation diffusion. Although most participants have been registered to Zap for at least a year, they have not used Zap often. Twelve months is a long period such that if the mobile payment solution was meant for pertinent needs of participants, the participants would have used it several times.

Most consumers expressed intention to use Zap in future only if the service is improved in the following ways: introduced to more people through mass media; given an assurance that money in Zap account is safe; improvement on the network instability; and recruitment of more Zap agents across the country. This implies that some participants are on the verge of deciding whether to stop or continue using Zap.

The participants in the study were knowledgeable on sending and receiving money as well as purchasing mobile phone units but were not conversant with other features of Zap. In addition, they felt that many people are not aware of Zap which could be due to poor awareness to potential consumers.

5   Conclusion

The problem of mobile network instability was a major concern from the consumers. Considering that mobile payments involve financial transactions, it is of paramount importance for the mobile network operator to improve the network so that consumers can build trust on the performance of the network.

In a situation where a Zap account holder sends electronic money to an Airtel customer who does not have a Zap, it is not possible for the recipient to get cash from the Zap agents. Zap has to be integrated with commercial banks in order to broaden the customer base since it will serve those that have bank accounts and those that do not have. In addition, Zap has to be integrated with payment of utilities such as water and electricity. Payments for these utilities are characterized with long queues which might be avoided by using mobile payment.

References

1. Au, Y.A., Kauffman, R.J.: The economics of mobile payments: understanding stakeholder issues for an emerging financial technology application. Electron. Commer. Res. Appl. 7(2), 141–164 (2007)
2. Camner, G., Pulver, C., Sjoblom, E.: What makes a successful mobile money implementation? - M-PESA in Kenya and Tanzania, Financial Sector Deepening (2009)
3. Carlsson, C., Walden, P., Bouwman, H.: Adoption of 3G+ services in Finland. Int. J. Mobile Commun. 4(4), 369–385 (2006)
4. Carr, M.: Mobile payment systems and services: an introduction (2007). http://www.mpf. org.in/pdf/Mobile%20Payment%20Systems%20and%20Services.pdf. Accessed 17 October 2010

5. Dahlberg, T., Mallat, N., Ondrus, J., Zmijewska, A.: Past, present and future of mobile payments research: a literature review. Electron. Commer. Res. Appl. **7**(2), 165–181 (2008)
6. Dewan, S.G., Chen, L.: Mobile payment adoption in the USA: a crossindustry, cross-platform solution. J. Inf. Priv. Secur. **1**(2), 4–28 (2005)
7. Donner, J., Tellez, C.A.: Mobile banking and economic development: linking adoption, impact, and use. Asian J. Commun. **18**(4), 318–332 (2008)
8. ECB: Eurpoean Central Bank: Paper Issues for ECB Conference on 10 November 2004: e-payments without frontiers (2004). www.ecb.europa.eu/pub/pdf/other/epaymentsconference issues2004en.pdf. Accessed 13 October 2010
9. FMB: FMB - Bringing banking closer to the people (2010). http://www.fmbmalawi.com/news22.html. Accessed 24 November 2010
10. Gans, J.S., Scheelings, R.: Economic Issues Associated with Access to Electronic Payments Systems (1999). http://www.mbs.edu/home/jgans/papers/cecs.pdf. Accessed 10 October 2010
11. Heeks, R., Jagun, A.: Mobile Phones and Development: The Future in New Hands?, University of Sussex. Institute of development studies (IDS) (2007)
12. Hofstede, G.: Culture's consequences (abridged edition). Sage, Beverly Hills (1984)
13. Hsu, C.L., Lu, H.P., Hsu, H.H.: Adoption of the mobile internet: an empirical study of multimedia message service (MMS). Omega **35**(6), 715–726 (2007)
14. Hughes, N., Lonie, S.: M-PESA: mobile money for the "Unbanked" turning cellphones into 24-Hour tellers in Kenya. Innovations: Technol. Gov. Globalization **2**(1–2), 63–81 (2011)
15. Humphrey, D.B.: Retail payments: new contributions, empirical results, and unanswered questions. J. Bank. Finance **34**(8), 1729–1737 (2010)
16. IndeBank: IndeBank (2010). http://www.indebank.com/sms_banking.html. Accessed 24 November 2010
17. ITU: World Telecommunication/ICT Indicators Database – Mobile Cellular Subcriptions (2011). http://www.itu.int/ITUD/ict/statistics/. Accessed 11 March 2011
18. Jarvenpaa, S.L., Lang, K.R.: Managing the paradoxes of mobile technology. Inf. Syst. Manage. **22**(4), 7–23 (2005)
19. Jonker, N.: Payment instruments as perceived by consumers–results from a household survey. De Economist **155**(3), 271–303 (2007)
20. Kadhiwal, S., Zulfiquar, A.U.: Analysis of mobile payment security measures and different standards. Comput. Fraud Secur. **2007**(6), 12–16 (2007)
21. Karnouskos, S., Fokus, F.: Mobile payment: a journey through existing procedures and standardization initiatives. IEEE Commun. Surv. Tutorials **6**(4), 44–66 (2004)
22. Khanje, T.: Zain Malawi launches mobile banking service (2010). http://www.bnltimes.com/index.php?option=com_content&task=view&id=1692. Accessed 24 November 2010
23. Kim, C., Mirusmonov, M., Lee, I.: An empirical examination of factors influencing the intention to use mobile payment. Comput. Hum. Behav. **26**(2010), 310–322 (2010)
24. Kim, J., Lee, I., Lee, Y.: Exploring the mobile Internet businesses from a user perspective: a cross-national study in Hong Kong, Japan and Korea. In: Proceedings of the First Mobile Roundtable (2002)
25. Laukkanen, T., Lauronen, J.: Consumer value creation in mobile banking services. Int. J. Mobile Commun. **3**(4), 325–338 (2005)
26. Mallat, N.: Exploring consumer adoption of mobile payments-A qualitative study. J. Strateg. Inf. Syst. **16**(4), 413–432 (2007)
27. Mallat, N., Rossi, M., Tuunainen, V.K.: Mobile banking services. Commun. ACM **47**(5), 42–46 (2004)

28. Mashni, R.: Zain expands 'Zap' mobile commerce service to Malawi, Niger and Sierra Leone (2004). http://www.ameinfo.com/220486.html. Accessed 9 April 2010
29. Must, B., Ludewig, K.: Mobile money: cell phone banking in developing countries. Policy Matters J. **7**(2), 27–33 (2010)
30. Myers, M.D.: Qualitative research in information systems. MIS Q. **21**(2), 241–242 (1997)
31. NBM: NBM: National Bank of Malawi (2010). http://www.natbank.co.mw/index.php? pagename=sms_banking. Accessed 24 November 2010
32. Pagani, M., Schipani, D.: Motivations and barriers to the adoption of 3G mobile multimedia services: An end user perspective in the Italian market, pp. 957–960 (2003)
33. PEEC: Diffusion of Innovation theory resources (2003). http://www.peecworks.org/PEEC/ PEEC_Gen/I00045B6A. Accessed 25 October 2010
34. Pousttchi, K.: Conditions for acceptance and usage of mobile payment procedures, pp. 201–210 (2003)
35. Rogers, E.M.: Diffusion of Innovations, 4th edn. Free Press, New York (1995)
36. Saunders, M., Lewis, P., Thornhill, A.: Research Methods for Business Students, 3rd edn. Prentice Hall, New York (2003)
37. SEEP: Expanding Outreach in Malawi: OIBM's Efforts to Launch a Mobile Phone Banking Program (2009). http://www.google.mw/gwt/x?q=sms+banking+in+Malawi&ei=lEDt TKDpEZSPjAeYn6LOAw&ved=0CBEQFjAF&hl=en&source=m&rd=1&u=http://www. opportunity.org/wpcontent/uploads/2010/07/Expanding-Outreach-in-Malawi-OIBMs-Efforts-to-Launch-a-Mobile-Phone-Banking-Program.pdf. Accessed 24 November 2010
38. Siau, K., Sheng, H., Nah, F., Davis, S.: A qualitative investigation on consumer trust in mobile commerce. Int. J. Electron. Bus. **2**(3), 283–300 (2004)
39. Stavins, J.: Effect of consumer characteristics on the use of payment instruments. New England Econ. Rev. **2002**(3), 19–31 (2001)
40. Tsiakis, T., Sthephanides, G.: The concept of security and trust in electronic payments. Comput. Secur. **24**(1), 10–15 (2005)
41. Wandawanda, B.: Business dexterity: Can mobile business solutions offer a sustainable competitive advantage? Masters dessertation. United Kingdom: University of Derby (2005)
42. Wu, J.H., Wang, S.C.: What drives mobile commerce?: an empirical evaluation of the revised technology acceptance model. Inf. Manag. **42**(5), 719–729 (2005)
43. Zain: Zain dials up mobile banking in Africa with Zap (2011). http://www.zain.com/muse/ obj/lang.default/portal.view/content/Media%20centre/Press%20releases/ZapLaunchAfrica. Accessed 8 March 2011
44. Zain: Zain expands 'Zap' Mobile Commerce service to Malawi, Niger and Sierra Leone (2010). http://www.zain.com/muse/obj/lang.default/portal.view/content/Media%20centre/ Press%20releases/ZapExpansion. Accessed 8 March 2011

Stakeholder Analysis and Sustainability of Telecenter Projects in Rural Malawi

Christopher Banda[1](✉) and Patrick Albert Chikumba[2]

[1] Malawi Communications Regulatory Authority (MACRA),
Private Bag 261, Blantyre, Malawi
chrisbanda@gmail.com
[2] Department of Computing and Information Technology,
University of Malawi-The Polytechnic, Private Bag 303,
Blantyre 3, Malawi
patrick_chikumba@yahoo.com

Abstract. Telecenters are meant to provide public access to information and communication services and technologies that are expected to contribute to development of the masses. Government of Malawi is implementing ICT for Sustainable Rural Development Project which seeks to provide ICT services to the rural and underserved areas of Malawi. By 2012, it had established about 50 telecenters across the country but it seems that the performance of some of these telecenters has been poor and not meeting expected goals. One of the factors which affect sustainability of telecenters is lack of meaningful stakeholder engagement and relationship in formulating and running such projects. Therefore, this paper discusses how stakeholder management is conducted in the telecenter project in Malawi and how that affects performance and sustainability of the project.

Keywords: Sustainability · Telecenter · Stakeholder · Stakeholder analysis · Telecenter performance

1 Introduction

Information and Communication Technology (ICT) developments remarkably bring about great changes in the quality of life and business in the world and had been identified as one of the enabler of change in the society [5, 8, 15]. ICTs include a range of technologies which facilitate communication, processing and transmission of information by electronic means [6]. According to [13], ICT is a tool to alleviate poverty in rural areas through new income earning opportunities, improved delivery of basic services, and enhance participation of rural communities in decision making processes. Despite these opportunities which ICT bring to communities; it has been recognized that diffusion of ICTs is rather slow in rural areas compared with the urban counterparts [4].

In this context, telecenters concept has been implemented by international organizations, governments and communities as a new tool to introduce new information technologies to remote areas of the country [4]. Telecenters are meant to provide

© Institute for Computer Sciences, Social Informatics and Telecommunications Engineering 2014
T.F. Bissyandé and G. van Stam (Eds.): AFRICOMM 2013, LNICST 135, pp. 188–197, 2014.
DOI: 10.1007/978-3-319-08368-1_23

public access to information and communication services and technologies that are expected to contribute to development to the masses that would otherwise lack [14]. In theory telecenters have the potential to empower the economically disadvantaged and provide ICT access to the rural communities [13]. It is for this reason that a number of governments in developing countries as well as their partners have been and are investing in telecenters [13].

Despite these interventions, telecenter projects are having challenges of sustainability [13]. According to [1, 2, 10], one of the factors which affect sustainability of telecenters is lack of meaningful stakeholder engagement and relationship in formulating and running such projects. Many authors [1, 12] stress the need for participation of the local community to foster activities such as assessment of information needs, planning and operations. According to [3], one of the best strategies for community participation is to find local champions who can increase the credibility and potential spreading of the telecenter initiative. Rajalekshmi [11] calls them local human intermediaries who make the telecenter a success and focuses on the role of trust between them and the citizens. There is a need to maintain strong links with key stakeholders and remembering the key role that intermediary community groups can have in promoting the use of telecenters in the community [3].

Government of Malawi is implementing the ICT for Sustainable Rural Development Project (ISRDP) which seeks to provide ICT services to the rural and underserved areas of the country. By June 2012, Government of Malawi through MACRA had established about 50 telecenters across the country with an investment close to one billion Malawi Kwacha since 2008 [7].

Despite these interventions, the performance of these telecenters has been poor and not meeting expected goals. According to [16] some telecenters in Malawi have closed; others are on the verge of being closed or have been recommended for a different shape of model. These telecenters are performing poorly due to various factors ranging from awareness, location, staff competence and the model [16]. Stakeholder involvement assists in the successful implementation of developmental projects [1, 9].

Using a case study approach, this study explored how stakeholder management is conducted in a telecenter project in Malawi and how that affects the performance and sustainability of the project. The research is aimed at seeking to understand and identify stakeholders who are involved in the project and how they influence the shape and sustainability of the projects. The study used multi-purpose community telecenters under the ISRD Project.

2 Telecenter Stakeholder and Sustainability

Gómez et al. [17] define telecenter as a physical space that provides public access to ICT notably the Internet for educational, personal, social, and economic development. Telecenters serve as avenues for providing universal access communications and multimedia services to rural communities since they provide access to telephones, faxes, computers, the Internet, photocopiers and other equipment and services [13].

According to [18] Multipurpose Community telecenters are generally seen as structures that can encourage and support communities to manage their own development through access to appropriate facilities, resources, training and services. These structures provide services same as any kind of telecenters but these are specially owned by the communities themselves, because of their potential to address the needs of people and mostly empowers the communities they serve.

While telecenters are different, their common focus is on the use of digital technologies to support community, economic, educational, and social development with aims of reducing isolation, bridging the digital divide, promoting health issues, creating economic opportunities, and reaching out to youth for example. Telecenters matter as they offer young people a first place to learn about computers and provide villages an access to government services. They also allow isolated communities to bridge the education and health gap and open up economic opportunity for small entrepreneurs.

Telecenter projects have been deployed in developed and developing countries; however the major challenge has been the sustainability of these projects. Researchers have grouped telecenter projects sustainability in four ways [1, 19]: (a) financial sustainability; (b) social sustainability; (c) political sustainability; and (d) technological sustainability.

According to [19], telecenter sustainability could also be looked into other aspect which other authors have referred them as salient factors that affect sustainability. These factors include: (a) telecenter and its internal organization which refers to how content, services and people are managed within the telecenter; (b) telecenter and its local context (i.e. the local community) which refers to relationship that telecenters have with the community in which they operate; (c) telecenter and its national/international context which refers to national commitment by policy-makers.

Freeman [20] defines stakeholders as those groups who are vital to the survival and success of the corporation. Freeman et al. [21] state that the organization itself should be thought of as grouping of stakeholders and the purpose of the organization should be to manage their interests, needs and viewpoints. Carroll and Buchholtz [22] define stakeholder as individuals and groups with a multitude of interests, expectations, and demands as to what business should provide to society.

Stakeholder management is one of the crucial issues that the organisation needs to consider if the organisation aims at meeting the expectations of the stakeholders. According to [22], the main objective of the stakeholder management is to see it that the primary stakeholders achieve their objectives and those other stakeholders are dealt with ethically and are also relatively satisfied. Carroll and Buchholtz [22] further emphasize that stakeholder management must address the five major questions which are: (a) Who are the firms' stakeholders? (b) What are the stakeholders' stakes in the firm? (c) What opportunities and challenges do the stakeholders present to the firm? (d) What economic, legal, ethical, and charitable responsibilities does firm have to the stakeholders? (e) What strategies or actions should the firm take to best manage stakeholder challenges and opportunities?

Conducting stakeholder analysis is useful as it helps to know who the key actors are, their knowledge, interests, positions, alliances, and importance related to the project and allows policy makers and managers to interact more effectively with key stakeholders and increase support for a given policy or project.

3 Methodology

Since the study was focusing on how stakeholders influence implementation and sustainability of telecenter projects which is subjective as different people perceive things differently, therefore, the philosophy of phenomenology was chosen in this research as it is usually used in the social world of business. It is argued that business is too complex to lend itself to theorizing by definite laws in the same way as it is done in physical sciences.

The research used the deductive approach. The researcher used an existing theory of stakeholder management to explore the area under study. The research was a qualitative cross-sectional exploratory study. The study was a cross-sectional as the investigation was done at once due to limitation of time. Exploratory research was appropriate as the researcher was examining and investigating a new interest in stakeholder management of telecenters and the subject of study itself was relatively new.

The study targeted two out of the four multipurpose community telecenters under the ISRD project which are Vikwa telecenter in Kasungu and Khudze telecenter in Mwanza. The researcher used non-probability sampling methods such as: (a) purposive sampling method during identification of stakeholders; (b) convenience sampling technique when choosing the multi-purpose community telecenters; (c) snowballing method when identifying the stakeholders during data collection.

Since the data was qualitative in nature there were continuous conducting additional interviews until data saturation (until all are reached). The semi-structured interviews was chosen in this research because they gave more room for interviewee (than structured interview) to provide his or her own point of view of the research subject. These types of interview also helped to maintain consistency for topics covered with each interviewee because a number of people were involved as participants.

Focus groups were used because they sample the experiences of a wide variety of subjects in a relatively easy fashion. Focus groups provide an opportunity for participants to report their individual experiences, and also respond to the experiences of other group members.

4 Stakeholder Involvement in Telecenter Project

Most of the stakeholders were identified at the initial phase of the telecenter project at the community level. However, the process excluded Area Executive Committee (AEC), Area development Committee (ADC) and Village Development Committee (VDC). These are the major primary stakeholders in the local community responsible for requesting and monitoring developmental projects within the community. This process was contrary to the provision in the Decentralization Policy and Local Government Act of 1998 which recognizes local communities with traditional leaders and District Assembly. The telecenter projects failed to follow the lied down government decentralization policies in implementing the project and it was against community practices, culture and expectation.

Furthermore, the process was centrally to the recommendations made by different authors and projects implementers who have strongly argued to include key stakeholders in the developmental projects and follow the cultural or political practice of the community. There was need for community participation of target groups and understanding of the local political context [9, 25, 26].

The stakeholder management process was stopped at the identifications stage and did not formally escalate to behavior explanation, coalition analysis, management and conflict management for both telecenters. Specifically, some of the stakeholders who were left out during initial stages were not included at the later stage. In addition, the process lacked characterization of the stakeholders with regards to contributions needed from them, the expectations they have concerning rewards for delivering the contributions and their power in relation to the telecenter project. This suggests that telecenter projects implementers are unable to take action in the interest of all stakeholders and design a strategy on how to manage them [20, 27]. Freeman [20] further suggests that an organisation which does not understand who its stakeholders are has no process for dealing with their concerns and has no set of transaction for negotiating with them.

Although traditional leaders were consulted in the initial phase of the telecenter project, they were no longer consulted during other phases of the telecenter project. Consequently, the community leadership felt that the telecenter was the business for few individuals but not the community. This was felt strongly at Khudze Telecenter where the local leaders have praised the initial approach to the project but there was lack of coordination with the local leaders. They have claimed that the telecenter is the business for few individuals but not the community. Furthermore, when traditional leaders request for general performance reports of the telecenters, the Local Management Committee feel these request are beyond their mandate. This was noticed at Vikwa telecenter and the possible reasons for these misunderstanding could be from twofold.

The initial consultations lacked full community participation. Community participation is an active process by which beneficiaries influence the direction and execution of a development project with view to enhancing their well-being in terms of income, personal growth, self-reliance or other values they cherish [28]. Chigona et al. [2] point out that stakeholder consultations sometimes could be used merely as a political maneuver and not really meant to get the views of the stakeholders. Due to these the telecenter projects lack ownership by the community which feels that telecenters benefit few individuals especially those who work directly with the project. Sabien [29] argues that strong links with key stakeholders is vital to sustainability of telecenters and critical to longer term survival of the telecenter, particularly where contracts for service delivery are involved.

The project adopted a top-down communication approach with the Rapid Rural Appraisal in order to consult local communities because it is simple and quick to engage the community in an ICT developmental projects but it has great negative impact on the project. The top down approach lacks engagement with local communities which leads to lack of ownership which results into low usage or patronage of the telecenter project hence the supporting activities for local communities tend to suffer. Mosha [30] states that imposition of policies, projects concepts into local communities is unfavorable to local people who reject what is seemed to be an imposition from above. It is important to create comprehensive telecenter projects concepts with an involvement of the local people. Similarly, Rapid Rural Appraisal tools are designed to provide a quick snapshot of the make-up of communities, including wealth and other ranked differences, and to open the way to social and economic change [31]. However, these tools were criticized as they are mostly quick, and narrowly focused to be used for rural developmental projects [32].

The project being new in these rural communities, there was a need to choose the best approach which could promote full participations of the communities without ignoring the political context of the communities. Pade-Khene et al. [9] suggests a holistic approach to rural developmental projects which considers the critical Success factors for sustainability of the rural developmental projects. The holistic approach clarifies how the telecenter project can relate to the rural community and it is not implemented in isolation of the information systems and activities that make up a community [9].

The aim of any developmental project is to empower the local people and for this to take place, the local stakeholders must be committed to an activity and have a sense of ownership of it, as evidenced by their taking on responsibilities for the activity and its outcomes [25]. Ownership is a processes where local stakeholders take control and responsibility for the design, implementation, and monitoring of an activity [25].

The community sense of ownership at these telecenters is poor. There is indication that at both telecenter there is no ownership of the project however this could be differentiated between the two telecenters looking at responsibilities taken for each telecenter. The traditional leaders, the LMC members and the staff felt that the project is owned by MACRA and not the community as even after two years of operation, mainly because the decision making is still in the powers of MACRA. Specifically, the community at Khudze telecenter was only involved in the site identification and possible selection of committee while other things such as bricks and other building material were sources by the contractors. The implementation of the telecenters project was monitored by MACRA through a committee and no updates were sent to local leaders. This meant that the communities were not empowered to fully partic-ipate in the construction of the telecenter project which has led to complete reliance on MACRA. This let the community disjointed with the telecenter project. In addition this has led LMC, staff and traditional leaders to work in isolation with no recognition of political culture during the operation of the telecenter. There was no coordination among LMC, staff and traditional leaders on any issues as things were reported directly to MACRA.

Nerveless, communities at both telecenters expect that the telecenter would benefit the community. For example, they expect that the funds from the telecenter could be used to construct a school block or a borehole so that those who do not use the telecenter could indirectly benefit. However these expectations have not been met as MACRA has advised the telecenter managers not to do that. The foregoing suggests that MACRA should limit roles in management of telecenters and empower the local community to own the telecenters. Ballantyne [25] states that the stakeholder par-ticipation needs to start from the beginning of any project. External players (actors) that traditionally lead design and formulation phases need to limit their direct roles and responsibilities. They need to encourage local stakeholders to participate and take the lead. Furthermore, Colle and Roman [33] suggest that broad-based community participation is part of a telecenters mandate. The participation concept should try to address the following (a) Why is participation important to this project? (b) Who should participate? (c) How might people participate? (d) How much participation should be sought? (e) When should participation take place? (f) What incentives can be offered? [33].

There is challenge in management of these telecenters emerging from different sources. Although the structure of local management committee comprises ten members with two ex-officials from MACRA and District Councils for each telecenter [24], the study revealed that district council representatives have never attended any meeting together with MACRA. Furthermore, there has been no clarity on how frequent would the two institutions participate in the meetings. As a result, the telecenter projects have been isolated from District Council activities. It is therefore necessary to continuously involve the District Council so that they could monitor the telecenter projects after MACRA hand over the project to the community. In addition, they need to be trained on how to monitor these telecenters and the role of local management committee need to be clearly stated and procedure for renewal of mandate documented.

The Local Management Committee comprises the villagers with the risk of having members from the same family which raises governance issues on the management of the telecenter. Furthermore, the telecenters lack local ICT champion and the committees lack knowledge and exposure to services offered at these telecenters despite being trained once at the initial stage of the telecenter projects. It is advisable to choose local ICT champions who could understand the applications of these services with entrepreneurship skills as which can help to develop awareness, innovations and belief in the project objectives. The role of a ICT champion should not be equated to that of a full-time paid staff member; usually the role is on a part-time or volunteer basis (IDRC, 2004).

The findings further reveal that there were many issues that affected the operation of the telecenter hanging on infrastructure availability, quality of services, leadership, awareness, local participation and literacy and political interference at these telecenters. Specifically, the road network at Khudze posed a challenge for users to access the telecenter especially during rainy season. This is due to the location of the telecenters as it is situated several kilometers off main road at the headquarters for Traditional Authority Kanduku. Although, the location for the Khudze Telecenter was obviously not ideal for the sustainability of the telecenter, the community chose the location which is close to the Headquarters of Traditional Authority while neglecting factors that could affect its sustainability. It could easily be concluded that the community chose the location due to either lack of knowledge of the telecenter or to honor or respect their Traditional Authority as these consultations meetings were being conducted at same place. To avoid such things [26] suggest that the community should be encouraged to participate in the following (a) determining the goals and benefits of the project, (b) selecting target groups that represent the social groups (women, youth, local leaders) in the community to participate in the planning, analysis, implementation and evaluation of the project, (c) discussing the limitations and risks of the project, especially with regard to the impact it has on the social and cultural norms of the community, (d) encouraging participation to empower the community to express their local needs and requirements with regard to ICT use as an enabler of development.

Some local people are afraid to use the telecenters due to the type of the building and furniture which is installed in these telecenters. The building is of high standard and the furniture which is installed has the high quality as such district councils wanted these structures to be in the town as they could change the face of the township instead of putting in the villages. Most locals are afraid to use even to touch a computer as it looks very strange. This shows that there were no consultations with the community on what type of the buildings could be constructed in terms of the standard and the furniture to put in place. Colle and Roman [33] suggest a research as a tool for finding out the needs for the community, participation and a systematic, persistent effort toward community awareness about telecenter and ICT.

5 Conclusion

There were different stakeholders identified at different levels at the initial stage of these telecenter projects. Different approaches were used to identify these stakeholders at both national and community levels. However, despite these approaches it was found that some key stakeholders were missed at the initial phase of the project. The stakeholders expressed different behaviour and expectations towards both telecenters. These ranged from the originality, the services ownership, consultations and the general management of the telecenters. The stakeholders were interacting at different stage of the project. However the general findings show that there was more inter-action at the initial phase of the project. Furthermore, as time went by, other stake-holders were being left out in the other phases of the project. The stakeholders were involved at different stage of the project. The involvement was being limited to few stakeholders as time went during the stages of the projects. The stakeholders expressed that some of the factors that could hinder sustainability of these telecenters that could be: (a) location of telecenter, (b) accessibility to the telecenter, (c) quality of Service offered at telecenter, (d) leadership at the telecenter, (e) awareness, (f) local participation, (g) level of literacy and (h) economic activities.

References

1. Bailur, S.: Using stakeholder theory to analyze telecenter projects. Inf. Technol. Int. Dev. 3(3), 61–80 (2006)
2. Chigona, W., et al.: Investigating the impact of stakeholder management on the implementation of a public access project: case of smart cape. S. Afr. J. Bus. Manag. 41(2), 39–49 (2010)
3. Colle, R.: Memo to telecenter planners. Electron. J. Inf. Syst. Dev. Countries 21(1), 1–13 (2005)

4. ITU.: World telecommunication/ICT development report 2010 – monitoring the WSIS targets, Geneva (2010). http://www.itu.int/pub/D-IND-WTDR-2010. Accessed 27 June 2012

5. Laudon, K.C., Laudon, J.P.: Management Information Systems, 11th edn. London Pearson Education LTD., London (2010)

6. Louis, F.: Enhancing the livelihoods of the rural poor through ICT: a knowledge map. South Africa Country Report, South Africa (2008). www.infodev.org/en/Document.516.pdf. Accessed 26 Jan 2013

7. MACRA.: ICT Policy implementation overview - telecenters status in Malawi. In: Telecenter Managers Workshop, Blantyre (2012)

8. McNamara, K.S.: Information and communication technologies, poverty and development: learning from experience. World Bank, Geneva. http://icttoolkit.infodev.org/files/1039_file_Learning_From_Experience.PDF (2003). Accessed 26, Jan 2013

9. Pade-Khene, C., Mallinson, B., Sewry, D.: Sustainable rural ICT project management practice for developing countries: investigating the Dwesa and RUMEP projects. Inf. Technol. Dev. 17(3), 187–212 (2011). http://www.tandfonline.com/doi/abs/10.1080/02681102.2011.568222. Accessed 29 Oct 2012

10. Perrini, F., Tencati, A.: Sustainability and stakeholder management: the need for new corporate performance evaluation and reporting systems. Bus. Strategy Environ. 308, 296–308 (2006). http://onlinelibrary.wiley.com/doi/10.1002/bse.538/abstract. Accessed 27 Jan 2013

11. Rajalekshmi, G.K.: E-governance services through telecenters : the role of human. Inf. Technol. Int. Dev. 4(1), 19–35 (2008)

12. Roman, R., Colle, R.: Themes and issues in telecentre sustainability. Institute for Development Policy and Management, p. 20 (2002). Available at: htt. Accessed 28 Oct 2012

13. UN-ESCAP.: Guidebook on developing community E-centres in rural areas: based on the Malaysian experience. Economic and Social Commission for Asia and the Pacific, New York (2006)

14. Wellenius, B.: Sustainable telecenters: a guide for government policy. The World Bank Discussion Paper (2003). http://rru.worldbank.org/Documents/PublicPolicyJournal/251Welle-121302.pdf. Accessed 26 Jan 2013

15. World Bank.: Information communication technology. Sector strategy Approach Paper (2011). http://siteresources.worldbank.org/INTICTSTRATEGY/Resources/2010-12-27_ICT_Sector_Strategy_Approach_Paper_EN.pdf. Accessed 17 Aug 2012

16. MCA.: Report on evaluation of the performance of telecenters in Malawi, Blantyre (2012)

17. Gómez, R., Hunt, P., Lamoureux, E.: Enchanted by telecentres: a critical look at universal access to information technologies for international development. In: New IT and Inequality. International Development Research Center (IDRC), University of Maryland (1999)

18. Jensen, M., Esterhuysen, A.: The community telecentre cookbook for Africa recipes for self-sustainability. United Nations Educational Scientific and Cultural Organization, Paris (2001)

19. Rega, I.: What do local people think about telecentres? University of Lugano (2010)

20. Freeman, E.R.: Strategic Management: A Stakeholder Approach. Cambridge University Press, New York (2010)

21. Freeman, R.E., Wicks, A.C., Parmar, B.: Stakeholder theory and the corporate objective revisited? Org. Sci. 15(3), 364–369 (2004). http://orgsci.journal.informs.org/cgi/doi/10.1287/orsc.1040.0066. Accessed 18 July 2012

22. Carroll, A.B., Buchholtz, A.K.: Business & Society, Ethics and Stakeholder Management, 8th edn. South-Western Cengage Learning, Mason (2012)
23. Bhattacherjee, A.: Social Science Research: Principles, Methods, and Practices, 2nd edn. Creative Commons Attribution, Zurich (2012)
24. MACRA.: ICT for Sustainable Rural Development (ISRD) Project - Malawi -Field Survey Activity Review of Research Findings Workshop, Blantyre (2006)
25. Ballantyne, P.: Ownership and partnership: keys to sustaining ICT-enabled development activities. IICD Research Brief no 8 (2003). http://editor.iicd.org/files/Brief8.pdf. Accessed 31 May 2013
26. Pade-Khene, C.: An investigation of ICT project management techniques for sustainable ICT projects in rural development. Rhodes University (2006). http://eprints.ru.ac.za/900/. Accessed 31 May 2013
27. Jepsen, A.L., Eskerod, P.: Stakeholder analysis in projects: challenges in using current guidelines in the real world. Int. J. Project Manag. 27(4), 335–343 (2009). http://linkinghub. elsevier.com/retrieve/pii/S0263786308000549. Accessed 6 Oct 2012
28. Paul, S.: Community participation in development projects. World Bank, USA (1987). http://www-wds.worldbank.org/servlet/WDSContentServer/IW3P/IB/1999/09/21/0001788 30_98101903572729/Rendered/PDF/multi_page.pdf. Accessed 2 June 2013
29. Sabien, B.: Some principles of financial sustainability based on telecentres and a telecentre network in Australia. J. Dev. Commun. (2001). http://telecentres.isoc.am/references/info/ jdc-sabien.doc. Accessed 2 July 2013
30. Mosha, L.: Imposition of architectural and spatial planning concepts into local dwelling culture. Prime J. Bus. Admin. Manag. (2011). http://www.primejournal.org/BAM/pdf/ 2012/jun/Livin.pdf. Accessed 31 May 2013
31. Chambers, R.: The origins and practice of participatory rural appraisal. World Dev. 22(7), 953–969 (1994). http://linkinghub.elsevier.com/retrieve/pii/0305750X94901414
32. Cooke, B., Kothari, U.: Participation the New Tyranny?. Zed Books, London (2001)
33. Colle, R.D., Roman, R.: The telecenter environment in 2002. J. Dev. Commun. 12 (2001). http://www.communicationforsocialchange.org/body-of-knowledge.php?id=2229

The NOAH Project: Giving a Chance
to Threatened Species in Africa with UAVs

Miguel A. Olivares-Mendez[1], Tegawendé F. Bissyandé[1,2]([✉]),
Kannan Somasundar[1], Jacques Klein[1], Holger Voos[1], and Yves Le Traon[1]

[1] SnT, University of Luxembourg, Luxembourg, Luxembourg
{miguel.olivaresmendez,tegawende.bissyande,somasundar.kannan,
jacques.klein,holger.voos,yves.letraon}@uni.lu
[2] FasoLabs, Ouagadougou, Burkina Faso

Abstract. Organized crime now targets one of the most precious wealth
in Africa, the wild life. The most affected by the poaching are the Big 5,
whose survival requires attention and efforts from everyone, in accordance
to his own expertise. Just as Noah (A patriarchal character in Abrahamic
religions) was tasked to save every species from the Genesis flood, we envision the NOAH Project to (re)make natural parks as a safe haven. This
endeavor requires efficient and effective surveillance which is now facilitated by the use of UAVs. We take this approach further by proposing
the use of ICT algorithms to automate surveillance. The proposed intelligent system could inspect a bigger area, recognize potential threats and
be manage by non-expert users, reducing the expensive resources that are
needed by developing countries to address the problem.

1 Introduction

It takes about 10 min for a poacher to kill and dehorn a rhino. This period of
time is too short that poachers are assured to strike continuously if significant
and effective efforts are not put in place to deter them. For example, just in
South Africa, two rhinos are dehorned everyday. Park rangers are indeed faced
with the challenges of efficiently surveilling a territory that can be extremely
large for careful and consistent patrol. South African Rangers now have eyes in
the sky thanks to Air Rangers, small Unmanned Aerial Vehicles (UAVs) that
are used to cover more land by providing live video feed of the terrain. While the
proposed approach can be improved by using more adapted technologies that
we will discuss, it opens the road for more efficient and cheaper systems using
ICT knowledge.

ICT4D projects have recently proven that they can leverage high-tech products
and sophisticated computer and communication algorithms to deliver
solutions to the problems of developing areas. Mostly such solutions aim at addressing the cost for achieving equivalent results with traditional means. In a previous
work [1] it was shown that ICT4D could also leverage directly the cultural model of
Africa to adopt technologies and paradigms that may appear inadequate in developed countries where they were born. We take further this notion in this paper to

© Institute for Computer Sciences, Social Informatics and Telecommunications Engineering 2014
T.F. Bissyandé and G. van Stam (Eds.): AFRICOMM 2013, LNICST 135, pp. 198–208, 2014.
DOI: 10.1007/978-3-319-08368-1_24

advocate the use of equipments that, at first glance, can appear to be a luxury for developing countries. Examples of such equipments are the Unmanned Aerial Vehicles (UAVs) which are now getting the front position in robotics research. Miniaturization and power increase of electronic components and sensors during the last decade has greatly participated to improve the usability of UAVs while leading at the same time to significant cuts in the cost for acquiring units of such vehicles. Consequently, in developing areas, NGOs and governments can now invest in these vehicles to address specific civilian issues.

1.1 Motivation

Human brigades cannot manage the thorough surveillance of very large national parks in Africa. The huge area of the wildlife reserves and their reduced budgets make it impossible to carry surveillance strategies that are efficient for protecting various animals against poachers. UAV capabilities as well as their affordability and improved usability make them an ideal tool for surveillance tasks. Indeed, the eye in the sky gives a big advantage against illegal hunters who now manage to evade traditional surveillance methods. A UAV can inspect a big area in few minutes, when the same area would be covered in more than one hour by humans. Another point in favor of unmanned fixed wings is the reduced noise that they produce during operation flying, contrary to army helicopters, drastically limiting the possibilities for being detected by poachers. Furthermore, autonomous flight and visual detection would reduce the dependency on expert knowledge to use this kind of vehicles. One of the aim of the NOAH project is that the aircrafts could be used by the current employees of the natural parks, being a simple system that can be used by non-expert users. The autonomous detection of potential poaching situations will also allow to simplify and reduce the need for humans to supervise the functionning of the system.

1.2 Constraints

The current state of art on vision algorithms allows to make autonomous detection based in color, edge and corner detection, optical flow, shape and other approaches. The big issue of the computer vision is to manage the light changes. There are some strategies to solve this problem attached to the specific task to solve. In our case the principal problem is not this, but it also have to take into account. The poachers would like not to be detected as animals or natural parks' guards. Because of this extra complexity of this specific scenario, the color detection could not be used. The visual algorithms that must be used in this approach have to be focused in the movement detection of people or trucks and the edge and corners detection of the poachers vehicles.

This paper. We discuss in this paper the need and objectives of the NOAH project, establishing the ground for ICT4D-oriented research on UAVs. We make different contributions including:

1. a brief description of UAVs and their capabilities for fighting poaching. We also discuss already implemented approaches using UAVs to mark their deficiencies and highlight the possibilities in ICT for addressing existing challenges.
2. a discussion on the different aspects of the NOAH project. In particular we provide in-depth details on how we envision an autonomous patrol system and how ICT will help to autonomously detect poaching events and track poachers as they flee the scenes of crime.

The remainder of this paper is organized as follows. Section 2 introduces information about related work and how the battle against poaching was revolutionized by the appearance of UAVs in the parks sky. Section 3 provides details on the NOAH project and what we hope to achieve as well as the ICT means and techniques that will be leveraged to address the different challenges of autonomous surveillance of natural parks. In Sect. 4 we outline different open questions for a successful course of the NOAH project. These questions are noted to create a research synergy around the use of ICTs to fight for a precious heritage in Africa with a high response time and reduced costs. Finally, Sect. 5 concludes this work.

2 Unmanned Aerial Vehicles and Anti Poaching

In this section, we introduce UAVs for civilian use nd provide general information about their characteristics. Subsequently we present the SPOTS-Air Rangers for anti-poaching with UAVs.

2.1 Unmanned Aerial Vehicles

Each day the use of UAVs is more prolific for civil applications. Cost reductions of sensors and the availability of new prototypes that are easier to control have indeed contributed to make UAVs affordable. In parallel, the research community in sensor detection and tracking, navigation and control have recently made great advances. Nowadays most UAVs are connected to a ground station that users rely on to send real-time commands to the aircraft so as to modify its trajectory or access the feed of the on board camera. Some of them can carry a CPU on board to process in situ the information acquired by embarked sensors and modify their trajectory accordingly. Some examples are [2,3] which use UAVs with rotary wings and vision to track objects, [4–7] which can perform autonomous landing tasks of a helicopter, or implement navigation and control systems for see-and-avoid tasks [8–10].

UAVs can be equipped with fixed or rotary wings. Just like their manned versions, each unmanned vehicle has its advantages and disadvantages that must be checked based on the mission to accomplish. In the specific case of UAV for anti poaching, the best solution is to use fixed wings, because they allow to cover a bigger area with less power or gas consumption. Furthermore, such wing type delivers reduced noise from the aircraft, constituting another advantage against the vertical take off and landing (VTOL).

There are today around the world numerous companies that manufacture UAVs with fixed wings. The specifications however are different from one company to another. Usually the fixed winds include one propeller that could be located at the front or the back part. The airframe of the UAV could be manufactured with different kinds of materials: some of them are flexible foam [?], fiber-reinforced polymer (FRP), glass-reinforced plastic (GRP) or balsa wood. On-board the UAV could be installed a set of sensors depending on the application. A basic set of sensors includes an inertial measure unit (IMU), GPS, pressure sensor and compas. Other sensors such as normal, thermal or omni-directional cameras, sonars, lasers, could also be included. Depending on the application, a certain equilibrium must be reached between the propeller power, airframe material, sensor on board and endurance, stability and sensing.

2.2 SPOTS-Air Rangers

To the best of our knowledge, the only working approach that relies on UAVs for fighting against poaching is the excellent initiative conducted by SPOTS-Air Rangers [11]. As is mentioned in their webpage, they are a *"registered Section 21 Conservation Company focussed purely on the conservation and the protection of any and all threatened species"*. The company is using the UAVs in Africa, specifically South Africa, for the specific task of poacher detection. They use fixed wings aircrafts equipped with a high quality thermal camera, among others sensors needed to fly. The aircrafts are provided by *Shadowview* which is also a non profit organization providing multiple UAS solutions for conservation and civilian projects [12]. The main goal of Air Rangers is to participate in the fight against poaching, through detection of potential poachers. The monitor of the capture cages with zero impact to the wildlife in the area. They also use the UAVs to track animals and thus improve the wildlife census system. Furthermore, this company applied their aircrafts for burn assessment and biomass management. Based on what we could extract from SPOTS' website, they are not using any software for autonomous detection of poaching situations, by e.g., detecting poachers, vehicles, camps and strange behaviors. No specific algorithms to increase the effectiveness of the patrol trajectories is shown in their website too.

The excellent work of this company and its project in Africa could be improved with the automation techniques that are discussed in our work and presented in this paper. Our objective is to increase the number of detected poachers, and improving the effectiveness and efficiency of autonomous flights.

2.3 Real-World Problem Statement

In this section we revisit the problems that practitioners face when trying to protect the wild life heritage of Africa. We show how human expert-controlled UAVs have shifted the challenges of natural parks, then highlight the introduced challenges as well as the shortcomings that we plan to address in the NOAH project. We discuss two dimensions of the real-world problems that could be alleviated by autonomous surveillance.

Can we assure surveillance Anytime, Anywhere? National parks in Africa cover very large bands of lands that can be hard to access in some parts. For example, the Kruger National Park covers an area of $19,480\,km^2$ where more than 2 rhino is killed everyday. To survey this park, rangers rely on airplane and helicopter patrols and on foot and vehicular patrols. The former is noisy, thus significantly reducing the element of surprise on poachers, while the latter is too slow and is aggravated by the vegetation which affects visibility. Furthermore, surveillance is drastically compromised during the night.

The introduction of UAVs greatly reduced the difficulties mentioned above by improving the capability for air rangers to quietly survey the areas, day and night, using cameras. Thus, with UAVs, such as the Air Ranger aircrafts, poachers can be detected before they act, and can be more efficiently tracked.

Nonetheless, to the best of our knowledge, these aircrafts can only survey parts of the national parks, i.e. only areas where the ground pilots are taking the UAVs. Furthermore, detection of poachers and poaching events is still performed by humans who visioned surveillance footage, and are thus prone to distraction and false alarms because of fatigue-caused confusion.

What response-time can the surveillance brigade guarantee? Surveillance by human brigades had the advantage of being near the crime scene when detection of poaching event or of the poachers occurs. Thus, they could readily strike. With UAVs, response-time has become critical as the people who actually "see" the poaching are located remotely and must manually use pilot the aircraft to follow the poachers until they are intercepted by park rangers.

There is therefore a need to automate the detection of poaching and the alert-system as well as the tracking of poachers to improve efficiency of anti-poaching task-force by increasing the response-time. Intelligent systems would indeed directly send positions of the crime scene, and of the poachers, as well as triangulate the best locations for interception, the whole autonomously.

How many people can we afford as surveillance personnel? To cover the 19 thousands km^2 of the Kruger park, authorities must train and involve a huge number of park rangers, who put their lives in danger while patrolling. In particular, during the night, a suitable time for poaching, park rangers cannot be efficient nor can they be safe.

The Air Rangers have leveled the field by reducing the need for human patrol during the night. An Air Ranger aircraft can perform the patrol in replacement of 80 human rangers at night. Unfortunately, each of these aircrafts still requires 1 technician and 1 camera operator for its flight. Since several aircrafts are necessary to cover the entire park, a new specific personnel, with expert training on UAVs, will be required. With automation, the current human rangers employed by the parks will be able to maneuver the system seamlessly.

3   Autonomous Aerial Surveillance for African National Parks

We present in this section the different parts of the autonomous aerial system that we envision for patrolling huge areas of National Parks in Africa. The system aims at reducing time and cost investments while increasing the effectiveness of the current surveillance system in such areas. First, we discuss the autonomous patrol system to improve the efficiency of the surveillance task. Then, we provide insights on the visual algorithms that could be used for the detection of poachers and potential poaching situations. We highlight points that will be underlined in the open research questions of Sect. 4.

3.1   Autonomous Patrol System

Nowadays the huge zones of National parks in Africa is inspected, in most of the cases, by a limited number of humans patrolling in group, using ground vehicles and binoculars and facing constant danger in face of unscrupulous poachers. One potential contribution of the NOAH project is to reduce the number of people needed to cover the different parts of the Natural Parks. Furthermore, the use of the UAVs will significantly reduce the amount of time needed to check if there are potential poachers in a specific sector of the Park. Finally, from a bird view it should be easier to detect potential poaching situations.

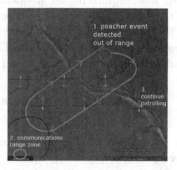

Fig. 1. Autonomous patrol flight plan - the entire area will be inspected in one round

Fig. 2. Covering a extended area the UAV come back to report an incident when the detection has done out of range

The autonomous patrol system consists in the use of any GNSS[1] signal to define a square area to patrol (Fig. 1). Given two or four GNSS positions in a map an automated UAV can patrol the area in an efficient way and provide a visual feedback from the sky of inspected area. In places where such signals are

---

[1] Global Navigation Satellite System.

lacking for navigating over the overflown area, an alternative would be to install beacons/antennas that will enable the UAVs to "know" their positions. During patrol, a supervisor who is checking the image from the onboard camera could select a specific position if any suspicious situation is detected. In this case the UAV will fly around this area to get more information. More than one position could be selected as highly suspicious areas (HSA) so that UAVs can modify their paths to focus on these areas. Then, once a poaching situation is detected the coordinates of its exact position will be stored, and the supervisor could send the command to the UAV to come back to the home position, or to stay on patrol above the crime scene, or to continue patrolling the rest of the initial selected area.

The system could flies autonomously covering a big area, being the UAV not always inside the communications range. In the case that the UAV detect autonomously a potential poaching event, it will come back suddenly inside the communications range to communicate the incident. After that it will continue patrolling from the place of the incident detected. An example of this behavior is shown in Fig. 2.

The use of dedicated aircrafts to track animals, as in the SPOTS project, could be performed to prevent poaching too. Indeed, it is possible to store in a database common paths of animals in the park in order to create a map of high risk areas (HRA). Furthermore, using GPS tracker signal of animals could also help specify flight plans for UAVs which will then be performing bodyguard tasks. HSA and HRA stored information could further be used as a set of map points that require higher frequency surveillance. This is a typical example of the traveling-salesman problem and there are a set of algorithms present in the literature that could be used to improve the effectiveness of the system, including the more recent Cross-Entropy method [13]. An example of a flight based on interest points (HSA and HRA) is shown in Fig. 3.

3.2 Autonomous Detection and Tracking of Potential Poaching Events

The second part of the NOAH project is to provide an autonomous system to detect potential poachers, their vehicles and camps. Once one of these items is detected the system will send an alarm signal to the ground/mobile station. The system will furthermore be able to track potential poachers autonomously if the aircraft is requested to do so. The best way to perform an autonomous detection of such kind of situation is to rely on a camera.

Advances in vision algorithms in the last decade have pushed cameras in front as the most suitable sensor in robotics. A camera gives a wide range view of the environment of the robot with a reduced equipment. Furthermore, similarities with the human vision sensor gives an advantage that information obtained from this sensor can be easily understood and analyzed, unlike other sensors such as sonars and lasers. The literature already includes various state-of-the art algorithms that can be easily adapted to suit the specific needs of the NOAH project.

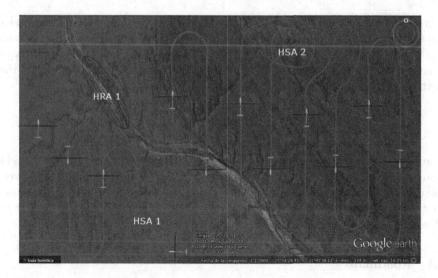

Fig. 3. Autonomous patrol focus on high risk areas (HRA) and high suspicious areas (HSA)

In general, poachers are more likely to kill animals during the night when animals are more vulnerable and ranger brigade cannot be efficient. For this reason the aircrafts in the NOAH project must integrate a thermal camera for the visual detection. With this kind of camera, it is easy to detect, recognize and track humans, vehicles or camps which emit thermal energy.

For the visual detection of object shapes, most of the algorithms are based on the RANSAC paradigm [14] and the Hough transform [15,16], and the generalization by Ballard of Hough transform for the detection of arbitrary shapes [17]. An issue with these techniques is the high computational cost that they imply. A common solution in computer vision is then to use one or more edge detection algorithm to reduce the image information to be processed by the shape detection algorithm. The most used algorithms for the edge detection are the Robert's Cross operator [18], Sobel operator [19], laplacian of gaussian filter [20] and the Canny's edge detection algorithm [21]. The latter is the one that is selected in most real time applications such as those that will be implemented in the NOAH project.

Use of edge detection increases the possibilities of detecting vehicles, camps (tent edges) and rifles, since straight lines reinforce edge and border detection. Furthermore, it is a known fact, that in most of the cases, objects with straight lines are productions of human activities, because there are very few cases of that sort in nature. Finally, detection of poacher is based on a simple difference between humans and animals: animals have two more legs than humans that can be easily differentiated on a thermal image acquisition.

Another important part of the NOAH project is to develop an easy human machine interface (HMI) so that the system could be used by non technician users. The different autonomous modules that will be developed will make easier the selection between one and the other by the HMI. The HMI will then give all the information needed for the user in real time as well as visual shortcuts to change to a new task or to modify the trajectory of the aircraft, making it the next best weapon that will be provided to park rangers.

4   Open Research Questions

The NOAH project envisions to fully automate the surveillance of parks to fight against poaching but also to participate in medical care of sick animals. However, to successfully complete this endeavor, there are various ICT research avenues that must be undertaken by a research task force that includes researchers from IT as well as veterinarians, rangers, etc.

4.1   Roadmaps

In this section we enumerate a few ICT research questions for the NOAH project:

Machine learning. For automating the recognition of poaching event, and of poachers about to act or after the crime, there is a need to train UAVs. With machine learning, algorithms can be developed to help UAVs autonomously recognize unusual events or aspects in the park. Furthermore, ad hoc heuristics must be implemented to empower UAVs to:

- differentiate between humans (e.g., between a hunter/poacher and a hiker/ tourist)
- differentiate a sick animal from a resting one

Indeed, while vision detection algorithms can help highlight anomalies, only machine learning will allow us to reduce the number of false alarms, and thus focus the allocated resources into the efficiency of a smart autonomous anti-poaching system.

Global Positioning. Good GPS coverage is not guaranteed in many parts of Africa. Yet, for UAVs to be able to alert human rangers on ongoing poaching events, they need to be able to provide the positions of the event so that the nearest brigade can move on site. To overcome the challenge of poor GPS coverage, we could setup and hide beacons in strategic places of the parks allowing UAVs to triangulate and confirm locally-comprehensive positions.

Air-Ground Liaison. Finally, a challenge remains in the way ground stations communicate with UAVs when those go too far to patrol autonomously and need to report a serious event without disrupting the course of their patrol. This challenge can be overcome by the use of long-range WiFi which is commonly used for low-cost, unregulated point-to-point connections. There is also a possibility to use the operator network to send SMS with coordinates which will be extracted and used by applications in a ranger's smartphone.

4.2 Reuse of Domain-Specific Knowledge

In the course of discussion for the kick-off of the NOAH project, we agreed that ICT alone, even with the most sophisticated techniques, cannot overcome the challenges of anti-poaching systems. There is a need to try to leverage knowledge from the context of developing regions and from the field of animal behavior. For example, simple heuristics to drive the autonomous patrol of UAVs can include taking into account details such as:

- the convergence of hyenas: these animals are known to be among the first to notice that another animal, even a much stronger one, is sick or in danger. If UAVs can spot such a convergence, they have an indication of where to focus patrol tasks.
- the divergence of animal herds: in the wild, animals usually move in groups. When a danger (e.g., a poacher) is flared, there is a general stamped which is more easily recognized by vision algorithms.

5 Concluding Remarks

Animal poaching is threatening various species in Africa, even those that are living in national parks. With the advent of UAVs for civil use, the fight against poachers has gained a new breath. With the NOAH project we plan to automate patrol with UAVs so as to cover a bigger area, require less expert personnel, and reduce costs while delivering effective detection of poaching events.

In this position paper we have motivated the NOAH project and discussed how it will serve to protect Africa's wild life heritage. Numerous challenges for a successful completion of the project were enumerated, and we have identified ICT research roadmaps that will be followed in the course of the project. With this paper, we hope to create a synergy of ICT research around a real-world development problem that is poaching.

References

1. Ouoba, J., Bissyandé, T.F.: Leveraging the cultural model for opportunistic networking in Sub-Saharan Africa. In: Jonas, K., Rai, I.A., Tchuente, M. (eds.) AFRICOMM 2012. LNICST, vol. 119, pp. 163–173. Springer, Heidelberg (2013)
2. Olivares-Mendez, M.A., Campoy, P., Martinez, C., Mondragon, I.: A pan-tilt camera fuzzy vision controller on an unmanned aerial vehicle. In: IEEE/RSJ International Conference on Intelligent Robots and Systems, IROS 2009, pp. 2879–2884, October 2009
3. Dobrokhodov, V.N., Kaminer, I.I., Jones, K.D., Ghabcheloo, R.: Vision-based tracking and motion estimation for moving targets using small UAVs. In: American Control Conference, 2006, p. 6, June 2006
4. Shakernia, O., Ma, Y., Koo, T.J., John, T., Sastry, S.: Landing an unmanned air vehicle: vision based motion estimation and nonlinear control. Asian J. Control 1, 128–145 (1999)

5. Saripalli, S., Montgomery, J.F., Sukhatme, G.S.: Vision-based autonomous landing of an unmanned aerial vehicle. In: IEEE International Conference on Robotics and Automation, 2002 Proceedings, ICRA '02, vol. 3, pp. 2799–2804 (2002)

6. Saripalli, S., Sukhatme, G.S.: Landing a helicopter on a moving target. In: Proceedings of IEEE International Conference on Robotics and Automation, pp. 2030–2035, Rome, Italy, April 2007

7. Olivares-Mendez, M.A., Mondragon, I.F., Campoy, P., Martinez, C.: Fuzzy controller for uav-landing task using 3d-position visual estimation. In: 2010 IEEE International Conference on Fuzzy Systems (FUZZ), pp. 1–8, July 2010

8. Olivares-Mendez, M.A., Mejias, L., Campoy, P., Mellado-Bataller, I.: Cross-entropy optimization for scaling factors of a fuzzy controller: a see-and-avoid approach for unmanned aerial systems. J. Intell. Robot. Syst. **69**, 189–205 (2013)

9. Zhihai, H., Lyer, R.V., Chandler, P.R.: Vision-based UAV flight control and obstacle avoidance. In: Proceedings of the American Control Conference, p. 5, June 2006

10. Beyeler, A., Zufferey, J.-C., Floreano, D.: Vision-based control of near-obstacle fight. Auton. Robots **27**(3), 201–219 (2009)

11. Spots-air rangers. http://www.spots.org.za/ (2013)

12. Shadowview. http://www.shadowview.org (2013)

13. De Boer, P.-T., Kroese, D.P., Mannor, S., Rubinstein, R.Y.: A tutorial on the cross-entropy method. Ann. Oper. Res. **134**(1), 19–67 (2005)

14. Bolles, R.C., Fischler, M.A.: A ransac-based approach to model fitting and its application to finding cylinders in range data. In: Proceedings of the 7th International Joint Conference on Artificial Intelligence - Volume 2, IJCAI'81, pp. 637–643, San Francisco, CA, USA. Morgan Kaufmann Publishers Inc. (1981)

15. Hough, P.V.C.: Method and means of recognizing complex patterns (1962)

16. Duda, R.O., Hart, P.E.: Use of the hough transformation to detect lines and curves in pictures. Commun. ACM **15**(1), 11–15 (1972)

17. Ballard, D.H.: Generalizing the hough transform to detect arbitrary shapes. In: Fischler, M.A., Firschein, O. (eds.) Readings in Computer Vision: Issues, Problems, Principles, and Paradigms, pp. 714–725. Morgan Kaufmann Publishers Inc., San Francisco (1987)

18. Chickanosky, V., Mirchandani, G.: Wreath products for edge detection. In: Proceedings ICASSP 1998, pp. 2953–2956 (1998)

19. Ying-Dong, Q., Cheng-Song, C., San-Ben, C., Jin-Quan, L.: A fast subpixel edge detection method using sobel-zernike moments operator. Image Vis. Comput. **23**(1), 11–17 (2005)

20. Kamgar-Parsi, B., Rosenfeld, A.: Optimally isotropic laplacian operator. Trans. Image Proc. **8**(10), 1467–1472 (1999)

21. Ding, L., Goshtasby, A.: On the canny edge detector. Pattern Recogn. **34**, 721–725 (2001)

Geographic Information System as a Tool for Enriching Drug Logistics Information at District Level in Malawi: Challenges on Data Quality

Patrick Albert Chikumba[✉]

Department of Computing and Information Technology,
University of Malawi-The Polytechnic, Private Bag 303, Blantyre 3, Malawi
patrick_chikumba@yahoo.com

Abstract. A well-functioning logistics management information system (LMIS) provides decision makers throughout a supply chain with accurate, timely, and appropriate data for managing and monitoring flow of supplies, accounting for products in supply chain, reducing supply imbalances, and improving cost-effectiveness but LMIS, whether manual or automated, seems to be one of the weakest links in the logistics chain in developing countries. District pharmacies in Malawi use a computerised information system to monitor the flow of products from a warehouse to health service delivery points and determine understocked or overstocked products at each health facility. Currently, all drug logistics information reports are in tabular forms. The Geographic Information System (GIS) can help health and drug logistics officers to get additional spatial information, such as locations of health facilities and environmental factors, to the existing reports in the form of maps. This paper discusses some challenges on quality of drug logistics data for decision making with emphasis on place and time utilities. It could be very important to use also maps from the GIS to enrich existing information especially when place and time are concerned since these utilities are very critical in logistics.

Keywords: Drug LMIS · GIS · Rights of LMIS · Place and time utilities · Feedback in drug LMIS · Quality of LMIS data · Problems in drug LMIS

1 Introduction

Improved availability of the essential drug supplies depends on effective logistics systems. A well-functioning logistics management information system (LMIS) provides decision makers throughout a supply chain with accurate, timely, and appropriate data for managing and monitoring the flow of supplies, accounting for products in supply chain, reducing supply imbalances, and improving cost-effectiveness. In Malawi, there is a well established logistics management system which is the medical supply system of inventory management and recording and reporting for health commodities which ensures that all Malawians are able to receive products they need, and receive quality treatment when they visit a health facility. Health commodities

© Institute for Computer Sciences, Social Informatics and Telecommunications Engineering 2014
T.F. Bissyandé and G. van Stam (Eds.): AFRICOMM 2013, LNICST 135, pp. 209–218, 2014.
DOI: 10.1007/978-3-319-08368-1_25

move from major stores down to health facilities while the drug logistics information moves from health facilities to upper levels.

Malawi like most other countries in Sub-Saharan Africa relies mainly on the public sector for delivery of health care services to its citizens. Ministry of Health (MoH), with the support of donors, has designed a health commodity delivery system aimed at improving service delivery to clients. Logistics management information system (LMIS), whether manual or automated, seems to be one of the weakest links in the logistics chain in developing countries which requires a lot of attention. There are so many problems that exist in the drug logistics management in developing countries which result in shortages and uneven distribution of drugs, among others.

Currently, district pharmacies use a computerised Information System named Supply Chain Manager which manages supply chain information in the health commodity logistics management. It helps drug logistics and health program managers determine which health facilities are understocked or overstocked among other information. Reports generated from this system are distributed to different users such as district health officers (DHO), regional medical stores (RMS) and stakeholders on monthly basis and on request. Although there is the well-established drug LMIS, it seems there are problems on the supply of drugs and other health commodities to health facilities. Information on reports generated from this system is only in a tabular form. It is necessary for drug logistics managers to have information about actual locations of health facilities, road networks and other spatial information for their day-to-day decision making. The Geographic Information Systems (GIS) can be used in this case to provide such information.

The Geographic Information Systems (GIS) can be used in the drug (LMIS) with the aim for enriching drug logistics information for drug logistics and health managers at a district level in Malawi. The managers can use the GIS to get additional information to existing reports in the form of maps, which would show actual locations of health facilities, and other spatial information including road networks. Therefore, this paper discusses whether, or not, the drug logistics information is in a form suitable for decision making with emphasis on place and time utilities and how maps generated by the GIS can enrich the drug logistics information.

2 Drug Logistics Management Information Systems

Drugs and medical supplies are essential commodity for delivery of health services. The lack of drugs has been shown to discourage utilization of public health facilities [11]. Availability of drug supplies is essential element in the delivery of quality, integrated health services [17]. The improved availability of affordable essential drugs, vaccines, and contraceptives depends on effective logistics systems to move essential commodities down the supply chain to the service delivery point, ultimately, to the end user [3]. Beith et. al. [2] emphasise that a good LMIS ensures the right quantity at the right time and at the right place.

Beith et. al. [2] defines the logistics system as the coordination of various organisations and functions to source, procure, and deliver goods and services to the customer. Macueve [13] defines the logistics management or system as the task of trying to place the right good, in the right quantities and conditions, at the right place, at the right time, for the right customer, in the most cost-effective manner. The main purpose of the logistics system is to deliver the *right* product to the *right* customer, in the *right* quantity, in the *right* condition, to the *right* place, at the *right* time, and for the *right* cost [4, 15, 16]. DELIVER [4] suggests six "rights" for LMIS data: the managers must receive the *right* data (essential data), in the *right* time (in time to take action), at the *right* place (where decisions are made), in the *right* quantity (having all essential data from all facilities), in the *right* quality (correct or accurate), and for the *right* cost (not spend more to collect information than spend on supplies).

The logistics adds a value to product by creating utility [10] and the more the logistics contributes to the value of a product, the more important the logistics management is [18]. The product refers to a set of utilities or characteristics a customer receives as a result of the purchase. The place and time utilities are directly affected by the logistics. The place utility is a value added to a product by making it available for purchase or consumption in the right place while as the time utility is a value added by making a product available at the right time.

The purpose of LMIS is to collect, organise, and report logistics data that will be used to make logistics decisions. The gathered information is used to improve customer service by improving quality of management decisions. A well-functioning LMIS provides decision makers throughout a supply chain with accurate, timely, and appropriate data for managing and monitoring flow of supplies, accounting for products in supply chain, reducing supply imbalances, and improve cost-effectiveness. Data from the LMIS are also useful for evaluating programs and supply chain operations.

Logistics reports, including summary and feedback, are used to move the essential data to logistics decision makers and data should be available to managers in a form suitable for decision making. The summary report contains all essential data items for a specific facility and for a specific time period (usually monthly or quarterly) in the form of simple report, aggregate summary report, or request report. The feedback reports inform the lower levels about their performance and even inform higher level managers about how the system is performing.

The LMIS, whether manual or automated, seems to be one of the weakest links in the logistics chain in the developing countries which requires a lot of attention. There are so many problems that exist in the drug logistics management in the developing countries which result in the shortages and uneven distribution of drugs, among others. According to some studies carried out in Jordan, Malawi, Mozambique, Nepal, Tanzania, Uganda, and Zambia, some of problems in drug LMIS include lack of accurate information, lack of staff training and support, weak supervision and monitoring, and shortage of human resources at all levels. The studies make some conclusions and one of them is: if data and information are properly collected and sent on a timely basis to decision-makers, it could potentially be helpful on deciding what drugs and medical supplies to deliver, how much, where and when.

3 Methodology

The framed experiment was the one used in this research with the focus on the following: (a) non-standard subject pool which consisted of pharmacy technicians, statisticians and pharmacy-in-charge; (b) experiences and information that the subject pool has with emphasis on the GIS and computer operations; (c) the GIS prototype treated as a new commodity to the drug logistics and health staff; and (d) demonstration of the GIS prototype to the subjects in their respective working places and subjects participated and provided feedback and comments.

The interviews were conducted with the aim of understanding working practices of the drug logistics staff and in the hierarchical manner starting from Regional Medical Stores in Blantyre, in the southern region of Malawi, down to its district pharmacies and district health offices in Blantyre and Mulanje districts, and then two health centres in each of the two districts. This was supplemented by analysis of data collection forms and some reports from the Supply Chain Manager and direct observation on its data entry and reporting at Blantyre district pharmacy aiming on finding out how it handles drug logistics data.

Interviewee at the regional level was the pharmacy in-charge focusing on information flow and feedback system between levels. At the district level, two pharmacy technicians (one from each district) were interviewed on data entry, processing and reporting using the Supply Chain Manager. Four health centre in-charges (one from each health centre) were interviewed on data collection and reporting at facility level.

Data was also collected through the evaluation of a GIS prototype whose spatial data was collected from the Department of Survey and Department of Roads Authority. The GIS prototype was demonstrated to pharmacy technicians and statisticians from the Blantyre DHO and the pharmacist-in-charge from RMS in their respective working places. It was performed by applying the DECIDE framework [19] and drug logistics and health data of September 2008 was used. The demonstration focused mainly on (a) reporting and analysis of drug logistics information and (b) integration of spatial, drug logistics and health data. After the demonstration participants were interviewed for their feedback on the proposed GIS.

4 Findings

4.1 Drug Logistics Management Information System

In Malawi, the drug logistics data is collected at a health facility level and processed at a district level (district pharmacy) using different tools in order to produce required logistics information for decision making. A responsible level reports in every month to its upper level which is supposed to send feedback to the lower level and concerned stakeholders (see Fig. 1).

By the end of each month, health facilities initiate a drug-ordering process by compiling monthly drug reports that are submitted to the district pharmacy. Then a district pharmacy technician assesses requirements of the health facility, completes the order part of drug report in accordance with given criteria and forwards it to

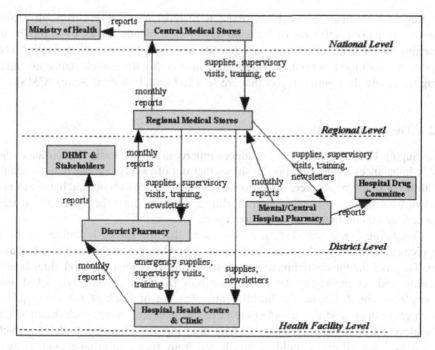

Fig. 1. Information flow and feedback between levels in drug LMIS

Regional Medical Stores (RMS). RMS supplies ordered drugs directly to the concerned health facility.

There are several forms that are used for recording and reporting of logistics data as part of LMIS. The forms include stock card, monthly LMIS reports, delivery note, district monthly aggregated order report, requisition for medical supplies, requisition and issue form, and requisition and issue voucher. Patient registers are also used in some health facilities for verifying drug logistics data when reporting.

A health centre-in-charge completes a LMIS form by using data from stock cards, in order to report information on stock balances, losses and adjustments, and quantity used by the health centre. Then the form is sent by fifth day of the month to the district pharmacy technician for assessments. The in-charge of health centre needs to make sure that the data on the LMIS form is valid all the time before sending to the district pharmacy. Some health centres use both registers and physical inventory to verify the collected data.

At the district level, LMIS reports are captured into the software system and then it calculates quantity required of each health commodity for each health facility and determines which facilities are adequately stocked, overstocked or understocked. It also reviews trends in consumption on a product-by-product basis and identifies facilities with potential inventory management problems. The software system generates stock status reports and other logistics reports that are used to review stock status of a particular health facility.

Regional Medical Stores (RMS) expects to receive all reports from all health facilities in its respective region by tenth day of each month. It uses these reports to determine what health commodity and quantity to be supplied to a health facility. The reports are also used to prepare reports such as monthly drug stock status, essential drug trace, and distribution report that are sent to Central Medical Stores (CMS).

4.2   The Proposed GIS

The Supply Chain Manager only produces reports in tabular form. For instance, the stock imbalances report (see Fig. 2) shows that out of twenty-one catchments health facilities in Blantyre, six were understocked and seven were overstocked but it was not known what happened to other eight health facilities, whether they were adequately stocked, or no consumption, or did not report.

Comparing Fig. 2 with Fig. 3, it was found that the spatial reporting can be a supplement to the original report which shows actual location of the health facility and how far it is from the district pharmacy. It shows that in September 2008, three health facilities did not report any data on SP and only five were adequately stocked. For example in Fig. 2, Chimembe health centre was out of stock of SP and required emergency supply and at the same time three health centres were much overstocked. Therefore, the map (see Fig. 3) would help drug logistics managers to decide which health facilities SP drugs could be transferred from, based on distance and accessibility between understocked and overstocked health facilities.

Supply Chain Manager Ministry of Health Blantyre District	**Stock Imbalances** Report Period: September, 2008 All Facility Type Health Centre					Run Date: Run Time: 04:19 PM Page: 1 of 1	
Facility	Product	Closing Balance	AMC	Months of Stock	Quantity Required	Status	
Chimembe HC	Sulphadoxine 500mg/pyrimetherine	0	4,000	0.0	12,000	Stocked Out	
Bangwe HC	Sulphadoxine 500mg/pyrimetherine	3,000	4,333	0.7	9,999	Below Minimum	
Dziwe HC	Sulphadoxine 500mg/pyrimetherine	5,000	6,000	0.8	13,000	Below Minimum	
Makata HC	Sulphadoxine 500mg/pyrimetherine	1,000	4,000	0.3	11,000	Below Minimum	
Soche HC	Sulphadoxine 500mg/pyrimetherine	2,000	4,000	0.5	10,000	Below Minimum	
Zingwangwa HC	Sulphadoxine 500mg/pyrimetherine	13,000	15,667	0.6	34,001	Below Minimum	
Chavala HC	Sulphadoxine 500mg/pyrimetherine	21,000	1,667	12.6	-15,999	Overstocked	
Limbe HC	Sulphadoxine 500mg/pyrimetherine	11,000	3,333	3.3	-1,001	Overstocked	
Lirangwe HC	Sulphadoxine 500mg/pyrimetherine	19,000	2,000	9.5	-13,000	Overstocked	
Lundu HC	Sulphadoxine 500mg/pyrimetherine	17,000	2,667	6.4	-8,999	Overstocked	
Madziabango HC	Sulphadoxine 500mg/pyrimetherine	10,000	333	30.0	-9,001	Overstocked	
Mpemba HC	Sulphadoxine 500mg/pyrimetherine	21,000	1,333	15.8	-17,001	Overstocked	
South Lunzu HC	Sulphadoxine 500mg/pyrimetherine	12,000	2,333	5.1	-5,001	Overstocked	

Fig. 2. Drug LMIS report from supply chain manager

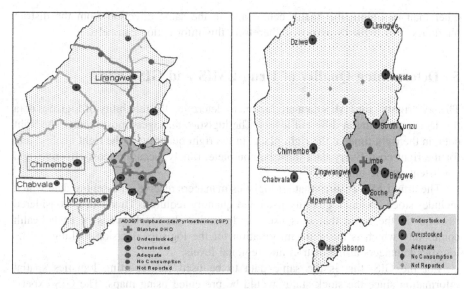

Fig. 3. Generated map from GIS prototype for stock status reporting

4.3   Enriching Drug Logistics Information

It is important that reports from the drug LMIS provide enough information for logistics managers to make sure that right quantity of required drug and medical supplies is delivered to health facilities which request the product. At the same time the product should be delivered on time, in good condition and to right clinic patients and other users. For instance, stock imbalances report (see Fig. 2) has very important information for the logistics managers, such as name of facility, product, stock balance, quantity required and stock status. In this case, (a) *product* represents which drugs and medical supplies should or not be delivered depending on the stock status (the *right* product); (b) *facility* shows which health delivery points the product should be delivered to (the *right* place); (c) *quantity required* indicates how much to deliver to the health facility (the *right* quantity); and (d) *stock status* can be used to determine how soon the product should be delivered to the health facility (the *right* time).

By considering the place and time utilities, this example report seems not to give complete information for decision making. The district pharmacy is responsible for handling all emergency orders from understocked health facilities as quickly as possible. The information about distances between the district pharmacy and concerned health facilities and how close they are to each other is very important in this circumstance. But the distance itself cannot help much due to poor road conditions in developing countries. It is important for the drug logistics managers to consider also the road conditions when making decision on the travel time to health facilities.

Using the map generated by GIS prototype (see Fig. 3), it can be observed that Zingwangwa, Bangwe and Soche health centres are very close to the district pharmacy as compared to Chimembe, Makata and Dziwe health centres. In terms of distances between health facilities, Dziwe and Makata health centres are much closer to each other than to Chimembe health centre and in the same direction from the district pharmacy. For logistics purposes, therefore, this information can help.

5 Determining Quality of Drug LMIS and GIS Data

The six "rights" for LMIS data are factors to determine the reliability of logistics data for decision making at different levels. The logistics managers must receive the right data, in the right time, at the right place, in the right quantity, in the right quality, and for the right cost. Every data must be complete, timely, accurate, cost-effective, and consistent among others.

The drug LMIS ensures that all logistics managers receive all essential data which includes stock on hand, quantity used and quantity required. This data is considered essential in the sense that it is used to determine the stock status of each health commodity which is the main information for the logistics decision making by the logistics managers at the district and regional levels.

For the GIS, this is the same data to be used for reporting logistics spatial information since the stock status would be presented using maps. The GIS experiment has shown that GIS would also require essential spatial data which includes administrative boundaries, health facilities, road networks and others.

The main challenge is the lack of personnel which results in work overload. This forces some health facilities to use other staff to collect logistics data. This brings the problem of the data quality because these people have not been trained on data collection. Currently, there is no logistics or health staff trained in the spatial data collection and updating for the GIS at the district level.

The essential data is supposed to be available in time for logistics managers to make decision. In the drug LMIS, this is achieved by setting deadlines for receiving reports from lower levels. Although there is "no report no drug" policy, there is still a problem of late or even not reporting from lower levels which affects the distribution of the health commodities to concerned health facilities.

If the pharmacy technicians receive data, including spatial data, in time, it means that the GIS subsystem will provide updated spatial information to the logistics managers and other users. It can be good for Ministry of Health to cooperate with other institutions that involve in spatial data management in the country so it can get all necessary updates on time. This cooperation is also important between departments in the Ministry of Health for easy spatial data sharing.

It has been observed that the essential logistics data is always sent to where decisions are made. The right place to send the spatial data is the district pharmacy because it is where the GIS subsystem would be used and other users would just get the spatial logistics information.

The district pharmacies make sure that all their respective health facilities report essential data every month so that they can have complete data. The policy of "no report no drug" forces the health facilities to report data with fear of not receiving health commodities. But this is not the case for some health facilities especially those not under government control.

From the research it has been observed that current spatial database misses some essential data of district, health facilities and their attributes. This gives an evidence of incompleteness of spatial data and that it is difficult to use.

The drug LMIS makes sure that all essential data is correct or accurate before using them which is achieved through supervision, physical inventory and training at all levels of the logistics management system. But still there is the lack of trust on the accuracy of the logistics data.

Sometimes some health centre-in-charges fill the LMIS reports right there at DHO when they come to perform other duties and this likely brings invalid data. Even the RMS experiences the same problem of some health facilities just guess or 'cook' figures. What they need is just a report being sent to the district pharmacy so that they get drugs and other health commodities. It is also necessary to make sure that the spatial data is accurate before using in the GIS application.

Every information system requires data collection and it is important not to spend more time on this process than on other duties. The software system used at the district pharmacies has simplified the work of pharmacy technicians to prepare reports in time. Much of the work is done at the health facilities where logistics data is collected manually. There is a long list of health commodities whose data should be filled in and this requires a lot of time.

As observed in the GIS experiment, it has been a requirement of collecting and then updating the spatial data. Although spatial data used in the GIS prototype was already prepared by other institutions it was necessary to update it for missing attributes, health facilities, districts and inaccurate road networks among others. This update exercise required a lot of time.

6   Conclusion

Reports from the Supply Chain Manager provide information that currently drug logistics managers use for decision making but the information is not enough for decision making. It has been found that it could be very important to use also maps from the GIS to enrich the existing information especially when place and time are concerned since these utilities are very critical in logistics. To make sure that the logistics data is rich enough for decision making, the "six rights" must be achieved. The logistics managers must receive the *right* data, in the *right* time, at the *right* place, in the *right* quantity, in the *right* quality, and for the *right* cost.

References

1. Bates, J., Rao, S.: Zambia: Implications of Health Sector Reform for Contraceptive Logistics. Family Planning Logistics Management (FPLM)/John Snow, Inc. (JSI), for the U.S. Agency for International Development (USAID), Arlington, VA (2000)
2. Beith, A., Quessada, N., Abramson, W., Sanchez, A., Olson, N.: Decentralizing and Integrating Contraceptive Logistics Systems in Latin America and the Caribbean, With Lessons Learned from Asia and Africa. DELIVER, for the U.S. Agency for International Development, Arlington, VA (2006)

3. Bossert, T.J., Bowser, D.M., Amenyah, J.K.: Is decentralization good for logistics systems? Evidence on essential medicine logistics in Ghana and Guatemala. Health Policy Plann. **22**, 73–82 (2007). (Oxford University Press in association with The London School of Hygiene and Tropical Medicine)

4. DELIVER.: The Logistics Handbook: A Practical Guide for Supply Chain Managers in Family Planning and Health Programs. John Snow Inc./DELIVER, for the U.S. Agency for International Development (USAID), Arlington, VA (2004)

5. DELIVER.: Malawi: Health Commodities Logistics Management System Standard Operating Procedures Manual. John Snow, Inc./DELIVER, for the U.S. Agency for International Development, Arlington, VA (2006)

6. DELIVER.: Tanzania: Final Country Report. DELIVER, for the U.S. Agency for International Development, Arlington, VA (2007a)

7. DELIVER.: Zambia: Final Country Report. DELIVER, for the U.S. Agency for International Development, Arlington, VA (2007b)

8. FAMILY PLANNING LOGISTICS MANAGEMENT (FPLM).: Nepal: Contraceptive and Drugs Logistics System, Review of Accomplishments and Lessons Learned (1993–2000). Family Planning Logistics Management (FPLM)/John Snow, Inc. (JSI), for the U.S. Agency for International Development (USAID), Arlngton, VA(2000)

9. Galimoto, M.S.: Integration of Health Information Systems, Case Study from Malawi. Master Thesis, University of Oslo (2007)

10. Lambert, D.M., Stock, J.R., Ellram, L.M.: Fundamentals of Logistics Management, International Editions. McGraw-Hill, Singapore (1998)

11. Lewis, M.: Tackling Healthcare Corruption and Governance Woes in Developing Countries – CDC Brief. Center for Global Development (2006)

12. Lufesi, N.N., Andrew, M., Aursnes, I.: Deficient supplies of drugs for life threatening diseases in an African community. BMC Health Services Research, BioMedical Central (2007)

13. Macueve, G.A.: Drugs Logistics Management Information System in Mozambique: Challenges and Opportunities. Master Thesis, University of Oslo (2003)

14. McGregor, K., Chandani, Y.: Experiences from the Field: Strategies for Skills Transfer in Supply Chain Management for Developing Countries. John Snow, Inc./Family Planning Logistics Management (FPLM), for the U.S. Agency for International Development, Arlington, VA (1999)

15. Owens, R.C., Warner, T.: Concepts of Logistics System Design. John Snow, Inc./ DELIVER, for the U.S. Agency for International Development (USAID), Arlington, VA (2003)

16. Population Information Program (PIP). Family Planning Logistics: Strengthening the Supply Chain (2002). http://www.infoforhealth.org/pr/j51/j51.pdf, Accessed 30-04-2008

17. Sowedi, M., David, V., Olupot, G., Ekochu, E., Sebagenzi, E., Kiragga, D., Ngabirano, T.: Baseline Assessment of Drug Logistics Systems in Twelve DISH- supported Districts and Service Delivery Points (SDPs). Delivery of Improved Health Services (DISH) II Project, Health Management and Quality Assurance Component, Uganda (2006)

18. Stock, J.R., Lambert, D.M.: Strategic Logistics Management, 4th edn. McGraw-Hill, Singapore (2001)

19. Sharp, H., Preece, J., Rogers, Y.: Interaction Design: Beyond Human Computer Interaction, 2nd edn. Wiley, New York (2007)

GrAPP&S, a Distributed Framework for E-learning Resources Sharing

Thierno Ahmadou Diallo[1,2]([✉]), Olivier Flauzac[2], Luiz Angelo Steffenel[2], Samba N'Diaye[1], and Youssou Dieng[3]

[1] Département d'Informatique, LMI, Université Cheikh Anta Diop,
5005, Dakar-Fann, Sénégal
{thierno80.diallo,samba.ndiaye}@ucad.edu.sn
[2] Laboratoire CReSTIC-Equipe SYSCOM,
Université de Reims Champagne-Ardenne, Reims, France
{olivier.flauzac,luiz-angelo.steffenel}@univ-reims.fr
[3] Département d'Informatique, Université de Ziguinchor,
523, Ziguinchor, Sénégal
ydieng@univ-zig.sn

Abstract. This article presents GrAPP&S (Grid APPlication & Services), a specification of an E-learning architecture for the decentralized sharing of educational resources. By dealing with different resources such as files, data streams (video, audio, VoIP), queries on databases but also access to remote services (web services on a server, on a cloud, etc.), GrAPP&S groups the resources of each institution in the form of a community and allows sharing among different communities. Educational resources are managed on a transparent manner through proxies specific to each type of resources. The transparency provided by proxies concerns the location of sources of educational data, the processing of queries, the composition of the results and the management of educational data consistency. Furthermore, the architecture of GrAPP&S has been designed to allow security policies for data protection, both within a community and between different communities.

Keywords: E-learning system · Proxies · Peer to peer system · Prefix routing

1 Introduction

An interesting idea that people actually consider that the pedagogical integration of ICTs to all education degrees improve clearly the quality of African education systems. Online learning (E-learning) and mobile learning (M-learning) help not only to strength the planning and the management of a democratic and transparent education, but also to extend the access to learning, to improve quality and ensure inclusion.

© Institute for Computer Sciences, Social Informatics and Telecommunications Engineering 2014
T.F. Bissyandé and G. van Stam (Eds.): AFRICOMM 2013, LNICST 135, pp. 219–228, 2014.
DOI: 10.1007/978-3-319-08368-1_26

Thanks to the opportunities they offer in terms of use or adaptation, in particular in environments where there are insufficient resources, free access educational resources constitute an excellent opportunity to achieve the goal of a education of quality for everyone. This is the first motivation of the project GRAPP&S. The objective of this project is to construct an E-learning architecture for sharing and decentralized management of all educational resources formats like files, streams (video, audio, VoIP) and resources from web services, cloud and distributed computing services. These resources are transparently presented to the user (student, teacher) thanks to the use of proxies adapters tailored for each educational resources.

Nowadays, it is very easy to share and learn using Internet. The Internet has contributed greatly to the education system by introducing the concept of E-learning. The latter is now accepted in the various educational institutions to improve the learning process for students and teachers or administrators. An important characteristic of E-learning systems is the sharing and use of educational resources between institutions.

Although most of E-learning repositories give free access to their repositories of educational resources, the integration process is still costly [11] as most learning repositories [2,3] rely on different standards to access the resources [1]. Furthermore, several systems rely nowadays on storage facilities on the cloud, which poses a problem to isolate localities due to the access speed.

Therefore, an intuitive approach is to regroup different local learning repositories from each institutes (schools, universities, repositories of research laboratories, etc.) in a "Community", which can foster the aims of reusing and sharing educational resources without costly duplicating them into local learning repositories. Through the use of communities, we can promote the goals of reuse and sharing educational resources. By extending the coverage to different educational resources (files, videos, data in a database, even a video stream for example when subscribing to TV channel for learning languages), we can integrate all tools to improve education in a single infrastructure, with a smaller cost. Following this approach, two major research challenges must be considered to ensure interoperability across the Web:

1. Compatibility between systems: if today most APIs (Dropbox, Google Drive, etc.) allow to handle simples files, it is less clear how to integrate complex data such as queries on a database, data streams or web services.
2. Decentralized data management: most platforms are migrating to the cloud, but at the expense of losing its proximity to the consumers, as well as poor access speed and privacy threats.

From these elements, we present GrAPP&S, an architecture designed to connect institutes interested on the sharing of educational data sources through the network. GrAPP&S brings therefore:

1. A decentralized solution for sharing all types of educational resources, not only files (text/xml) but also databases, streams (video, audio), and resources

from remote services such as web services and distributed computing, all integrated through the use of data proxies.

2. A simpler way to connect a large number of institutes interested into resource sharing. This is obtained through the aggregation of resources from each educational institute in the form of a "community". This will allow quick access to resources due to the proximity to consumers, unlike most of the E-learning solutions based on cloud storage when consumers are penalized because of the slow access speed.

3. The possibility to define security policies for the protection of educational resources within a community, and access policies between different communities through the establishment of *Service-Level Agreements (SLAs)*.

The remaining sections of the paper cover: Sect. 2 discusses the related work. Section 3 presents an overview of GrAPP&S architecture and describes the different elements of this architecture, while Sect. 4 describes the lookup algorithm used to locate resources inside GRAPP&S. Finally, Sect. 5 concludes this paper.

2 Related Work

Because GRAPP&S aims at the decentralized management of resources, it seems natural to identify peer-to-peer (P2P) works in this area. Indeed, an architecture for sharing educational resources among different learning institutions is proposed in [1]. This architecture, called LOP2P, aims at helping different educational institutions to create course material by using shared educational resource repositories. Nonetheless, resources of different formats cannot be easily integrated in this platform. Similarly, [7] develops a P2P based E-learning system that uses the video for learning. This system divides multimedia data into fragments managed by assigned agents, and this system allows the sharing of multimedia data, but it cannot deal with other data types.

Several E-learning systems based on cloud are being proposed, like [4] or [5]. In [4], an E-learning ecosystem based on cloud computing and Web 2.0 technologies is presented, and the article analyses the services provided by public cloud computing environments such as Google App Engine, Amazon Elastic Compute Cloud (EC2) or Windows Azure. It also highlights the advantages of deploying E-Learning 2.0 applications for such an infrastructures, and identify the benefits of cloud-based E-Learning 2.0 applications (scalability, feasibility, or availability) and underlined the enhancements regarding the cost and risk management. In addition, [5] is used to run web 2.0 applications, such as video teleconferencing, voice over IP, and remote management, over handheld devices and terminals. As [5] Leopard Cloud is targeted towards military usage, it has a multi-level security and the network infrastructure is encrypted.

It is quite evident that the cloud-based system would help the educational institutes or universities to share and disseminate knowledge among students, teachers and researchers, but the use of Cloud Computing in the educational system presents many risks and limitations: not all applications run in cloud, there are risks related to data protection, security and accounts management. Also, the access speed to cloud infrastructures may be a critical factor, amplified by the lack of a stable Internet connection that may affect the work methods in some isolated areas.

3   The GrAPP&S Architecture

The GrAPP&S framework is an E-learning solution for the decentralized sharing all types of resources. It allows pooling of data each institution in the form of community, and allow different communities to share resources based on pre-defined access rules. For this reason, GrAPP&S can also be extended to other areas of the school, by creating a community in the administrative part, separated from the education part, with safety rules and resource protection. In the following sections, we present the different elements of our framework GrAPP&S for the decentralized sharing of educational resources.

3.1   Model

We consider a model of communication represented by an undirected and connected graph $G = (V, E)$, where V denotes the set of nodes in the system and E denotes the set of communication links between nodes. The model used for this system is studied in [6]. Two nodes u and v are said to be adjacent or neighbors if and only if u, v is a communication link of G. $u_i, v_j \in E$ is a bidirectional channel connected to port i for u and to port j for v. Thus nodes u and v can mutually send and receive messages. Nodes communicate by using asynchronous messages.

A message m in transit is denoted $m(id(u), m', id(v))$ where $id(u)$ is the identifier of the node that sends the message, $id(v)$ is the identifier of the receiving node and, m' the message content. Each node u of the system has a unique id and has two primitives: **send(message)** and **receive(message)**.

3.2   Nodes of GrAPP&S

In order to present our architecture, we introduce some notations first. A community (C_i) is an autonomous entity, which includes educative resources sharing some properties: same location (resources institute, university, research laboratory), same administration authority, or same application domain (administrative resources vs teaching resources). A community contains one communicator process noted (c) and at least one *Resource Manager* process noted RM and one process *Data Manager* noted DM and these processes are hierarchically organized in the Community.

Communicator (*c*) nodes play an essential role that is related to information transmission and interconnection between different communities, such as when passing messages through firewalls. A Communicator is the community entry point and assures its security towards the outside, through establishment of *Service-Level Agreements (SLAs)* with other communities. The communicator also defines the security rules (access) for the protection of educational resources inside the community (for example the administration community can see the data on the educational system, but not the reverse, thanks to this access rules defined by the communicator).

Resource Manager (*RM*) processes ensure indexing and organization of educational resources in the community. The RM_i processes are involved in the search and indexing of data in the community c_i, and by receiving queries from its neighbors communities. Given the important role of RM processes in research and indexing of resources, we choose a RM among ordinary nodes that have good performance levels in both CPU, memory size and communication speed.

Data Manager (*DM*) processes interact with sources of educational data such as databases, file, email servers, WebDAV servers, FTP servers, disks, or cloud services. A DM node is a service that has the following components (see Fig. 1):

- a proxy interface adapted to the various formats of educational data,
- a query manager that allows to express queries on local or global educational resources, and
- a communications manager that allows the DM node to communicate with the RM node to which it is connected.

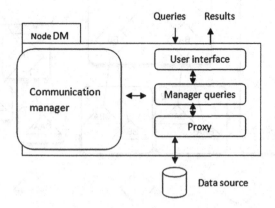

Fig. 1. DM node architecture

3.3   Management of the Community

GrAPP&S can be deployed in several ways, depending on the placement of the nodes. For example, we can find the following deployment topologies;

1. Nodes can be grouped into a single physical machine (see Fig. 2a). This is an example of a machine of a student or a teacher who wants to host a community of architecture.
2. The nodes are organized in a server farm such as a cluster, which is characteristic of an HPC network (Fig. 2b).
3. Nodes can be distributed over different machines, which corresponds to a grouping of educational resources in a university or a school with remote sites. These resources share the same administration entity (see Fig. 2c).

Each node on GrAPP&S has its own unique identifier (ID). The IP or the MAC addresses are not sufficiently accurate because they do not identify uniquely different nodes that can reside on a same machine (e.g. RM and DM). Thus, we rely on the identification method proposed by JXTA [12], which uses a string of 128 bits. Each node has a unique and string $ID - local$, as "$urn : name - community : uuid : string - of - bit$". As GRAPP&S is hierarchically structured, the expression of hierarchical addressing is done by concatenating the IDs as a prefix, i.e., ID c_i node is equivalent to its $ID - local$, the node ID is formed by RM_i $ID\text{-}c_i/ID\text{-}RM_i$, and DM_i node ID has the form $ID\text{-}c_i/ID\text{-}RM_i/ID\text{-}DM_i$.

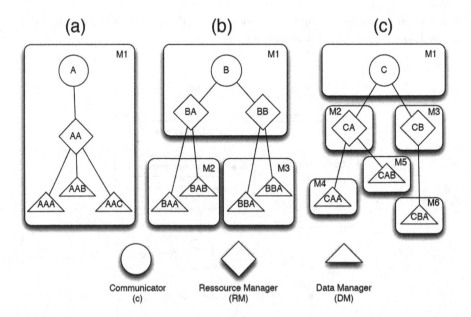

Fig. 2. Organization of the nodes in a machine (a), in a cluster (b) and in a network (c)

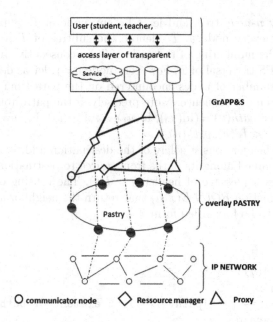

Fig. 3. Deployment of nodes GrAPP&S on Pastry

An advantage of using an addressing model specific to GrAPP&S is that it is independent of the overlay network addressing model that is implemented. Indeed, Fig. 3 presents an illustration of GRAPP&S implemented over the Pastry [10] P2P middleware. Thus, two communities GrAPP&S implemented on different middleware can still be compatible, once the connection is established between their communicators.

4   Accessing the Resources

A GrAPP&S community is an hierarchical network with an addressing system independent from the underlying network. This addressing scheme is used to help data lookup and also to help route data during transfers. This hierarchical addressing also simplifies the integration to another network community. In the following paragraphs, we will propose a routing algorithm and a method of data lookup in our system.

4.1   Routing Algorithm

Let T be the tree of a community GRAPP&S. Thanks to the results of Fraigniaud and Gavoille [8]; Thorup and Zwick [9] we can construct a routing scheme in the tree T. For each message m for a vertex y, the current vertex x sends m on a shortest path in T.

Let T be any *n-node* tree, and let r be any node of T. Suppose that T is rooted at r. For every node u, T_u denote the subtree of T rooted at u. We define $Id(u)$ as the numbering of the node of T by consecutive integers in $[1, n]$ obtained by a DFS traversal of T. For every node $u \neq r$, let as define $path(u)$ as the sequence of number of nodes encountered on the path from r to u. We set $path(r) = ()$, the empty sequence. More precisely, if the path from r to u is $r = u_0, u_1, \ldots, u_k$ then $path(u) = (Id(u_0), Id(u_1), \ldots, Id(u_k))$. For every node x of T the address $l(u) = < Id(u), path(u) >$.

The message header consist solely of the destination address of the message and it not be modified along its paths from source to destination. Assume that a node x receives a message of header $h = l(y)$. The routing decision at x is described by a function $ROUTE(x, h)$ that return the neighbor w of x on which the message has to be forwarded form x.

```
ROUTE (x,l(y))
BEGIN
  IF Id(x) = Id(y)
        Return x;
  ELSE IF (Id(y) == p= (|path(x)|-1)-th element of path(x) Then
          Return p;
  Else Return (|path(x)|+1)-th element of path(y);
END
```

4.2   Lookup Algorithm

The search for a resource in a community GrAPP&S is illustrated in Fig. 4, and the procedure works as follows:

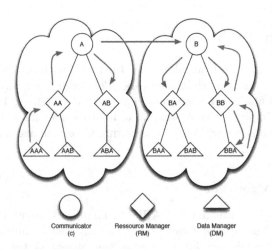

Fig. 4. looking for a resource in a routing GrAPP&S

1. User comes into contact with a DM_i proxy.
2. Node $DM_i \in C_i$ sends the request to its $RM_i \in C_i$.
3. RM_i checks in its index among its neighbors if there's a DM that contains the searched resource.
4. If so, then the node returns to RM_i DM node a list of nodes that contain DM information searched.
5. Otherwise, RM_i node forwards the request directly neighbors $RM_k \in C_i$, either to the node c_i to retransmit other $RM_k \in C_i$.
6. When node $RM_k \in C_i$ found the correct answer, then the query will be returned to transmitter node DM_i following the opposite path.
7. If the data sought is not in the community C, then c_i node forwards the query to other community.

The user has two options for accessing the resource either through a direct connection (if the network support is) or a routed connection (if the user is in another different network node that owns the resource).

5 Conclusions and Future Works

In this article we present an E-learning architecture specification named GrAPP&S, which is a decentralized solution for managing and sharing educational resources. GrAPP&S has been constructed as an hierarchical network to allows a pooling resources of each institute under the concept of "community", and to take advantage of the proximity of data and the users (students, teachers, administrative, etc.). One can even extend the use of a community of GrAPP&S to other sectors of an institute such as a community just for the administrative departments, separated from the educational users. In addition, GrAPP&S uses security rules to protect the resources of each community, and defines access policies between different community. The use of proxies for each specific type of data allows sharing a transparent manner not only files but also databases, streams (video, audio, VoIP), resources from the web services, cloud services, distributed computing.

The next step towards the validation of this specification is its use under real situations. We are starting to develop a prototype of GrAPP&S that will be used for testing and deployment on educational institutions. This prototype uses P2P Pastry underlying network to distribute the nodes of a community (local network institution) of GrAPP&S as illustrated in Fig. 3. The choice of Pastry allows a community GrAPP&S a P2P network, which will allow a community institute include a large number of nodes and to perform scaling tests.

References

1. de Santiago, R., Raabe, A.L.A.: Architecture for learning objects sharing among learning institutions LOP2P. IEEE Trans. Learn. Technol. **3**(2), 91–95 (2010)
2. Cheng-Zhong, X., Rao, J., Bu, X.: URL: a unified reinforcement learning approach for autonomic cloud management. J. Parallel Distrib. Comput. **72**(2), 95–105 (2012)
3. Fardoun, H.M., Lopez, S.R., Alghaz-zawi, D.M., Castillo, J.R.: Education system in the cloud to improve student communication in the institutes of C-LearniXML++. Procedia Soc. Behav. Sci. **47**, 1762–1769 (2012)
4. Ouf, S., Nasr, M., Helmy, Y.: An enhanced e-learning ecosystem based on an integration between cloud computing and Web2.0. In: Proceedings of the IEEE International Symposium on Signal Processing and Information Technology (ISSPIT), pp. 48–55 (2011)
5. Cayirci, E., Rong, C., Huiskamp, W., Verkoelen, C.: Snow leopard cloud: a multinational education training and experimentation cloud and its security challenges. In: Jaatun, M.G., Zhao, G., Rong, C. (eds.) Cloud Computing. LNCS, vol. 5931, pp. 57–68. Springer, Heidelberg (2009)
6. Chalopin, J., Godard, E., Métivier, Y., Ossamy, R.: Mobile agent algorithms versus message passing algorithms. In: Shvartsman, M.M.A.A. (ed.) OPODIS 2006. LNCS, vol. 4305, pp. 187–201. Springer, Heidelberg (2006)
7. Hayakawa, T., Higashino, M., Takahashi, K., Kawamura, T., Sugahara, K.: Management of multimedia data for streaming on a distributed e-learning system. In: 2012 26th International Conference on Advanced Information Networking and Applications Workshops (WAINA), pp. 1282–1285 (2012)
8. Fraigniaud, P., Gavoille, C.: Routing in trees. In: Orejas, F., Spirakis, P.G., van Leeuwen, J. (eds.) ICALP 2001. LNCS, vol. 2076, p. 757. Springer, Heidelberg (2001)
9. Thorup, M., Zwick, U.: Compact routing schemes. In: 13th Annual ACM Symposium on Parallel Algorithms and Architectures (SPAA), pp. 1–10. ACM Press, July 2001
10. Rowstron, A., Druschel, P.: Pastry: scalable, decentralized object location, and routing for large-scale peer-to-peer systems. In: Guerraoui, R. (ed.) Middleware 2001. LNCS, vol. 2218, pp. 329–350. Springer, Heidelberg (2001)
11. Yu, H.Q., Dietze, S., Li, N., Pedrinaci, C., Taibi, D., Dovrolls, N., Stefanut, T., Kaldoudi, E., Domingue, J.: A linked data-driven & service-oriented architecture for sharing educational resources. In: 1st International Workshop on eLearning Approaches for Linked Data Age (Linked Learning 2011), 8th Extended Semantic Web Conference (ESWC2011), 29 May 2011, Heraklion, Greece (2011)
12. Ahkil, B.T.: Project JXTA 2.0 Super-Peer Virtual Network (2005)

Y Nut, a Phonetic-Based Learning System for Spoken Languages

Omer L. Nguena Timo[1] and Tegawendé F. Bissyandé[2](✉)

[1] LaBRI, University of Bordeaux - CNRS, Talence, France
nguena@labri.fr
[2] SnT, University of Luxembourg, Luxembourg, Luxembourg
tegawende.bissyande@uni.lu

Abstract. Communication between humans is of importance for our societies. It requires constant learning of new languages, e.g., by travellers whose extended stay in foreign locations facilitate learning. When a language possesses a written form, much of the meaning necessary for its learning is directly provided by the text. In spoken languages however, the meaning is only vehicled by the sounds. Nonetheless, learning spoken languages can take advantage of linguistic contents available in audio or video media which abound on the Internet and the social networks. We open a discussion and describe a system that enables to enrich a phonetic database so as to ease learning of basic expressions of spoken languages. Such a system could be useful for the survival of the plethora of spoken languages in Africa. The purpose of such a system is to provide within a reasonable period, automatic syntactic translation services.

1 Introduction

By the year 2100, 50–90 % of the current 7,000 languages spoken across the world will be extinct [1]. Recent statistical summaries[1] have reported that most of the still alive languages are actually spoken in developing regions in Africa (30 %) and Asia (30 %) where the loss of *spoken languages*, aka *oral languages*, will actually significantly harm cultural diversity. Today, spoken languages in African developing areas are endangered because of the cultural/political/economic hegemony of the West [1]. Nonetheless, there is currently a momentum of (re)learning languages that estranged populations now value in various contexts. For example, a song in *Lingala*[2] broadcasted over the internet may spark the interest of an expatriate congolese, while old recordings of historical speeches by African elders may need to be valued.

Thanks to video-sharing sites and web-based music streaming services, an abundance of multi-media content now proliferates on the internet. Because it originates from all parts of the world, this content features a considerable number of spoken languages. And because the internet can be accessed from all around

---

[1] http://www.ethnologue.com/statistics/area
[2] Bantu language spoken in Congo.

© Institute for Computer Sciences, Social Informatics and Telecommunications Engineering 2014
T.F. Bissyandé and G. van Stam (Eds.): AFRICOMM 2013, LNICST 135, pp. 229–233, 2014.
DOI: 10.1007/978-3-319-08368-1_27

the globe, we are presented with ample opportunity to leverage its multimedia content to learn languages in an adequate socio-technical environment.

It is commonly accepted that the difficulty for learning a language is correlated to the difficulty for the learner to recognize the sounds, i.e. phones [3], made when speaking the language. Furthermore, in a given language, several phones can actually be perceived as equivalent although they are not identically pronounced (e.g., the 'k' sound is aspirated in the word 'kit' and unaspirated in 'skill'). Such a set of phones is known as a *phoneme* and will be transcribed identically. As a result, transcribing phonemes of a given language is an important step towards providing a corpus for its learning.

State of the art. In previous work, Nguyen Thi Minh has studied the phonetic transcription of Vietnamese [4]. This work was facilitated by the fact that Vietnamese is a written language and already possesses an alphabet. Purely spoken languages present distinct challenges for phonetic transcriptions. Our endeavour however involves the transcription of such languages which are the majority of endangered languages in developing regions. Work on phonetic transcriptions has mainly relied on two basic techniques:

- **Rule-based approaches:** such approaches require the implementation of transcription rules, and are thus adapted for languages that are already equipped with such rules. The simpler and precise the rules are, the faster and precise the transcription is. Ordean *et al.* have implemented *Grapheme-to-Phoneme* trancription rules that were integrated in the text processing component of a text-to-speech system for Romanian [5].
- **Statistical approaches based on learning:** These approaches are used with an initial lexicon that is progressively enriched by applying statistical techniques to infer new transcriptions. This method is particularly adapted for the extension to new languages. Besling has also used a statistical approach to derive phonetic transcriptions independently of the languages, building upon background lexica [2].

This paper. We propose in this paper the Ynut system for providing a socio-technical environment for the transcription of spoken languages. The contributions of this paper are:

1. we introduced a new research avenue for African researchers in the learning of spoken languages using multimedia content.
2. we propose a collaborative approach to learning, which is likely to benefit from the cultural model of Africa.
3. we discuss the design of the Ynut system for enriching the huge amount of multimedia content on the internet with phonetic transcriptions that will help learning.

The remainder of this paper is structured as follows. Section 2 introduces domain-specific terms that are necessary to understand our approach. Section 3 then details the Ynut system, describing each module and what service it delivers. We conclude in Sect. 4.

2   Preliminaries

This section introduces the preliminaries to understand the scope of our research project, and how realistic our endeavour is. We first detail different concepts that are necessary to grasp the challenges of phonetic transcriptions. Then, we discuss the abundance of multimedia content and the opportunities that they provide.

Phonetic systems and units. **Phonemes** are the basic linguistic units of languages' phonology. Substituting a phoneme for another one modifies the listening and the meaning of the speech. In written languages, each phoneme can be represented with a combination of symbols of an **alphabet**. Each symbol of an alphabet is also called a **grapheme**. One grapheme also represents one phoneme. Written languages are equipped with **dictionaries** that enumerate the **root words** of the languages. Root words are represented with sequences of graphemes. Written languages also provide rules for creating and composing new valid words and phrases.

Multimedia broadcasting services. With the latest advances on data storage systems and the improvement of Internet connection across the world, multimedia broadcasting services such as Youtube, Dailymotion and Netflix for video or Deezer for audio, the traffic on the Internet mostly deals with multimedia content. Social networking paradigm has enabled user experience of videos to be more inclusive by allowing a single video clip to be passed over and shared by thousands in a matter of days. Such epidemic spread of multimedia content, their lifetime on the web, and their random origins from anywhere on earth, make them a very good medium to assess the flourishing of various spoken languages. Unfortunately, listening and watching videos is even more useful for a non-native of the spoken language when there are accompanying subtitles. However writing subtitles for a multimedia content is a daunting, solitary, and sometimes unrewarding task. For spoken languages, the challenges are aggravated by the limited number of subtitles that must be transcribed in a foreign alphabet.

3   The Ynut System

Ynut is a pilot project for a more effective learning of spoken languages leveraging multimedia content that is available on the Internet and that potential learners already stream everyday. The Ynut system thus aims at enabling users to enrich audio and video media with transcription items refered to as *yphemes*. Yphemes are representations of morphemes in the Ynut systems. A ypheme is based on written languages and each instance of ypheme obeys to the phonetic system of the associated written language. It allows us to represent speeches of a spoken language. Intuitively, since spoken languages are not equipped with dictionaries, people that have rudiment (approximative or exact writing) knowledge about written languages can represent the speeches in spoken languages with morphemes of those written languages. The Ynut system is compromised of five modules, each delivering a specific service that will contribute to improve collaborative learning of spoken languages. As a collaborative system, Ynut relies on users to contribute with the yphemes for spoken languages and the associated written language that they understand.

3.1   The Yphemes Recording Module

The first module of the Ynut system is a recording Module for construction of a knowledge database. The yphemes Recording Module is in charge of recording yphemes provided by a contributor. Before he starts recording new yphemes for a given spoken language, the contributor must associate an input written language, (a part of) video/audio media, the translations of the yphemes into another written language or optionally into the international phonetic system. Thus the created corpus will contain information for linking sounds from a spoken language and their transcriptions for reading into a written language.

3.2   The Phonetic Transcription Module

The second module is internal to Ynut and does not require interaction with users. It is a phonetic transcription module which automatically transcripts recorded yphemes into the phonetic system of the associated written language or the international phonetic system. Example 1 illustrates an example of translation between Ynut's yphemes and the International Phonetic Alphabet (IPA).

Example 1. Here is a translation of two yphemes into the English IPA[3].

ypheme	IPA
y nut	ˈwaɪˈnət
why not	ˈwaɪˈnɑt

We observe from the above example that the two IPA phonemes are very similar although the yphemes look more different, thus highlighting how the Ynut systems addresses the challenge having contributors recording distinct yphemes for the same heard sound.

3.3   The Search Module

The Search module uses information retrieval techniques to enable the search for yphemes or words according to similarity criteria. In Ynut, these similarity criteria may include syntactic similarity between the yphemes or phonetic similarity.

3.4   The Automatic Media Transcription Module

This module is in charge of automatically inferring ypheme representations of speeches contained in audio or video content. It's implementation is possible using machine learning approaches that will use as training data the initial database of yphemes transcriptions that human contributors have recorded.

---

[3] http://project-modelino.com/english-phonetic-transcription-converter.php

3.5   The Automatic Translation Module

Finally to implement the final opportunity of the Ynut system, we leverage the corpus built by contributors and enriched automatically by Ynut to provide automatic translation capabilities between spoken languages and written languages.

4   Concluding Remarks

We opened a discussion regarding a learning system for spoken languages. The main idea of the system is the enrichment of a phonetic database based on the phonetic alphabet of written languages. The linguistic contents may come from several sources such as audio/video databases and social networks. Then we have proposed an architecture for our system and we have presented its main functionalities and the research challenges for each functionality.

Further development will consider the implementation of a generic platform that may be used by any community that intend to promote its spoken language. Then we will consider the enrichment of phonetic data-base for the authors native spoken languages.

References

1. Austin, P., Sallabank, J.: The Cambridge Handbook of Endangered Languages. Cambridge University Press, Cambridge (2011)
2. Besling, S.: A statistical approach to multilingual phonetic transcription. Philips J. Res. **49**(4), 367–379 (1995)
3. Crystal, D.: Linguistics (1971)
4. Nguyen, P.-T., Vu, X.-L., Nguyen, T.-M.-H., Nguyen, V.-H., Le, H.-P.: Building a large syntactically-annotated corpus of vietnamese. In: Proceedings of the 3rd Linguistic Annotation Workshop, ACL-IJCNLP '09, pp. 182–185, Stroudsburg, PA, USA. Association for Computational Linguistics (2009)
5. Ordean, M., Saupe, A., Ordean, M., Duma, M., Silaghi, G.: Enhanced rule-based phonetic transcription for the Romanian language. In: 2009 11th International Symposium on Symbolic and Numeric Algorithms for Scientific Computing (SYNASC), pp. 401–406 (2009)

Modeling Diffusion of Blended Labs for Science Experiments Among Undergraduate Engineering Students

Raghu Raman[✉], Krishnashree Achuthan, Prema Nedungadi,
and Maneesha Ramesh

School of Engineering, Amrita Vishwa Vidyapeetham Amritapuri,
Kollam 690525, Kerala, India
{raghu,krishna,prema,maneesha}@amrita.edu

Abstract. While there is large body of work examining efficacy of Virtual Labs in engineering education, studies to date have lacked modeling Blended Labs (BL) – mix of Virtual Labs (VL) and Physical Labs (PL) for science experimentation at the university engineering level. Using Rogers theory of perceived attributes, this paper provides a research framework that identifies the attributes for BL adoption in a social group comprising of (N=246) potential adopter undergraduate engineering students. Using Bass model the study also accounts for the interinfluence of related group of potential adopter faculties who are likely to exert positive influence on students. The results revealed that acceptance of BL as an innovation and its learning outcomes are strongly associated with innovation attributes like Relative Advantage, Compatibility, Ease of Use, Department and Faculty support. Learning outcomes are very positive under BL when compared to PL, though within BL, ordering of PL and VL was not significant. For certain innovation attributes gender differences were significant. Overall students expressed much more positive attitude to adopt BL model for learning than using only PL.

Keywords: Virtual labs · Blended learning · Innovation diffusion · Experiments · Engineering · Interinfluence

1 Introduction

With growing acceptance of educational technologies, significant emphasis is placed on the underlying pedagogical approach to attain desirable learning outcomes [1]. One of the recent emerging approaches to learning is known as blended learning. Blended learning involves a combination of online or virtual instruction in tandem with face-to-face sessions. According to [2] Blended Learning is an innovation if it is 'perceived as new by an individual or other unit of adoption. If the idea seems new to the individual, it is an innovation'. An educational innovation like BL will not occur in isolation in an environment where two interrelated potential adopters namely faculties and students influence each other and both have to adopt for the innovation to be successful.

Physical experimentation in labs has been a critical component in science and engineering education. Specifically, imparting practical skills as well and obtaining

© Institute for Computer Sciences, Social Informatics and Telecommunications Engineering 2014
T.F. Bissyandé and G. van Stam (Eds.): AFRICOMM 2013, LNICST 135, pp. 234–247, 2014.
DOI: 10.1007/978-3-319-08368-1_28

first-hand knowledge of challenges incurred in real environments can only be learnt in a physical lab. Research has shown that in spite of the important role physical experimentation has, the conceptual understanding of a phenomenon from practical lab experience alone is poor and ineffective in provoking student's innate creativity [3]. A combination of both learning environments did show enhancement in student understanding [4] and in some cases further improvements with virtual labs [5]. The level of visualization, flexibility, the repetitive practice that virtual labs allow, makes them far more effective learning tools. On the other hand, there are limitations to virtual labs in providing critical experiences of performing an experiment, the inability to grasp specific aspects of knowledge (for e.g. assumptions, measurement errors etc.) as in a physical lab [6]. These challenges can be surmounted by adopting a blended learning approach to lab education. The advantages of largely individualistic learning with virtual labs in combination with pragmatic skill development from physical labs are necessary to invoke motivation, enhance understanding and extend retention of complex phenomena. On the other hand, if all concepts were demonstrable in a laboratory our surmise is that it would in fact widen experiential learning and provide deeper understanding. This ideal scenario is nearly impractical for the exorbitant cost to host wide variety of instrumentation and difficulty in dovetailing them into the curricula under the constraint of limited allotted time and infrastructure for labs in most institutions. This paper provides directions to circumventing the challenges of current physical lab practices by introducing blended labs in mainstream under graduate engineering education. More importantly this paper provides the theoretical framework for the diffusion and the adoption patterns for blended labs using Rogers [2] theory of perceived attributes and takes into account the important intergroup influence of faculty on students.

2 Literature Survey

2.1 Diffusion of Educational Technologies

Roger [2] in his perceived theory of attributes writes that 'the perceived attributes of an innovation are one important explanation of the rate of adoption of an innovation'. The theory states that an innovation is perceived based on its relative advantage, compatibility, complexity, trialability, and observability. In order for an innovation to undergo a faster rate of diffusion the potential adopters must perceive that innovation (1) to have advantage relative to other innovations (2) to be compatible with existing practices and values (3) is not very complex (4) can be tried on a limited basis before adoption (5) offers observable results. According to Dayton [7] of these five attributes, relative advantage, compatibility and complexity influence the most when it comes to decision by potential adopters [8] focused on the importance of studying the adoption and diffusion of innovation in field of educational technology. The proportion of potential adopters who have adopted the innovation determines the success of any innovation. Over the years researchers have empirically confirmed that the rate of diffusion forms an S-shaped curve which represents a cumulative distribution of adopters. The shape of the curve rises slowly at first, because there are few adopters initially and accelerates to a maximum value till the point of inflection is reached. Thereafter the curve's rate of increase slows down until the remaining individuals have adopted. The two-segment structure with asymmetric influence which assumes the existence of influentials and imitators was studied by [9] which is very relevant to high-technology, healthcare care products can also be seen in the context of educational innovation involving faculties and students.

2.2   Blended Learning and Blended Labs

Web based networked technologies have provided the foundation for creation of new lab frameworks for science education in a blended learning context. There have been studies comparing the conceptual understanding in students when exposed to both physical and virtual labs. A framework for blending physical and virtual experiments was proposed by [5] based on specific learning outcomes such as cognitive, affective and psychomotor related objectives. The inference from this work was that blending physical and virtual labs did enhance student's conceptual understanding. Much of the literature talks about the importance of blended learning and hybridization of online and face-to-face instruction that could include a mixture of instructional modalities and methods [10]. The survey of the thesis's from a decade of research in blended learning portrayed insufficient emphasis on the impact of student motivation and engagement in blended learning environments [11]. Olympiou [12] in his work described the patterns of collaborative problem solving in an online experimental environment where groups of students conducted physical labs and online experiments collaboratively. The results indicated students performed better when the level of collaboration is high and when they were exposed to virtual labs prior to the physical labs. These results do not still indicate if individual learning has been progressive with this approach. When considering the use of VLs in a blended mode, one should anticipate its use by a growing scientific community of students that may be present at multiple locations. It becomes imperative to build scalable blended labs to accommodate a large number of students.

2.3   Virtual Labs for Engineering Education

One of the largest projects that have successfully built over 1500 virtual experiments as part of over 150 labs in nine disciplines of science and engineering to complement physical labs can be viewed at (www.vlab.co.in). The three fold objectives of VLs included: bridging digital divide and disparity in quality education across higher educational institutes, use of ICT in creating as nearly an experience of a lab to a remote learner and aligning content to complement the undergraduate and graduate curricula. These virtual labs cover different flavors of experiments from interactive animations, modeling and simulations with user interfaces mimicking reality to remote triggering equipment's made available over the web. As part of this mission, The Virtual Amrita Labs Universalizing Education project (VALUE) developed over 250 VL experiments in several areas including biotechnology, physics, chemistry, mechanical engineering and computer science [13]. An in-depth study on the development of VL [14, 15] showed how diverse areas of biotechnology that may be either protocol intensive or computationally demanding could both be incorporated in VLs.

3 Case Study: Factors Affecting Diffusion of Blended Labs

3.1 Research Model and Hypothesis

In the diffusion model of blended lab technology for learning we chose student positive behavior intention as the dependent variable. The blended lab's rate of adoption was investigated by assessing two groups of characteristics, which were the independent variables - innovation characteristics and environment characteristics (Fig. 1).

Employing Rogers [2] framework, Bass [16] proposed mathematical model as a nonlinear differential equation for diffusion of an innovation in a group of size M. In such a scenario [17] adoption of innovation is due to two influences viz. external influence (mass media) which is a linear mechanism and internal influence (word-of-mouth) which is a non-linear mechanism. The differential equation giving the diffusion is

$$\frac{dN(t)}{dt} = (p + qN(t))(M - N(t)) \tag{1}$$

where N(t) is the cumulative number of adopter-students who have already adopted by time t, M is total number of adopter-students who will eventually use the innovation, p is the coefficient of external influence and q is the coefficient of internal influence.

In terms of the fraction F(t) of potential adopter-students

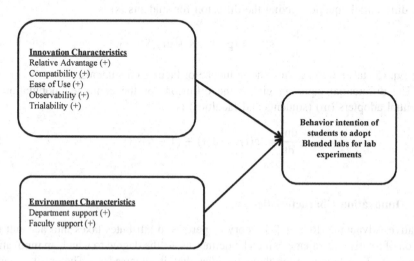

Fig. 1. Research model for diffusion of Blended Labs

$$F(t) = \frac{N(t)}{M} \tag{2}$$

the Bass model can be rewritten as

$$\frac{dN(t)}{dt} = (p + qMF(t))(1 - F(t)), F(t = 0) = F_0 \tag{3}$$

Equation (3) yields the S-shaped diffusion curve. It is assumed that the carrying capacity M of the adopter-students remains constant.

Now we extend the Bass model to account for the interinfluence of faculty on students. We define the following terms.

- p_1 external influence for the adopter-faculties
- q_1 internal influence for the adopter-faculties
- F total number of adopter-faculties who will eventually adopt the innovation
- f cumulative number of adopter-faculties who have already adopted by time t
- p_2 external influence for the adopter-students
- q internal influence for the adopter-students
- S total number of adopter-students who will eventually adopt the innovation
- s cumulative number of adopter-students who have already adopted by time t
- m total number of adopters who will eventually adopt the innovation
- μ relative importance students give to faculties for their support ($0 \le \mu \le 1$)
- α proportion of faculties in the total population of potential adopters ($0 \le \alpha \le 1$).

The differential equation giving the diffusion for faculties (f) is

$$\frac{df}{dt} = f(t) = (p_1 + q_1 f)(F - f). \tag{4}$$

The differential equation giving the diffusion for students (s) is

$$\frac{ds}{dt} = s(t) = (p_2 + q_2 s + \mu f)(S - s). \tag{5}$$

The Eq. (5) takes into account the influence of faculty on students.

The differential equation giving the diffusion for the combined population of potential adopters (m) (students and faculties) is

$$\frac{dm}{dt} = m(t) = \alpha f(t) + (1 - \alpha)s(t). \tag{6}$$

3.2   Innovation Characteristics

Relative Advantage: Rogers [2] theory of perceived attributes takes into account the notion of relative advantage, which he defines as − 'the degree to which an innovation is perceived as being better than the idea that it supersedes'. The most obvious advantage of BL is in the mixing of both PL and VL to offer best of both worlds.

Our hypothesis is Relative advantage of BL positively affects student's intention to adopt it (H1).

Compatibility: [2] defines compatibility as 'the degree to which an innovation is perceived as consistent with existing values, past experiences, and needs of potential adopters'. In terms of compatibility, BL learning approach is compatible in its functionality with the learning approach of PL. Our hypothesis is Compatibility of BL positively affects student's intention to adopt it (H2).

Complexity: Any innovation quickly gains a reputation as to its ease or difficulty of use [2]. In this context an important question is to what extent BL is perceived by users as complicated to use. In specific, the idea of complexity, as described by [2] was formulated from an "Ease of use" perspective in this study whereas the notion of adoption was substituted with the notion of attitude towards use. Our hypothesis is Ease of Use of BL positively affects student's intention to adopt it (H3).

Trialability: Trialability is "the degree to which an innovation may be experimented with on a limited basis" [2]. Innovations that potential adopter can experiment with on a trial basis are more easily adopted because an innovation that can be tried presents less risk to the potential adopter. Our hypothesis is Trialability of BL positively affects student's intention to adopt it (H4).

Observability: Another aspect of [2] is related to − the degree to which the results of an innovation are visible to others. Sometimes, observability refers to the ease with which the innovation is communicated to potential adopters. Our hypothesis is Observability of BL positively affects student's intention to adopt it (H5).

Department Support: More often teachers and students are motivated to consider technology decisions that are sanctioned and supported by the management since those will have adequate support resources. Department head who is the final decision maker for technology decision can play a pivotal role in encouraging students to use BL for learning. Our hypothesis is Department Support for BL positively affects student's intention to adopt it (H6).

Faculty Support: Since faculties play a pivotal role in implementing educational innovations, their perception of the innovation will strongly influence their students thinking. In other words, for the innovation to be successful, the personal willingness of faculty to adopt and integrate innovation into their classroom practice is crucial. The faculty has a positive interinfluence effect on the students. Our hypothesis is Faculty Support for BL positively affects student's intention to adopt it (H7).

4 Research Methodology

4.1 Participants

In this study, 246 students participated (54 % male, 46 % female). All students were either typical undergraduate engineering students who were enrolled in the engineering curriculum of Computer Science, Mechanical Engineering or integrated Master of Science majors in Physics and Chemistry. They were all in the first year of their study and had physical labs as part of their curriculum. None of the students had any exposure to these experiments prior to this study.

4.2 Implementation Methodology

The students were randomly divided into three groups. All measurements targeted individuals and not the groups.

- PL: Physical Labs Only. This group of students performed experiments only under the Physical lab (PL) condition.
- BLEND1: Blended Labs. The second group performed experiments under Blended Lab condition (PL followed by VL).
- BLEND2: Blended Labs. The third group performed experiments under Blended lab condition (VL followed by PL).

In BL students were given a complete orientation on how to perform experiments under VL. The orientation included showing pages that listed the objectives of the experiment followed by the procedural sequence to performing the experiment and concluding with the assignment. Pointers to the critical features such as viewing the video that had an overview of the experiment followed by interactive animation, if available and use of online help were presented. All of the students had fair amount of experience using computers on a day-to-day basis. Similarly in the case of PL, students were given written description of the experiment, objectives and its background. The procedure was then described. Each student had an opportunity to perform one or two iterations of the experiment to collect the necessary data. The number of iterations students did in PL and VL were held constant. The post lab assessment questions were almost identical in most cases. In cases where physical measurements were taken (for e.g. of the bar magnet) in PL, this data was given for VL students. More flexibility and additional variable factors were available in VL, so students got deeper understanding of the physical concepts and the impact of variables. The feedback was collected from students from both the BLEND1, BLEND2 groups. The Likert scaled feedback questions were modified based on a pre-survey study of five students (2 males and 3 females). A total of 33 questions were given to them and discussions with them were held to ensure that the questions were unambiguous and more importantly pertinent to their experiences with the blended lab approach. The total count of questions was reduced to 26 after this initial pre-survey study.

4.3 Measures

The post lab questions administered to the students tested their scientific grasp of the experiments. Both in PL and VL, students tabulated data in identical formats. Mathematical manipulations were required after data collection to arrive at the stipulated results. No auto-calculation facility was provided in VL and derivations needed to be done on paper as in PL. The results from both PL and VL were graded.

4.4 Research Procedure

Experiments that pertained to characterization techniques in three distinct areas related to magnetism, mechanics and optics were chosen in this study.

Deflection & Vibration Magnetometers: This experiments involved understanding the magnetic dipole moment of bar magnets and the horizontal intensity of earth's magnetic field. This required several trial data to be collected for the period of oscillation of the bar magnet as a function of its size using the vibration magnetometer and then on the deflection magnetometer, where the directions of the magnets were varied between tanA, tanB and tanC directions to calculate the ratio of the dipole moment to the earth's horizontal intensity. In the VL scenario, a complete animation sequence showing the entire experiment is provided. The animation allows students to get a full feel of the experiment after reading the theory (Fig. 2). Using the simulation engine of the VL experiment, students were allowed to vary a set of factors as in the physical lab like the size of the magnet, stop watch, rotation of the graduated scale that seats the compass box and the orientation of the magnet. To note the compass readings a tabular spreadsheet allows the students to immediately the values they see on the stop watch, the compass and the scale. Other than feeling the weight of the magnet and other components, every other aspect of the experiment was successfully replicated on the VL experiment.

At the end of both PL and VL experiments, the students calculated the moment of inertia of the magnet, the dipole of the magnet, and horizontal intensity of the magnetic field. On the VL experiments, additional questions were asked to observe variations from using magnets of different sizes.

Determining Young's Modulus of a Material: The learning objectives of this experiment included deciphering the young's modulus of a material using uniform bending technique and the factors that influence it (Fig. 3). The material of the beam could be wood, aluminum, copper or steel. The beam is supported on two knife edges. The parameters that can be varied include: (1) the distance between the knife edges (2) the addition of weights to the two hangers suspended symmetrically from the beam (3) the distance between the suspended weights. By focusing a microscope on the small

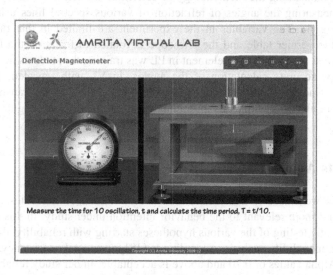

Fig. 2. Virtual Lab for Deflection Magnetometer

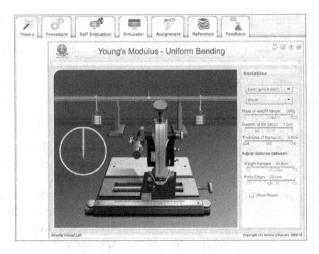

Fig. 3. Virtual Lab for Young's Modulus

deflections from bending and measuring it, the Young's modulus is calculated. In VL experiments, as in the PL, the microscope knobs can be adjusted to focus the crosswire on the pin mounted on the beam. The zoom feature allows accurate measurement of the beam deflection. There are two key distinctions between the PL and VL experiments in this case. They are (1) the beam width and thickness can be varied in VL and (2) the environment of the experiment with varying gravities can be easily changed in the VL. In PL, the beams are not varied and the experimental environment is a constant.

Measure Refractive Index using Prism Spectrometer: The learning objectives included understanding the methodology to determine the refractive index of a glass prism by measuring the angles of refraction of various spectral lines using a spectrometer (Fig. 4). The variables in the experiment are limited in that the prism is placed on the vernier table and the telescope is rotated to focus on the transmitted light. The most time consuming element in PL was training the students in the process sequence for accurate calculation of the angles. In VL with repeated attempts of changing the incident light and looking for the spectral lines of the transmitted light students were able to identify this minimum angle effortlessly and plug them into the Snell's law.

5   Results Analysis

SPSS and R were used to analyze the data. Some innovation attributes emerged as dominant and more relevant to the behavior intention under study. In this section we do a systematic testing of the various hypotheses starting with reliability, discriminant and convergent validity analysis. According to [18] for internal consistency, reliability Cronbach Alpha values of 0.70 and above is acceptable. In our study reliability of the seven factors had values ranging from 0.89 to 0.94. For discriminant validity analysis

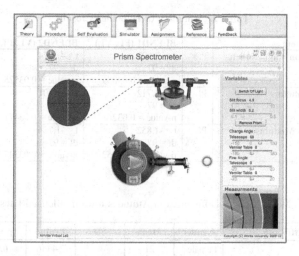

Fig. 4. Virtual Lab for Prism Spectrometer

we confirmed that Average Variance Extracted (AVE) between the attributes were larger than off-diagonal elements and AVE's were well above the recommended 0.50 level. Regression analysis was performed using all the 7 independent variables. Results are summarized in the Table 1. There is strong support for Hypothesis H1 (Relative Advantage), H2 (Compatibility), H3 (Ease of Use), H6 (Department Support) and H7 (Teacher support). The regression model was statistically significant ($p < 0.0001$) and accounting for 81 % of the variation in intention to adopt ($R^2 = 0.81$).

Further analysis of the two BL conditions (BLEND1, BLEND2) against the PL yielded interesting results (Table 2). Regardless of the order sequence of PL and VL within the BL, student learning outcomes under BL condition were better.

According to the independent t-test results to determine gender differences (Table 3), Male students were found more positive about adopting BL than Female students. The gender difference was significant for innovation attributes like Ease of Use, Relative Advantage and Trialability.

Table 1. Summary of Hypothesis results

Attributes		Beta	t-values	Result
Relative Advantage*	H1	0.41	3.56	Accepted
Compatibility*	H2	0.34	3.29	Accepted
Ease of Use*	H3	0.29	2.89	Accepted
Trialability	H4	−0.25	−2.14	Rejected
Observability	H5	−0.42	−2.45	Rejected
Department support*	H6	0.54	3.41	Accepted
Faculty support*	H7	0.49	2.94	Accepted
R^2		0.81		
Adjusted R^2		0.76		

*$p < 0.0001$

Table 2. Summary of Hypothesis results

Experiment		BLEND1 (PL, VL)	BLEND2 (VL, PL)
Deflection magnetometer	PL	t = -1.823 df = 97 p-value = 0.03859	t = -1.674 df = 97 p-value = 0.03525
Spectrometer	PL	t = -1.712 df = 97 p-value = 0.03261	t = -1.701 df = 97 p-value = 0.03471
Young's Modulus	PL	t = -1.852 df = 97 p-value = 0.03452	t = -1.734 df = 97 p-value = 0.03347

Table 3. Gender Differences in Attitudes towards Blended Labs

Attribute	Gender	Mean	SD	t value	p-value
RA Relative Advantage	Female	21	4	2.4446	**0.007**
	Male	22	4		
COM Compatibility	Female	10	2	1.027	0.15
	Male	10	2		
EOU Ease of Use	Female	13	2	3.2853	**0.0005**
	Male	14	2		
OBS Observability	Female	13	2	1.31	0.14
	Male	14	3		
TRI Trialability	Female	13	2	2.7099	**0.003**
	Male	14	2		
DS Department Support	Female	11	2	0.5743	0.283
	Male	11	2		
FS Faculty Support	Female	13	2	2.2287	0.14
	Male	14	3		

Since student's perception of faculty support emerged as a significant factor for adoption of Blended Labs, we looked at the shape of the resulting diffusion curve using intergroup influence adoption diffusion equations. It is intuitive to assume that the proportion of teachers is much less than that of the students. To illustrate different types of diffusion patterns we plot the m(t) (Eq. 6) along with its two parts $\alpha f(t)$ and $(1 - \alpha)s(t)$ for different set of parameter values of p's, q's, α and μ (Table 4).

In Fig. 5, Case (1) deals with the situation of high faculty support for students and results in a bell shaped diffusion curve. Case (2) deals with the situation of very low faculty support which results in delayed start of adoption by students but still results in a bell shaped diffusion curve. Case (3) where there is low faculty support results in a bimodal diffusion curve as faculties have reached their peak adoption levels before the students start adopting. It is easy to observe that low values of faculty support results in delay of diffusion among students.

Table 4. Set of parameters for different diffusion patterns with varying levels of faculty support

Case	Faculty parameters	Student parameters	Level of faculty support (μ)	Proportion of faculty (α)
1	$p_1 = 0.02$ $q_1 = 0.4$	$p_2 = 0.005$ $q_2 = 0.2$	0.3 (high)	0.2
2	$p_1 = 0.02$ $q_1 = 0.4$	$p_2 = 0.005$ $q_2 = 0.2$	0.005 (very low)	0.2
3	$p_1 = 0.02$ $q_1 = 0.4$	$p_2 = 0.005$ $q_2 = 0.2$	0.05 (low)	0.2

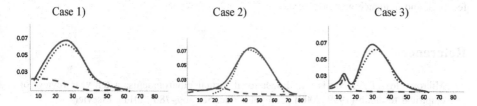

Fig. 5. Diffusion patterns based on students perception of varying levels of faculty support

6 Conclusions

Diffusion of Innovations framework when applied to blended learning in the context of lab education from this study showed its perception as a novelty and therefore an innovation by potential-adopter students. They ranked innovation attributes like Relative Advantage, Ease of Use, Compatibility, Department support and Faculty support as dominant factors. The Blended Labs innovation was better than the previous approach of using only Physical Labs or Virtual Labs (Relative Advantage); it was compatible with previously adopted idea of Virtual Labs (Compatibility); the concept was relatively easy to understand and use (Ease of Use); Students were able to try it out on a limited basis (Trialability), and finally the students could observe the results on the new Blended labs approach (observability). An interesting finding from our work is the emergence of Faculty support as a dominant factor for adoption of Blended Labs which confirms that for an educational innovation to diffuse both faculty and student adopters have to be targetted. Low levels of faculty support generally results in delayed diffusion among students. Our study results also indicate strong positive learning outcomes under BL when compared to PL though within BL, order sequence of PL and VL was not significant. For certain innovation attributes like Relative Advantage, Ease of Use and Trialability gender differences were significant. Unlike the difficulties faced with blended courses due to lack of teacher adoption [19] the data in this paper shows acceptance of blended approach to lab experiments by students. [20] noted 'Blended learning should be viewed as a pedagogical approach that combines the effectiveness and socialization opportunities of the classroom with the technologically enhanced active learning possibilities of the online environment'. The blended labs combine the best elements of physical labs and virtual labs.

An activity like lab experiment, whether done through Virtual Labs or Physical Labs is reasonably equally effective if the students performing them are cognitively active by constructing the experiments. Such a constructivist learning is supported by Blended Labs. The value of enhancing students skills by integrating virtual labs with physical labs not only provides improved conceptual learning but provides an ideal strategy to scale laboratory infrastructure easily.

Acknowledgements. This project derives direction and ideas from the Chancellor of Amrita University, Sri Mata Amritanandamayi Devi. This work is in part funded by Amrita University and National Mission on Education through ICT (NME ICT), Govt. of. India. The authors would like to acknowledge the contributions of faculty and staff at Amrita University whose feedback and guidance was invaluable.

References

1. Mikropoulos, T.A., Natsis, A.: Educational virtual environments: a ten-year review of empirical research (1999–2009). Comput. Educ. **56**, 769–780 (2011). Elsevier
2. Rogers, E.M.: Diffusion of Innovations, 5th edn. The Free Press, New York (2003)
3. Feisel, L., Rosa, A.: The role of the laboratory in undergraduate engineering education. J. Eng. Educ. **94**, 121–130 (2005)
4. Toth, E.E., Morrow, B.L., Ludvico, L.R.: Designing blended inquiry learning in a laboratory context: a study of incorporating hands-on and virtual laboratories. Innovative High. Educ. **33**(5), 333–344 (2009)
5. Zacharia, Z.C.: Comparing and combining real and virtual experimentation: an effort to enhance students' conceptual understanding of electric circuits. J. Comput. Assist. Learn. **23**, 120–132 (2007)
6. Corter, J.E., Esche, S.K., Chassapis, C., Ma, J., Nickerson, J.V.: Process and learning outcomes from remotely-operated simulated, and hands-on student laboratories. Comput. Educ. **57**, 2054–2067 (2011)
7. Dayton, D.: A hybrid analytical framework to guide studies of innovative IT adoption by work groups. Tech. Comm. Q. **15**(3), 355–382 (2006)
8. Surry, D.W., Farquhar, J.D.: Diffusion theory and instructional technology. J. Instr. Sci. Technol. **2**(1), 24–36 (1997)
9. Van den Bulte, C., Joshi, Y.V.: New product diffusion with influentials and imitators. Mark. Sci. **26**, 400–421 (2007)
10. Drysdale, J.S., Graham, C.R., Spring, K.J., Halverson, L.R.: An analysis of research trends in dissertations and theses studying blended learning. Internet High. Educ. **17**, 90–100 (2013)
11. Barros, B., Read, T., Verdejo, M.F.: Virtual collaborative experimentation: an approach combining remote and local labs. IEEE Trans. Educ. **51**, 242–250 (2008)
12. Olympiou, G., Zacharia, Z.C.: Blending physical and virtual manipulatives: an effort to improve students' conceptual understanding through science laboratory experimentation. Sci. Educ. **96**(1), 21–47 (2012)
13. Achuthan, K., Sreelatha, K.S., Surendran, S., Diwakar, S., Nedungadi, P., Humphreys, S., Sreekala, S., Pillai, Z., Raman, R., Deepthi, A., Gangadharan, R., Appukuttan, S., Ranganatha, J., Sambhudevan, S., Mahesh, S.: The VALUE @ Amrita Virtual Labs Project. In: proceedings of IEEE Global Humanitarian Technology Conference Proceedings, pp. 117–121 (2011)

14. Diwakar, S., Achuthan, K., Nedungadi, P., Nair, B.: Invited chapter - biotechnology virtual labs: facilitating laboratory access anytime-anywhere for classroom education. In: Agbo, E.C. (ed.) Innovations in Biotechnology InTech, ISBN: 978-953-51-0096-6 (2012)
15. Nair, B., Krishnan, R., Nizar, N., Rajan, K., Yoosef, A., Sujatha, G., Radhamony, V., Achuthan, K., Diwakar, S.: Role of ICT-Enabled Visualization-Oriented Virtual Laboratories in Universities for Enhancing Biotechnology Education – VALUE Initiative: Case Study and Impacts, FormaMente, Vol. VII, no. 1–2, ISSN 1970-7118 (2012)
16. Bass, F.M.: A new product growth for model consumer durables. Manag. Sci. **15**, 215–227 (1969)
17. Karmeshu, Pathria, R.K.: Stochastic evolution of a nonlinear model of diffusion of information. J. Math. Soc. **7**, 59–71 (1980)
18. Nunnally, J., Bernstein, I.H.: Psychometric Theory, 3rd edn. McGraw-Hill, New York (1994)
19. Mehmet, A.O.: Why are faculty members not teaching blended courses? Insights from faculty members. Comput. Educ. **56**, 689–699 (2011)
20. Dziuban, C., Hartman, J., Moskal, P.: Blended learning. EDUCAUSE Rev. (7) (2004)

The Impact of Internet Banking on Service Quality Provided by Commercial Banks

Angeline Liza Ndachiphata Chima
and Vanwyk Khobidi Chikasanda[⊠]

University of Malawi –The Polytechnic, P/Bag 303 Blantyre, Malawi
vchikasanda@poly.ac.mw

Abstract. Information technology has become the most important factor in the present and future development of banking, influencing business strategies of banks. One of the popular technologies is the internet which has changed operations of businesses. E-developments are rapidly emerging in all financial intermediation and markets but the phenomenon has not been researched in Malawi. This study investigated the impact of internet banking on service quality in one of the commercial banks in Malawi. The study measured service quality attributable to internet banking and explored ways of improving its delivery. The research employed a structured deductive approach in which the IBM and SERVQUAL theories were tested using a descriptive survey of 235 users of internet banking chosen from all the Blantyre branches of the bank. Results revealed that users of internet banking were generally satisfied with quality of service. The users were satisfied with internet banking variables such as security of information, ease of use, site organization, speed of transaction, ability to correct transactions, accessibility, information availability, problem solution and affordability. The study recommends further research to understand implications of internet banking on service quality in all banks in Malawi.

Keywords: E-banking · Information technology · Commercial banks · Malawi · Service quality

1 Introduction

Information technology (IT) has become the most important factor in the present and future development of banking, influencing marketing and business strategies of banks (Luštšik, 2003). One of the most popular technologies of our time is the internet which has essentially changed the operations of many businesses, and has become a powerful channel for business marketing and communication. E-developments are rapidly emerging in all areas of financial intermediation and financial markets leading to e-banking (electronic banking) a new service delivery platform in the banking sector.

Banan (2010) defines e-banking as the use of computer technology to give the option of bypassing the time-consuming, paper-based aspects of traditional banking. In other words, e-banking is an umbrella term by which a customer performs banking transactions electronically without visiting their bank. It encompasses the following channels though the list is not exhaustive:

© Institute for Computer Sciences, Social Informatics and Telecommunications Engineering 2014
T.F. Bissyandé and G. van Stam (Eds.): AFRICOMM 2013, LNICST 135, pp. 248–259, 2014.
DOI: 10.1007/978-3-319-08368-1_29

- Mobile banking (cell phone banking). In this channel, customers carry out banking transactions on their cell phones.
- Internet banking (online banking): Customers carry out bank transactions using their computers. This is real time and on line. This means that the accounts are updated as the customer is transacting.
- Telephone banking (Tele banking): Using this channel, customers do not carry out bank transactions themselves, but issue instruction to their bankers for example, asking for an account balance or requesting for funds transfer.
- Point of sale (POS): It is a device on which customers use debit cards to purchase items in shops rather than moving around with cash.
- Automated Teller Machines (ATMs): ATMs are machines where customers do some bank transactions like cash withdrawal, balance inquiry, printing min statements etc using a card.

According to Zarifopoulos and Economides (2009), out of the channels listed above, internet banking and mobile banking are the most popular and widely used. Laukkanen (2007) claims that out of these two channels, mobile banking stands out as a wireless service delivery channel providing increased value for customers' banking transactions. However, despite its many advantages, the use of mobile phones in banking services is still in its infancy and internet banking retains its position as the leading channel in the series of technological wonders of the recent past.

The new phenomenon in banking has not been researched in Malawi. Therefore, this study investigated the impact of internet banking on service quality in one of the commercial banks in Malawi. The objective of the study was to measure service quality attributable to internet banking and to explore ways of improving the delivery of internet banking and two major specific objectives arose and viz: to measure service quality that Internet Banking brings about to Standard Bank customers; and to suggest ways of improving internet banking in order to enhance service quality.

2 Related Literature

In recent years a large number of research studies have been conducted investigating the characteristics of banks that adopted internet banking (Jenkins, 2007). Sohail and Shaikh (2008) claim that much of the research in the context of internet banking has focused on investigating service quality attributes. Not only this but also a large number of empirical studies have been conducted with respect to the customer perception and acceptance of internet banking services (Durkin, 2004; Lee et al., 2005; Gerrard et al., 2006; Wang et al., 2000; Polatoglu and Ekin, 2003). In addition, there are also studies that looked at the benefits of internet banking. But, such studies have centered on the benefits of internet banking to banks and not to customers (Jenkins, 2007; Oliver, 1998). Most of the studies found out that by introducing internet banking, banks benefited a lot through cost cutting. The current researcher agrees with Johnsson and Gunnarson (2005) who found out that 'applying the internet with solely focusing on cost reduction may lead to high supply chain effectiveness while potential customer value opportunities may be ignored'. This is the reason Sohail and Shaikh

(2008) still maintain that no studies have paid sufficient attention in examining what customers (the actual users of the channel) perceive as the impact that internet banking has on service quality. However, even Sohail and Shaikh (2008) they too in their research had their own limitations. For instance, their sample included people who were not using internet banking. This might also have affected their findings. The question still remains unanswered 'by introducing this new channel, has service quality changed whether positively or negatively?' It is this gap that this research would like to fill.

2.1   Conceptual Framework

This research adopted internet banking model (IBM) as expounded by Mäenpää (2006); Sohail and Shaikh (2008); Safeena et al. (2011). These researchers came up with IBM variables as follows; ease of use, site organization, security concerns, speed of transactions, availability of internet, accessibility, information availability, problem solution, and affordability (see Fig. 1).

While most firms are keen to provide good service, many do not know how to manage customer expectations effectively because of its inherently intangible nature

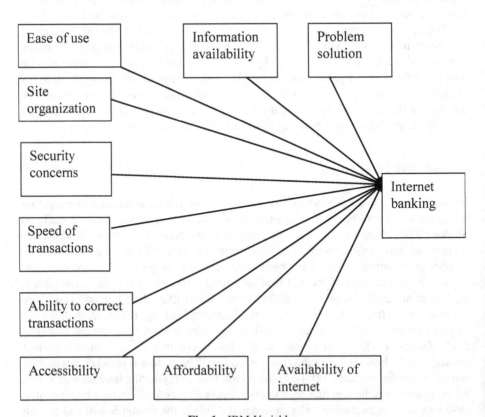

Fig. 1. IBM Variables

that makes it difficult to define service quality (Kandampully in Chua and Komoran, 2002). Early studies during 1980s focused on determining what service quality meant to customers and developing strategies to meet customer expectations (Parasuraman et al., 1988). The early pioneers of services marketing in Europe, especially the Nordic School, argued that service quality consists of two or three underlying dimensions. Lehtinen and Lehtinen (1985) referred to physical and interactive quality while Grönroos (1984) identified a technical dimension, a functional dimension and the firm's image as a third dimension. In later years, Parasuraman, et al. (1988) published empirical evidence from five service industries that suggested that five dimensions more appropriately capture the perceived service quality construct. Not only this, but some researchers have also conceptualized service quality as a gap between consumers' expectations and perceptions (Parasuraman, et al., 1988). In this paper, the writer adopted SERVQUAL instrument as developed by Parasuraman et al. and other researchers. This uncertainty hampers our understanding of service quality and casts doubts over the use of the SERVQUAL instrument in future research. It also shows that a considerable amount of research still needs to be done concerning the dimensionality of perceived service quality in general and SERVQUAL in particular, as called for by its developers (Parasuraman et al. 1991).

Service quality has been a frequently studied topic in various marketing literature. Much of the research done has focused on measuring service quality using SERV-QUAL instrument. The importance of service quality cannot be overemphasized. Akan (1995) stated that as competition increases, delivering better service becomes of more important nowadays than before. He further added that service quality is becoming a differentiating characteristic. Gronroos in Svensson (2004, p. 278) came up with seven ways in which service differs from physical goods as follows:

- Services are intangible and heterogeneous.
- The production, distribution and consumption of services are simultaneous process.
- Services are an activity or process.
- Service is a core value created in buyer – seller interactions.
- Customers participate in the production of service.
- Services cannot be kept in stock.
- There is no transfer of ownership in service.

Svensson (2007) further challenges "service quality is an important construct in service marketing; industrial marketing; relationship marketing as well as consumer marketing". Delivering quality service is essential for success and survival in today's competitive banking environment. (Yonggui et al., 2003). The author thinks this improves customer loyalty and retention and hence increases financial performance and profitability.

The major challenge of internet banking is how banks can manage service quality as this self service technology brings significant change in customer interaction and behaviour (Broderick and Vachirapornpuk, 2002). For a long time the customers have been used to visit branches and are served by bank's employees. With the coming of internet banking, the service is from their PCs, what a change! Service quality is therefore an important research topic in view of its significant relationship to costs, profitability, customer satisfaction, customer retention, service guarantee, and competitive capabilities. Service quality has also become a driver of corporate marketing and financial performance (Oliveira *et al.* 2002). One of the recent studies conducted by Al-Hawari and Ward (2006) further claim that service quality impacts on customer satisfaction which in turn affects the financial performance of banks.

Banking institutions often attempt to make their services more tangible by using different strategies to distinguish them from their competitors. Kassim and Abdulla (2006) claim that the problem of making services more tangible is particularly complex when they are provided not in a physical premise, with its own atmosphere, design or personal contact, but over the internet.

Al-Hawari et al., (2005), mentioned that numerous models have been developed to measure customer perceptions of service quality. Most of these models utilized face-to-face interaction between customers and the employees of service providers to conceptualize a service quality measurement models. However, developments in information and communications technology have provided a platform by which companies can design, develop and deliver services that can be perceived by customers as superior. Despite an agreement among researchers on the need to develop scales for assessing internet service quality, Sohail and Shaikh (2008) argue that literature has seldom addressed the measurement of customer perceptions of electronic service quality. The two also mentioned other scales such as; WEB-QUAL; IS-QUAL; SITEQUAL; E-S-QUAL; E-service quality and E-SERVQUAL. This researcher decided to use the SERVQUAL scale as developed by Parasuraman, et al. (1988).

SERVQUAL provides a technology for measuring and managing service quality (SQ). Since 1985, when the technology was first published, its innovators Parasuraman, et al., have further developed, promulgated and promoted the technology through a series of publications (Parasuraman et al., cited in Buttle, 1995).

SERVQUAL has traditionally been used as a generic instrument for measuring service quality of service providers with modifications to suit individual needs (Sohail and Shaikh 2008). This was echoed by Kang et al. (2002) who said that the SERVQUAL instrument has been the predominant method used to measure consumers' perceptions of service quality. Although many researchers have exposed deficiencies and inconsistencies regarding the validity of SERVQUAL, the scale remains the most widely accepted and used. Jabnoun and Khalifa (2005) explained five reasons that make SERVQUAL popular:

- It is accepted as a standard for assessing different dimensions of service quality.
- It has been shown to be valid for a number of service situations.
- It has been demonstrated to be reliable, meaning that different readers Interpret the questions similarity.
- The instrument is parsimonious in that it has a limited number of items...
- It has a standardized analysis procedure... page number if not paraphrased.

Parasuraman, et al. (1991) (cited in Rod et al. 2009) came up with a list of ten determinants (reliability; responsiveness; competence; access; courtesy; communication; credibility; security; understanding the customer; and tangibles) of service quality as a result of their focus group studies with service providers and customers which subsequently resulted in the development of the SERVQUAL instrument with these ten determinants distilled into five overall dimensions of service quality. The five dimensions of SERVQUAL as discussed by Rod et al. (2009) include reliability, responsiveness, assurance, empathy, and tangibles. The purpose of this paper was to examine the relationships among three dimensions of SERVQUAL that influence overall internet banking service quality just as Rod, et al. (2009) did. The three dimensions chosen are: assurance, empathy, and reliability.

3 Research Design

The research employed a structured deductive approach in which the IBM and SERVQUAL theories were tested. A descriptive survey using a self-completion questionnaire was used to generate the data. A self-service department of the bank provided email addresses of customers who were using internet banking. After getting their consent, a questionnaire was sent through email and allowed respondents to think about relevant key issues before completing the same at their convenience. The respondents sent their responses via the same email. The total population was 785 out of which 235 were chosen as a sample representing 30 % of the population and these were from all the Blantyre branches of the bank.

4 Results and Discussion

Results revealed that users of internet banking were generally satisfied with quality of service provided through the channel. The users were satisfied with most internet banking variables such as security of banking information, ease of use, site organization, speed of transaction, ability to correct transactions, accessibility, information availability, problem solution and affordability.

4.1 Ease of Use and Security Concerns

The study revealed that many respondents (over 50 %) find it easy to use internet banking. Standard bank customers also rated how they perceive the organization of the bank's internet banking site. Many respondents (67 %) agreed and 18 % strongly agreed that the site is well organized while 12 % neither agreed nor disagreed whereas only 3 % disagreed. Security concerns involve online safety and trustworthiness. Customers should feel that their money is safe and that no third parties have access to their finances as well as financial information. From Fig. 2, a collective total of 82 % respondents agree that their funds are safe even when they use the internet banking channel. There is nothing to worry about as far as security is concerned.

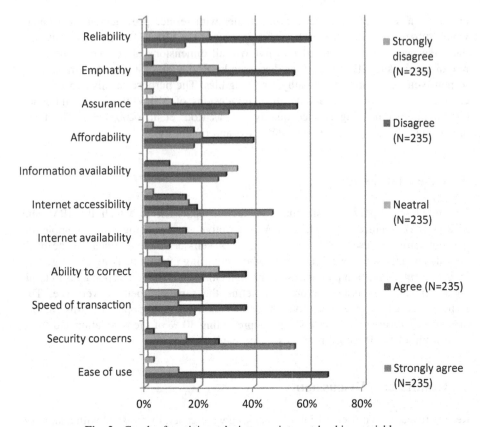

Fig. 2. Graph of participants' views on internet banking variables

4.2   Speed of Transactions and Ability to Correct Transactions

This refers to prompt processing of transactions. One thing that customers hate is to be kept waiting for a transaction or stand on a queue for a long time. Results presented in Fig. 2 show that a collective total of 55 % of the respondents agreed that carrying out transactions on internet banking was fast. This represents more than half of the respondents. 33 % disagreed while 12 % neither agreed nor disagreed.

Even though nobody likes mistakes, people still make mistakes any way. In traditional banks mistakes are made when the customer is filling the paper work. These mistakes are corrected by either crossing out and signing for the change or tearing the paper and filling in a new one altogether. It is therefore vital that customers are confident to use internet banking with an assurance that they will be able to cancel a transaction if they made a mistake. It was revealed that 58 % of the respondents agreed that there is room to correct transaction mistakes on internet banking. This is against a total of 15 % which disagreed.

4.3 Availability of Internet

This speaks to the uptime of internet. Internet banking channel is supposed to be a solution of convenience to traditional banking. Availability plays a crucial role. This channel is expected to be up 24 hours 7 days weekly but this is impacted by persistent power outages. However, only a collective total of 42 % agreed while a collective total of 24 % disagreed. The responses show that the customers agree that internet banking is available when a customer needs it.

4.4 Accessibility and Information Availability

Accessibility entails the evenness of the website. Does it crash most of the time? Just like internet availability the results percentages are slanted towards strong agreements that internet banking has been accessible. Guidance should be prearranged to customers on each and every step they take on the website. All essential information for the customer should be given on the website to such an extent that the customer does not have to ask for assistance over and over again. Collectively 57 % of the respondents agreed that information is readily available on internet banking while 9 % disagreed (See Fig. 2).

4.5 Problem Solution

As an internet banking provider, the bank has to arrange for problem solution options for the customer. They could have well trained personnel at the customer care centre to be contacted during the day as well as an online pop up guidance for the night hours. Many respondents (34 %) were undecided. Notwithstanding though, findings given in Fig. 2 skew to agreement as a total of 58 % were in agreement versus a total of 21 % in disagreement.

4.6 Affordability

It is general anticipation from the customer that e-banking channels should be rationally priced as compared to alternatives in order for customers to easily adopt them. Internet banking is one of the e-banking channels. For instance the pricing must catch the attention of the customer to prefer using internet banking to traditional banking. 87 % agreed.

4.7 Assurance, Empathy, Reliability of Internet Banking

Assurance, empathy and reliability of internet banking are dependent variables that were rated by the customers. Most respondents (67 %) agreed that internet banking promotes assurance compared to 6 % that disagreed. Like assurance, results on empathy also tend to lean towards agreement. A collective total of 88 % agreed against 12 % in disagreement. A collective total of 88 % agreed that internet banking is reliable. Only 3 % disagreed while 9 % were not sure.

4.8   Inferential Statistics

This research collected data which is non-parametric. The data is categorical and ranked. Saunders et al. (2008) assert that such type of data can be analyzed by calculating the Spearman's Rank Correlation Coefficients. These coefficients signify how the variables are correlated. The correlation are tested to be either significant or not by comparing the p-values with a chosen α-value such as $\alpha = 0.05$ or 0.01. If the p-value is smaller than the α-value, whether on a one-tailed or two-tailed test, the researcher either accepts or rejects the null hypotheses. In this research, the null hypothesis says there is a relationship between internet banking and service quality and the alternative hypothesis says there is no relationship between internet banking and service quality. This means that no matter what the result of the research could be, it would fall in either of the two hypotheses. Thus, it follows a one-tail test concept. Therefore, the results of the research, as in Table 1, below, were done in order to come up with the one-tailed test for which the Spearman's Rank Correlation Coefficients could be based.

Table 1 below shows the correlation coefficients for the independent against dependent variables. After getting the coefficients from SPSS, the data was exported to Excel in order to eliminate the one half unnecessary values so that the outcome could only have the other needed half. The respondents' attributes were also taken out so that the comparisons could only be made against independent and dependent variables for which two concepts will be related and concluded.

Table 1 shows the correlation coefficients at two α-levels ($\alpha = 0.01$ and $\alpha = 0.05$). Many independent variables show correlation with the dependent variables. Taking $\alpha = 0.05$, all the independent variables show that there is correlation with empathy, a dependent variable. The dependent variable (Reliability) also shows that there is correlation to all independent variables except affordability. However, the dependent variable (assurance) shows there are few correlations with independent variables. For example, site organization, ability to correct transactions and problem solution show correction with assurance, the rest of the independent variables show no correlation with assurance. Despite one variable (assurance) showing no correlation to most of the independent variables, the other two (reliability and empathy) show significant correlation with independent variables. Therefore, in general, the dependent concept is more correlated to the independent concept.

The null hypothesis was that there is a relationship between internet banking and service quality, while the alternative hypothesis stipulated that there is no relationship between internet banking and service quality as perceived by standard bank customer in Blantyre city. Since the independent variable is correlated to the dependent variable, then the null hypothesis holds. Therefore the researcher accepts the null hypothesis at $\alpha=0.05$. Therefore, there is a relationship between internet banking and service quality and the bank needs to strengthen the service with appropriate instruments.

Table 1. Non-parametric correlations for internet banking and service quality

Spearman's rho		Site_Organisation	Security_concerns	Abilit_to_Correct	Speed	Interne_Availability	Internet_Accessibility	Info_Availability	Problem_Solution	Affordability	Assurance	Empathy	Reliability
Ease_of_Use	Cor. Coef.	.552**	.347*	.414**	.500**	.321*	.345*	.518**	.387*	0.273	0.043	.310*	.388*
	Sig. (1-tailed)	0.001	0.026	0.009	0.002	0.036	0.029	0.001	0.014	0.069	0.407	0.042	0.014
	N	32	32	32	32	31	32	32	31	32	32	32	32
Site_Organisation	Cor. Coef.		.462**	.415**	.508**	.378*	.418**	.592**	.523**	.401*	.465**	.502**	.523**
	Sig. (1-tailed)		0.003	0.008	0.001	0.015	0.009	0	0.001	0.011	0.003	0.001	0.001
	N		33	33	33	33	32	33	33	32	33	33	33
Security_concerns	Cor. Coef.			.665**	.438**	.316*	.299*	.682**	.378*	0.148	0.068	.323*	.538**
	Sig. (1-tailed)			0	0.005	0.037	0.048	0	0.015	0.21	0.353	0.033	0.001
	N			33	33	33	32	33	33	32	33	33	33
Abilit_to_Correct	Cor. Coef.				.492**	0.288	0.126	.646**	.664**	0.154	.354*	.324*	.646**
	Sig. (1-tailed)				0.002	0.052	0.246	0	0	0.2	0.022	0.033	0
	N				33	33	32	33	33	32	33	33	33
Speed	Cor. Coef.					0.227	.443**	.725**	.351*	0.224	0.186	.543**	.446**
	Sig. (1-tailed)					0.102	0.006	0	0.022	0.109	0.15	0.001	0.005
	N					33	32	33	33	32	33	33	33
Internet_Availability	Cor. Coef.						.554**	.531**	.342*	0.077	0.208	.308*	.416**
	Sig. (1-tailed)						0.001	0.001	0.026	0.337	0.122	0.041	0.008
	N						32	33	33	32	33	33	33
Internet_Accessibility	Cor. Coef.							.595**	.343*	0.288	0.075	.429**	.334*
	Sig. (1-tailed)							0	0.027	0.058	0.341	0.007	0.031
	N							32	32	31	32	32	32
Info_Availability	Cor. Coef.								.529**	.368*	0.184	.437**	.492**
	Sig. (1-tailed)								0.001	0.019	0.152	0.005	0.002
	N								33	32	33	33	33
Problem_Solution	Cor. Coef.									0.279	.496**	.403*	.472**
	Sig. (1-tailed)									0.061	0.002	0.01	0.003
	N									32	33	33	33
Affordability	Cor. Coef.										0.264	.472**	0.127
	Sig. (1-tailed)										0.072	0.003	0.244
	N										32	32	32

**. Correlation is significant at the 0.01 level (1-tailed).
*. Correlation is significant at the 0.05 level (1-tailed).

5   Conclusion and Recommendations

Internet banking provides banks with a competitive advantage, by improving the quality of customer services and reducing the operational costs. However, banks should not apply the internet solely focusing on cost reduction while potential customer value opportunities are being ignored. In Malawi, little attention has been given to understand the impact of internet banking on service quality and it is unknown how customers perceive and evaluate electronically delivered services. This research has revealed that it is not enough to look at internet banking from the banker's view only. The customer's view also needs to be taken into account as well. The current research has therefore unearthed this existing knowledge gap related to internet banking in Malawi. It has identified the impact of internet banking on service quality as perceived by standard bank customers who have adopted the technology and revealed that they agree with most of the internet banking variables there is some concern on accessibility and security of the internet banking. While the customers' position may be attributed to national state of ICT infrastructure and general lack of knowledge of its usage, the bank needs to put policies in place to enable self service units support customers use of the facility. The study recommends further research to understand implications of internet banking on service quality in all banks in Malawi.

References

Al-Hawari, M., Ward, T.: The effect of automated service quality on Australian banks' financial performance and the mediating role of customer satisfaction. Mark. Intell. Plan. **24**(2), 127–147 (2006)

Al-Hawari, M., Hartley, N., Ward, T.: 'Measuring Banks' automated service quality: a confirmatory factor analysis approach. Mark. Bull. **16**(1), 1–19 (2005)

Banan, M.R.: E-banking and managerial challenges. Georgian Electron. Sci. J. Comput. Sci. Telecommun. **1**(24), 13–23 (2010)

Broderick, A.J., Vachirapornpuk, S.: Service quality in internet banking: the importance of customer role. Mark. Intell. Plan. **20**(6), 327–335 (2002)

Buttle, F.: SERVQUAL: review, critique, research agenda. Eur. J. Mark. **30**(1), 8–32 (1965)

Chowdhary, N., Parakash, M.: Prioritizing service quality dimensions. Managing Serv. Qual. **17**(5), 493–509 (2007)

Chua, C.C., Komaran, R.: Managing service quality by combining voice of the service provider and voice of their customers. Managing Serv. Qual. **12**(2), 77–86 (2002)

Durkin, M.: In search of internet banking customers; exploring the use of decision style. Int. J. Bank Mark. **22**(7), 484–503 (2004)

Gerrard, P., Cunningham, J., Devlin, J.: Why consumers are not using internet banking: a qualitative study. J. Serv. Mark. **20**(3), 160–168 (2006)

Jenkins, H.: Adopting internet banking services in a small island state: assurance of bank service quality. Managing Serv. Qual. **17**(5), 523–537 (2007)

Kang, G., Jeffrey, J., Alexandris, K.: Internal service quality: application of the SERVQUAL battery to internal service quality. Managing Serv. Qual. **12**(5), 278–291 (2002)

Kassim, N.M., Abdulla, A.: The influence of attraction on internet banking: an extension of the trust relationship commitment model. Int. J. Bank Mark. **24**(6), 424–442 (2006)

Laukkanen, T.: Internet Vs mobile banking: comparing customer value perception. Bus. Process Manag. J. **11**(4), 788–797 (2007)

Lee, E., Kwon, K., Schumann, D.W.: Segmenting the non-adopter category in the diffusion of internet banking. Int. J. Bank Mark. **23**(5), 414–437 (2005)

Luštšik, O.: E-banking in Estonia: Reasons and Benefits of Rapid Growth, vol. 3, pp. 24–35. Kroon & Economy, Taru (2003)

Mäenpää, K.: Clustering the consumers on the basis of their perceptions of the internet banking services. Internet Res. **16**(3), 304–322 (2006)

Oliveira, P., Roth, A.V., Gilland, W.: Achieving competitive capabilities in e-services. Technol. Forecast. Soc. Change **69**(7), 721–739 (2002)

Oliver, C.: Quality assuring an internet-based service. Managing Serv. Qual. **8**(2), 85–87 (1998)

Parasuraman, A., Berry, L.L., Zeithaml, V.A.: Refinement and reassessment of the SERVQUAL scale. J. Retail. **67**(4), 420–50 (1991)

Parasuraman, A., Zeithaml, V.A., Berry, L.L.: SERVQUAL: a multiple-item scale for measuring service quality. J. Retail. **64**(1), 12–40 (1988)

Polatoglu, V.N., Ekin, S.: An empirical investigation of the Turkish consumers' acceptance of internet banking services. Int. J. Bank Mark. **19**(4), 156–165 (2001)

Rod, M., Ashill, N.J., Shao, J., Caruthers, J.: An examination of the relationship between service quality dimensions, overall internet banking service quality and customer satisfaction: A New Zealand study. Mark. Intell. Plan. **27**(1), 103–126 (2009)

Safeena, R., Date, H., Kammani, A.: Internet banking adoption in an emerging economy: indian consumer's perspective. Int. Arab J. e-Technol. **2**(1), 56–64 (2011)

Saunders, M., Lewis, P., Thornhill, A.: Research Methods for Business Students, 4th edn. Financial Times Pitman Publishing, London (2007)

Svensson, G.: Interactive service quality in service encounters: empirical illustration and models. Managing Serv. Qual. **14**(4), 278–287 (2004)

Wang, Y., Wang, Y., Lin, H., Tang, T.: Determinants of user acceptance of internet banking: an empirical study. Int. J. Serv. Ind. Manag. **14**(5), 501–519 (2003)

Zarifopoulos, M., Economides, A.A.: Evaluating mobile banking portals. Int. J. Mob. Commun. **7**(1), 66–90 (2009)

Power Instability in Rural Zambia, Case Macha

Consider Mudenda[1], David Johnson[2], Lisa Parks[3], and Gertjan van Stam[1(✉)]

[1] Macha Works, Choma, Zambia
consider.mudenda@machaworks.org,
gertjan.vanstam@worksgroup.org
[2] Council of Scientific and Industrial Research, Cape Town, South Africa
djohnson@csir.co.za
[3] Center for Information Technology and Society, and Department of Film
and Media Studies, University of California, Santa Barbara, USA
parks@filmandmedia.ucsb.edu

Abstract. This paper provides insights on the nature of electricity supply in the rural village Macha, Zambia. It reports on case study research.
Use of Information and Communication Technologies and access to
e-services are constrained by the availability of electricity. In Zambia's
rural areas, 3.5 % of households have access to electricity supply. This
paper shows such electricity supply can be erratic. When supply is available, it follows a diurnal pattern. The electricity supply varies considerably, including voltage dips and brown outs. It can cause equipment to
enter into unstable states, to fail or to damage. Qualitative engineering
aspects interact also with social factors, especially in rural Africa. Interventions must be sensitive to the complex array of challenges for people
to be able to appropriate the benefits of ICT and e-services.

Keywords: Rural electrification · Power outages · Community
development

1 Introduction

This paper reports on engineering and ethnographic case study research from
within the rural community of Macha, Zambia. The work encompassed literature
review, interviews, and technical measurements between 2009 and 2013.

Zambia harbours a range of indigenous energy sources, including hydropower,
coal, woodlands and forests, and renewables. The country's hydropower resource
potential stands at an estimated 6,000 Mega Watts (MW) while the installed
capacity is a mere 1.9 MW [1]. Hydroelectric plants represent 99 % of electricity
production in the country with the major sources being Kafue Gorge, Kariba
North Bank and Victoria Falls Power Stations, and developments at Kafue Gorge
Lower, Itezhi-tezhi and Kalungwishi.

The major electricity users are the mines, which consume up to 68 % of the
total load. Industry and commerce account for 4 %, households for 19 %, and
agriculture and forestry consume 2 % of the supply. Government services use

© Institute for Computer Sciences, Social Informatics and Telecommunications Engineering 2014
T.F. Bissyandé and G. van Stam (Eds.): AFRICOMM 2013, LNICST 135, pp. 260–270, 2014.
DOI: 10.1007/978-3-319-08368-1_30

the remaining 7% [2]. Woodland and forests cover about 66% of the Zambia's land area and provide about 70% of its energy requirements. Zambian households mostly consume wood-fuel. This leads to deforestation to serve the (urban) demands for charcoal [3].

Zambia's developments have been guided by the Fifth National Development Plant, published in 2006 [4], and the Sixth National Development Plan in 2012 [1]. The plans position access to electricity equal to the need for shelter and water for every Zambian on a daily basis.

A 2009 ZESCO investigation assessed the degree of electrification in Zambia and determined the percentage of those with direct access to grid electricity and isolated electric systems. In 2009, 22% of all Zambian households had direct access to grid electricity, a small increase of 2% since 2005 [1]. Isolated electric systems serve a mere 0.03% of the population while the remaining 78% of the population has no access to electricity supply [5].

2 Zambia's Production Capacity

The Zambian electricity system is part of an interconnected regional power system that links it with its neighbors. The Zambian electricity supply industry was predominantly run by a single state owned company, the Zambia Electricity Supply Corporation (ZESCO). ZESCO was created in 1970 through the Zambia Electricity Supply Act. The Electricity Act, the Factories Act, and the Energy Regulation Act are the main governing legislation for electricity suppliers.

Liberalization in 1995 aimed to attract private sector companies to participate in the generation, transmission and distribution of electricity in Zambia. In order to promote this policy, the government set up the Energy Regulation Board (ERB) and the Office for the Promotion of Private Power Investors (OPPPI). The ERB regulates operations and pricing and the OPPPI promotes new players within the electricity market.

Three major players dominate in electricity provisioning in Zambia:

- ZESCO generates, transmits, distributes and supplies electricity throughout Zambia
- Copperbelt Energy Corporation (CEC) distributes electricity purchased from ZESCO through a network to the mining industry based in the Copperbelt
- Lunsemfwa Hydro Power Company, an independent power producer, generates about 48 MW of power and sells it to ZESCO

The Rural Electrification Authority (REA) focuses on increasing access to electricity in rural areas. Other participants in the industry include small-scale generators and hydro and solar based energy service enterprises supplying power in a limited number of rural areas. Examples are providers in Zambezi and Mwinalunga districts, which are located far from the national electricity grid.

2.1   Distribution Systems

The main transmission system runs at 66 kV, 88 kV, 132 kV, 220 kV and 330 kV (Fig. 1). All three companies use the transmission system which is operated by ZESCO and CEC. The Zambian Transmission System connects with Tanzania and Botswana on 66 kV, Namibia on 220 kV, with the Democratic Republic of Congo on 220 kV and Zimbabwe on 330 kV.

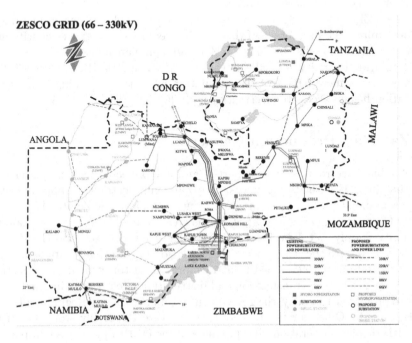

Fig. 1. ZESCO power grid [6]

The ERB licenses the transmission companies. The transmission grid is operated and monitored by the control centres of the various owners of the systems. Each of the companies has its own control and operations center, and monitors the performance of their respective transmission networks. There is no supervising or independent transmission systems authority. The Zambia Electricity Supply Act guides the cooperation. Additionally, like members of the Southern African Power Pool, the electricity suppliers operate within international operating guidelines.

3   Rural Electrification

Zambia strives for universal access to clean, reliable and affordable energy. Its development is consistent of the country's national development goals of sustained growth, employment generation and poverty reduction [4].

3.1   Definition of Rural Areas

There is no standard definition of the term *rural* [7]. In Zambia, 93.9 % of the surface is designated as customary, rural land [8]. Others texts estimate that 61.2 % of Zambia's population live in rural areas [9]. In 2005, Zambia reported that 6,268 (83 %) out of 7,576 schools were located in rural areas [10]. In 2008, Zambia operated 1,564 health facilities, of which 1,029 were classified as a rural health centres [11].

The definition of a rural community is "the smallest spatial group which encompasses the principal features to society, being a group of people interacting socially, with common ties or bonds with the geographic limited rural territory in which they live" [7]. Rural areas are often defined as 'non-urban areas', and that includes geographically isolated communities that are separated from central clusters (i.e. towns) and are deprived of modern amenities available in an urban or peri-urban environments. Zambians commonly designate these areas as 'deep-rural', distinguishing them from urban or peri-urban areas.

3.2   Rural Electrification Plan

The passage of the Rural Electrification Act of 2003 provides a platform for rural electrification efforts in Zambia. Rural electrification became the responsibility of the Rural Electrification Authority (REA), which manages the Rural Electrification Fund.

REA prepared a detailed Rural Electrification Master Plan (REMP) that serves as a blueprint for Zambia's electrification efforts for the period 2008 – 2030. The REMP indicates the electrification targets, the roll out sequence, and the methods, timing and budgets required. The REMP sets ambitious targets for increasing access to electricity by 2030. The plan identified a total of 1,217 'growth centers' in rural areas throughout Zambia. These are the targets for electrification during the plan period. The target is to increase the electrification rate in rural areas, from the current 3.5 % of households to 51 % by the year 2030. The plan targets three principal methods of electrification:

1. extension of the national electrical grid
2. creation of stand alone electricity systems supplied from renewable sources such as Mini Hydro Power Stations and Biomass Generation
3. implementation of solar energy systems

The REMP focuses on system extension as the main vehicle for expansion of access. The total investment required to achieve its target is estimated at USD 1.1 billion. This translates into an annual expenditure of USD 50 million (ZMW 250 billion) between 2008 and 2030.

4   Electricity in Rural Macha

In Zambia, most rural areas do not have electricity. If at all available, electricity supply is not stable because of frequent power cuts, and brown outs caused in part by load shedding. Regularly, the power fluctuations damage electrical equipment. Repairs result in extra costs for maintenance, shipping and replacement of parts that are not found easily in the province or country [12,13].

Macha is located in the Southern Province of Zambia, 70 km from the nearest town of Choma and 350 Km by road from the capital city of Lusaka. The topography of the area is undulating, primarily open savannah woodland averaging 1,100 m above sea level. The climate is tropical. The Macha area is populated by traditional Tonga villagers, living in small scattered homesteads which usually consist of one extended family. There are no corporate farmers or industries in the area. The primary livelihood is subsistence farming with maize being the main crop. There is an estimated population of 135,000 within an approximate 35 Km radius around Macha. Overall population density in this area is 25 per square kilometre. 50 % of the population is under 12 years of age. In the areas surrounding Macha, the average income for a person in the village is less than the equivalent of USD 2 per day.

5   Measuring Electricity

In Macha, since 2009, there were many dedicated attempts to measure the quality of the grid electricity supply for research purposes. Sourcing and installing measuring equipment took two years, with difficulties in funding, acquiring and transporting of such equipment to this remote area. Fluke measuring equipment was supplied through a research cooperation with UC Santa Barbara. However, the equipment broke down within several hours of the start of measurements. Replacement involved an other period of sourcing and transporting issues. At last, longitudinal quantitative measurements started in 2011. These measurements include a sample every second. They confirm the general community experience that the quality of power varies drastically.

Figure 2 shows a time line of power failures during in Macha during 2011. The y-axis shows the duration of the power failure. Figure 3 shows that, on average, the period between power failures is about 1 day, but this is skewed by the fact that when power is restored there are often repeated failures. The cumulative distribution function (CDF) of duration of power failures in shown in Fig. 4.

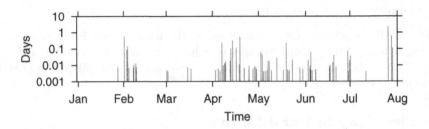

Fig. 2. Timeline of power failures in Macha.

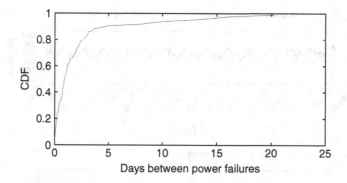

Fig. 3. CDF of time elapsed between power failures in Macha

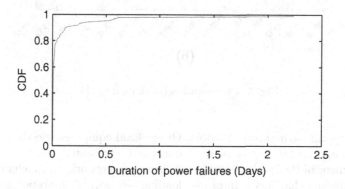

Fig. 4. CDF of duration of power failures in Macha

The average duration is approximately 1 h but 10 % of power failures do last longer than 12 h. The longest power failure in the data set was 2 days.

Figure 5(a) shows the measurements in a sample two week period in 2012. The x-axis plots time in days and the y-axis plots voltage. The gray areas on the plot indicate periods of a power outage. Voltage is sampled each minute with recording of the maximum and minimum voltage. The standard voltage in Zambia is 230 V. Measurements show the voltage varies from 150 V to 240 V, with frequent power failures. Furthermore, there are long periods of power brown-outs in which electricity is available, but the voltage is continuously low. Three brown-outs are clearly seen in this diagram. They have the much potential to put e-infrastructure in an unstable state. Voltage tends to follow a diurnal pattern with voltage dips most noticeable during evening periods when electrical stoves are used for cooking. These patterns are typical of a system that is overloaded.

Relatedly, Internet availability is shown in Fig. 5(b). It is clear that there is often no connectivity to the outside world even when power is available. The lack of Internet connectivity is often due to upstream problems in the grid or

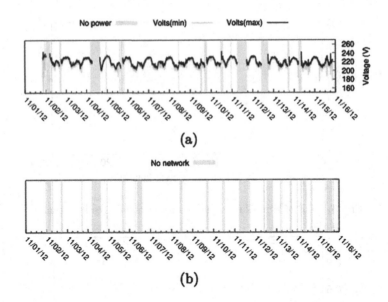

Fig. 5. Power and network quality [14]

connectivity infrastructure in Zambia. Often, local equipment needs to be reset after becoming unstable after power failures or brown-outs.

Assessment of the implementation of electricity networks in Macha buildings shows additional challenges. Improper loading and wiring, improper grounding, bad connections, improperly sized wire used, overloaded circuits, and insufficient supply all resulted in power sagging effects, especially due to 'in surge' currents from heavy equipment loads. Sagging effect are amplified when wiring is too small and when the feeding lines are too long.

6   Equipment Quality

In practice, there are many different standards and levels of quality of electronic and electrical equipment arriving in rural areas. Assorted batches of donated Information and Communication Technologies (ICT) equipment arrive with all kinds of levels of ruggedness and susceptibility to dirty power. Standard Uninterrupted Power Supplies (UPS), meant to protect equipment from energy disruptions, are easily damaged in the first line of defence. In Macha, out of over 40 high quality UPS systems, only 5 remained after one year of operation. Most UPS systems failed within the first month of use. Clearly, for rural areas, equipment that is rugged enough to withstand dirty power is a key issue that warrants further research.

7   Social Practice

It is not only the availability of the electricity source, but also the issue of *sharing* of electricity that plays a significant role. When bringing electricity in an area that was previously without electricity, priority areas need to be thought through carefully. For instance, meeting the needs for electricity of the chief might be regarded of a higher priority than use for ICT or the needs for an existing school or rural health center. Back up procedures also raise issues related to the prioritizing of access to electricity in the community. For example, when the main power supply is interrupted, why would only ICT equipment be provided with uninterrupted power and not the health clinic or the schools? The question of which constituencies in the community should be connected to the electrical grid is not only a pragmatic issue but can pose social and political challenges as well.

8   Alternative Energy Supplies

In practice, solar equipment proves difficult to source. Solar technology is plagued with battery issues as they falter due to high temperatures and abuse. Battery replacement requires much effort in the sourcing of funding, acquiring the right batteries, travelling to remote places. Solar installations typically involve equipment that necessitates specific training of engineers. Further, solar panels are vulnerable to physical damage or theft. Representatives of UC Santa Barbara donated 60 small solar-powered LED lights in July 2013 to assess their viability and utility among those who are not connected to the electrical grid. These solar powered lights were designed by the Institute for Energy Efficiency at UC Santa Barbara. It is anticipated that they will be very useful in Macha given that so few homes are connected to the electrical grid and given low incomes many cannot afford to purchase candles as often as they are needed.

9   Discussion

It is impossible to think about or use the Internet or mobile phones for e-Governance, e-Infrastructure, and e-Business in Macha (or anywhere) without thinking about electricity. Zambia currently is short of power, power goes on and off unpredictably almost every day in Macha. This paper shows that fluctuations and inconsistencies in the voltage occur. They can cause damage to electronic devices such as computers, large appliances such as refrigerators and can even causes dangerous fires in homes and other buildings. Power outages regularly interrupt Internet and mobile phone services, and thus access to services[1].

---

[1] Other common causes of Internet downtime in Zambia are: adverse weather conditions, low or shared bandwidth, and poor quality of copper cables/telephone connections [15, p. 24].

Rural communities such as Macha are particularly vulnerable to load shedding, the centralized practice of shutting off services to one area to support demand in another area – often urban areas or neighbouring countries. Almost every day the power goes out in the community at unpredictable times, sometimes for a few minutes but often for hours. Most Internet users expressed frustration with this situation and described their use as punctuated by these frequent disruptions. Web browsers are used for services such as web-based email, social networking or other cloud services and frequent disruption of Internet access interrupts work flow and becomes debilitating. Far from being a universal service, homogeneous in its durations, the dynamism of access to e-services is contingent upon the harnessing of resources, the timed flow of electrical currents, and the regulation of voltage.

The integration of Information and Communication Technologies within daily, rural lives is contingent upon the conversion of water, sun, fossil fuels and other materials into electrical power. While most rural households and community facilities live 'off the grid', ZESCO charges ZMW 75,000 (USD 15,000) to connect electricity to a school. In view of these high costs, most people in rural villages power their devices in other ways. Some use power outlets at the outdoor market in the village center to charge their electronics and pay a fee to do so. Some use solar panels to power up radios, lights, and other small appliances. Others jerry-rig car batteries to energize TV sets and stereo systems. Thus, consumer electronics are fueled by the manual labour of people who take time and energy each day to devise ways of empowering their devices on or off the grid [16].

It is important to recognize that the digital economy is layered upon the resource economy. The success of e-Governance, e-Infrastructure, and e-Business relies upon electricity and a multitude of other physical and social resources. Each of these resources presents challenges in its deployment and/or use. For ICT services to be sustainable in rural Africa, attention to all these factors is crucial, and access to electricity supply, in all its facets, should be a central priority.

For rural areas, deeper understanding of priority areas for electrification based on community input is required in order to avoid the situation of supplying IT equipment before supporting other vital areas such as a health clinic or the community's chief. Reviewing Information Systems implementations in Malawi, Mpazanje et al. confirmed that project success is achieved only when stakeholder interests are strongly interwoven with the project's needs [17]. The incorporation of electricity provisioning in rural areas must take into account the characteristics of local cultures, including social habits, employment, language and cuisine. Apart from well-trained engineers at the power utilities, the training of the rural electricians is crucial since they will be responsible for laying power cables in a village from transformers or alternative energy supplies to other sites. Their proper training will help to ensure that correct gauge cable and cable lengths are used for the expected load. However, currently there are no obvious places for formal apprenticeships of electricians in rural areas.

There are a number of alternative energy options. However, in Macha, none of the alternative energy implementations remained operational for an extended period due to various constraints. A robust UPS is required for rural areas, one that can handle dirty power. Research and development are needed to assess which components in the UPS are vulnerable to unstable rural power. Further, there are opportunities for smart local grids that protect equipment by disconnecting sections of the grid when voltage discrepancies are detected.

10   Conclusion

Description of the current context and observations on electricity is scarce in rural Africa. Electricity in rural areas is notoriously unstable. It has caused serious damage to equipment and can shorten its life span due to frequent power outages. However, electricity is a foundational resource that is necessary for any application of ICT and access to e-Infrastructure and services. This paper provides input through cross-sectional analysis of information gathered in rural Macha, Zambia by Macha Works and other researchers working in the community.

Quantitative engineering mixes with social factors, and we find that both play key roles. Research, development, and evaluation must be sensitive to a complex array of challenges if all rural areas are to receive usable access to electricity and ICTs.

References

1. Government of the Republic of Zambia. Sixth National Development Plan 2011 2015. Ministry of Finance and National Planning, Lusaka (2011)
2. Government of the Republic of Zambia. Vision 2030, A prosperous Middle-income Nation By 2030. Government of the Republic of Zambia, Lusaka (2006)
3. Kalapula, E.S.: Woodfuel situation and deforestation in Zambia. Amibo **18**(5), 293–294 (1989)
4. Government of the Republic of Zambia. The Fifth National Development plan (FNDP) 2006–2011. Ministry of Finance and National Planning, Lusaka (2006)
5. ZESCO. General Description of the Electricity System (2009)
6. Sisala, R.P.: Challenges and possible solutions in the power sector. Technical report, ZESCO (2008)
7. Gregory, D., Johnston, R., Pratt, G., Watts, M., Whatmore, S. (eds.): The Dictionary of Human Geography. Wiley-Blackwell, Chichester (2009)
8. Adams, M.: Land Tenure Policy and Practice in Zambia: Issues Relating to the Development of the Agricultural Sector. Mokoro, Oxford (2003)
9. Central Statistics Office Zambia. 2010 Census of Population and Housing Preliminary Report (2011)
10. Government of the Republic of Zambia. Educational Statistical Bulletin. Ministry of Education, Lusaka (2005)
11. Government of the Republic of Zambia. Annual Health Statistical Bulletin. Ministry of Health, Lusaka (2008)

12. Matthee, K., Mweemba, G., Pais, A., van Stam, G., Rijken, M.: Bringing Internet connectivity to rural Zambia using a collaborative approach. In: IEEE/ACM International Conference on Information and Communication Technologies and Development (ICTD2007), Bangalore, India. IEEE (2007)

13. van Stam, G., Johnson, D.L., Pejovic, V., Mudenda, C., Sinzala, A., van Greunen, D.: Constraints for information and communications technologies implementation in rural Zambia. In: Jonas, K., Rai, I.A., Tchuente, M. (eds.) Fourth International IEEE EAI Conference on eInfrastructure and eServices for Developing Countries (Africomm 2012), Yaounde, Cameroon. Springer (2012)

14. Zheleva, M., Paul, A., Johnson, D.L., Belding, E.: Kwiizya: local cellular network services in remote areas. In: MobiSys13, Taipei, Taiwan (2013)

15. Mulozi, D.L.: Rural Access: Options and Challenges for Connectivity and Energy in Zambia. eBrain Forum of Zambia/IICD (2008)

16. Parks, L.: Water, energy, access: internet and mobile phone infrastructure in rural Zambia. In: Parks, L., Starosielski, N. (eds.) Signal Traffic: Critical Studies of Media Infrastructures. University of Illinois Press, Urbana Champaign (2014)

17. Mpazanje, F., Swechurran, K., Brown, I.: Rethinking information systems projects using actor-network theory: a case of Malawi. EJISDC **58**(1), 1–32 (2013)

Considering Misconceptions in Automatic Essay Scoring with A-TEST - Amrita Test Evaluation and Scoring Tool

Prema Nedungadi[1,2(✉)], Jyothi L[2], and Raghu Raman[1]

[1] Amrita CREATE, Amrita University, Vallikavu, Kollam, India
{prema,raghu}@amrita.edu
[2] Department of Computer Science, Amrita University,
Vallikavu, Kollam, India
amritajyothi8@gmail.com

Abstract. In large classrooms with limited teacher time, there is a need for automatic evaluation of text answers and real-time personalized feedback during the learning process. In this paper, we discuss Amrita Test Evaluation & Scoring Tool (A-TEST), a text evaluation and scoring tool that learns from course materials and from human-rater scored text answers and also directly from teacher input. We use latent semantic analysis (LSA) to identify the key concepts. While most AES systems use LSA to compare students' responses with a set of ideal essays, this ignores learning the common misconceptions that students may have about a topic. A-TEST also uses LSA to learn misconceptions from the lowest scoring essays using this as a factor for scoring. 'A-TEST' was evaluated using two datasets of 1400 and 1800 pre-scored text answers that were manually scored by two teachers. The scoring accuracy and kappa scores between the derived 'A-TEST' model and the human raters were comparable to those between the human raters.

Keywords: Feature extraction · Essay scoring · Text analysis · Text mining · Latent semantic analysis (LSA) · SVD · Natural language process- NLP · AES

1 Introduction

The advancement in internet technologies has increased the reach of web based assessment and tutoring to tens of thousands of users. However in most systems the process of evaluation and grading is limited to objective questions that are not enough to evaluate a student in more complex tasks. Scoring text answers has challenges as there are multiple right and wrong answers. This often requires machine learning of a large number of humanly evaluated answers and using similarity of essays to high scoring essays to grade the essays.

This paper proposes a text evaluation tool called 'A-TEST' (Amrita Text Evaluation & Scoring Tool), which learns from a text corpus. We describe the architecture of the system and evaluate the accuracy of the system with two datasets of 1400 and 1800 pre-scored essays.

© Institute for Computer Sciences, Social Informatics and Telecommunications Engineering 2014
T.F. Bissyandé and G. van Stam (Eds.): AFRICOMM 2013, LNICST 135, pp. 271–281, 2014.
DOI: 10.1007/978-3-319-08368-1_31

The main contributions of this paper are

1. Design and develop an automatic essay scoring system that learns from previously scored essays and training materials.
2. Propose a novel approach based on LSA to not only identify key concepts but also to learn from common misconceptions.
3. Generate the summary of the learnt concepts and misconceptions for the set of essays.
4. Use multiple regression to model a scoring formula using similarity with good concepts and similarity with misconceptions, and other factors such as spelling errors and word count.

2 Background and Related Works

A system for automated assessment saves cost and time for teachers and is consistent with manual scoring. Recently there has been a lot of research and studies in the area of Automated Essay Scoring. Researchers were successful to a great extent in using the essays as the most significant tool for assessing students' learning outcomes, their ability to recall, organize and integrate ideas, express oneself in writing and the ability for application of data.

The performance of the Latent Semantic Analysis in various Information Retrieval tasks apart from automated essay grading has been analyzed [1]. LSA has proved to be one of the most successful methods for content-based essay grading. Studies show that LSA-based systems can perform as well as the human grader while other studies [2, 13] used Probabilistic Latent Semantic Analysis (PLSA). PLSA adds a stronger probabilistic model to LSA based on a mixture decomposition derived from the latent class model. In fact, the results achieved with PLSA are quite similar of those achieved with LSA. However, over fitting problems can be avoided by the generalization of maximum likelihood model [4].

According to [1, 2], the four quality criteria for an automated essay grading system are accuracy, defensibility, coachability and cost-efficiency. An accurate system is capable of producing reliable grades measured by the correlation between a human grader and the system. In order to be defensible, the grading procedure employed by the system must be traceable and educationally valid. Coachability refers to the transparency of the grading method. For example, if the grading is based on simple methods that ignore content, students can circumvent the system to obtain higher grades than they deserve. Hence content assessment should be key criteria in grading.

3 A-TEST

Spell checkers, word count and such features are important but are limited to providing feedback on errors in the surface features. LSA is a powerful Information Retrieval technique that uses statistics and linear algebra to discover underlying "latent" meaning of text and has been successfully used in English language text evaluation and retrieval [8–10]. To assess knowledge, A-TEST uses Latent Semantic Analysis (LSA) to measure the student's knowledge based on analyses of a set of textual information on the subject domain and the student's answer and then validates the model using similarity measures. A-TEST learns from a corpus of manually scored answers using NLP and LSA techniques and from direct entries from the subject matter expert to determine an optimal evaluation and scoring model for each question with a text response. NLP is used to detect the features during the evaluation and LSA is used to compare the new essay by comparing with the ideal set of essays to determine the similarity with such essays. However, this does not incorporate common misconceptions that can be learnt from low scoring essays. For example, in an essay about Turtles, a common misconception is as follows.

> **fact :** Turtles are reptiles.
>
> **misconception :** Turtles are amphibians.

The set of highest scoring essays for turtles will have reptiles in it, while the lower scoring ones may have amphibian. Hence, an essay with amphibian may be given a lower score by a human teacher, but may be ignored as an irrelevant keyword by AES systems that only learn from the corpus of best essays. A-TEST performs LSA by learning from the lowest scoring essays and then removing the concepts that are common from the best scoring essays. This is because the low scoring essays may have a few correct concepts along with incorrect or irrelevant ones. Only the ones which are learnt as misconceptions are maintained.

4   A-TEST Architecture

The main component of the system includes the Pre-processor, LSA, Grade definition and other feature selection modules. The base forms of words in the input documents as well as the pre-processing stages are functioned. In the Scoring model, Word by Context matrix is processed with LSA and creates reduced representation of WCM. Figure 1 depicted below abstracts the broad level architecture of the proposed A-TEST system.

The system consists of mainly two phases: Analysis and Grading phase. In the Analysis phase, a series of algorithms is followed such as: pre-processing, dimensionality reduction, weighting schemes, and similarity measure. In the Grading phase, the essays are graded according to the scoring model created in Analysis phase. The system learns the key concepts from the course materials such as passages from lecture notes, textbooks or pre-graded essays.

4.1   Analysis Phase

Pre-processing: The pre-processing stages used are spelling correction, stop word removal, stemming, force word removal and term weighting. A word by context matrix (WCM) is created, which represents the course materials. In the scoring model,

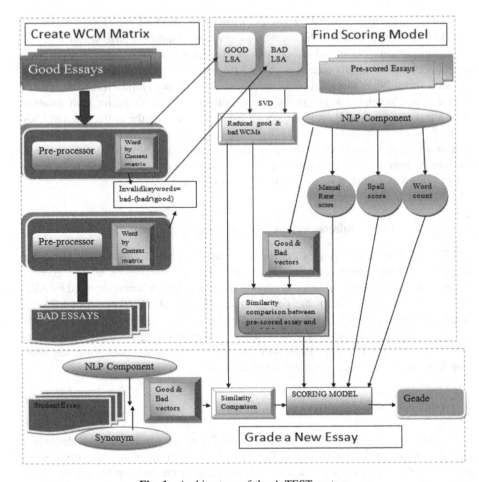

Fig. 1. Architecture of the A-TEST system

the WCM is processed with LSA which results in a reduced representation of WCM by removing items the details which are not required.

Latent Semantic Analysis: LSA is a complex statistical technique that can be applied to automated essay grading [10]. LSA might be described as comprising of the training, test and result phase.

A_k matrix obtained after the dimensionality reduction consists of keywords as rows and documents as columns, where each element S_{ij} in the matrix is the value corresponding to the semantic dimension with respect to the most dominant value from the singular matrix. The final weight W_{ij} for each term is obtained as follows

$$Wij = tfij * idfj, \quad idfj = log(n/dfj) \tag{1}$$

where n is the total number of documents, df_j is the number of times the term j occurs, tf_{ij} is the number of occurrence of jth term in doc i, idf_j is the inverse document frequency of term j.

The matrix A is factored into the product of three matrices using the singular value decomposition (SVD) [12]. U is the term-to-concept similarity matrix, V is the concept-to-document similarity matrix and Σ represents the strength of each concept and has with positive and decreasing singular values [7].

The process increases the dependency between contexts and words, making the underlying semantic structure evident by reducing the noise in the data. Given an m x n matrix A, where without loss of generality m x n and rank (A) = r, the singular value decomposition of A, denoted by SVD (A), is defined as [3, 8],

$$A = U \sum V^T \tag{2}$$

Similarity. The cosine similarity comparison is performed between the document vector of the new student essay with the reduced WCM and the student essays with highest weight values along with their corresponding scoring of the best matches is used as an independent variable in the scoring model. The cosine similarity between vectors A and B of length n can be obtained as [5],

$$cosim(A, B) = \frac{\sum_{i=1}^{n}(A_i \times B_i)}{\sqrt{\sum_{i=1}^{n} A_i^2} \times \sqrt{\sum_{i=1}^{n} B_i^2}} \tag{3}$$

where A_i & B_i are the contribution of word i to the vector A and B and n is the number of distinct words.

4.2   Learning Phase

The input to the A-TEST system is represented as a matrix with keywords as rows and documents as columns. Keywords are extracted from the dataset and the matrix is generated on the basis of occurrence of each keyword in the documents. Each essay is independently scored by two raters on a scale from 1 (lowest) to 6 (highest). The documents with the highest score of 6 are used as the input.

Algorithm 1: Learn key concepts from training material and best essays
Input: Essays multiple documents containing texts of which weight has to be calculated.
Output: The Algorithm returns (Keyword, weight) pairs.
Generate the matrix A m×n from the essay.
1. Decompose A into U, V and $\sum$ (singular value decomposition)
2. Represent each word and document is as a vector of length k.
3. Apply weight function on the matrix obtained after the dimensionality reduction.
4. Return (keyword, weight)

The time complexity of Algorithm 1 is as follows: Let m be the total number of keywords, n be the number documents to create the word-document matrix A. In Step 1, we first construct the word-document matrix and this requires time complexity of O $(\min\{mn^2, m^2n\})$ operations. In Step2, SVD is performed to reduce the dimensionality where U and V are the orthogonal matrices containing the left and right singular vectors of A and Σ is the diagonal matrix containing the singular values of A where r is the $\min(m,n)$. As we truncate the SVD to an optimal value $k \leq r$, the time complexity of this step is O (mnk). By summing up these we get the time complexity of A1 algorithm as O $((\min\{mn^2, m^2n\}) + mnk)$.

4.3   Scoring Model

The following algorithm is used for learning concepts of pre-scored essays.

Algorithm 2: Learning concepts of pre-scored essays
Input: Learn pre-score essays
Output: Essays with scores, content count, spell count and word count are stored.
Step1:
        for all human rated essays in training set
        {
find vectors of both valid keywords/phrases and misconception in the essay;
    correct_similarity = highest cosine similarity value of best matched essays;
    misconception_similarity = highest cosine similarity to the misconceptions vectors
        save content_count, spell_score, and word_count of best matched essays and similarity_correct and similarity_misconception.
        }
    Step2: find the scoring model based on the factors found in step1 using multiple regression.

4.4   Evaluating a New Essay

The following algorithm evaluates a new essay.

Algorithm3: Evaluating a new Essay
Input: new Essay
Output: Score calculated by A-TEST of new Essay
1. Pre-process essay such as removing spelling errors
2. Compute valid keywords from the submitted essay
3. Derive the vector of valid concepts from the submitted essay that are in the Master list of concepts and in the Misconception list.
4. Find cosine similarity between the valid_concepts vector and best_similarity vectors to find the essay with the highest similarity score.
5. Compute the dot product of the similarity of the misconceptions to each misconceptions vector to find the highest similarity value
6. Use both the similarity values and the other factors such as spelling errors and word count in the scoring model derived in Algorithm 2 to compute the score.

---

5 Experiment

We used a dataset from a competition on kaggle.com, by the William and Flora Hewlett Foundation [15]. The data consists of 8 sets of essays in ASCII text, written by students from Grade 7 to Grade 10. Essay set 1 and 2 were used in the study. The theme of the first dataset1 of essays learnt was the effect of computers on people. Each essay has one or more human scores and a final resolved score. Each essay is approximately 150 to 550 words in length. For dataset2 we used 60 essays to train the system and tested the model using 306 of the 1800 pre-scored essays.

Based on a bag of features, we used unigram, frequency and presence of features to perform the task with different combinations. Finally a multiple regression analysis is performed to determine the grade based on the concepts learnt, the spelling errors and the word length.

We selected two metrics to evaluate the accuracy of our predictions: grades based on the exact inter-rater agreement and grades based on the exact and adjacent (scores differ by exactly 1) inter-rater agreement between the system generated grades and the human-rater grades. Both kappa and multiple-quadratic kappa were used to determine the inter-rater agreement.

6 Scoring Models Using Multiple Regression

Grades are determined using multiple regression model using the score of the essay with the highest cosine similarity weight of the concept keywords, grade of the best match, the highest cosine similarity weight of the misconception_keywords, spelling errors, the total number of words and the grade given by the human rater1. The following factors were found to be significant by the usage of multiple regression analysis and the grade of rater1 as the training labels. These two models derived with multiple regression analysis are shown below.

$$Score_{withoutmisconceptions} = scorebestmatch * 0.145 + spellerr^{\frac{1}{4}} * 1.08 + \\ diffinspellerr * 0.45 + wordcount * 0.0023 \tag{4}$$

$$Score_{considering\_misconceptions} = scorebestmatch * 0.179 + spellerr^{\frac{1}{4}} * 1.265 + \\ diffinspellerr * 0.689 + wordcount * 0.001 - \\ misconception_{similarity} * .0415 \tag{5}$$

7 Discussion

Kappa scores and quadratic kappa scores are used to measure inter-rater agreement between the two manual scores and the scores from our model and we find a moderate agreement. A kappa of 1.0 means that two raters show perfect agreement, a kappa of -1.0 means that they show perfect and consistent disagreement, and a kappa of 0 means that the two raters show no relationship between their ratings. When kappa and quadratic weighted kappa are applied to the same agreement table, the value of weighted kappa is higher than the value of kappa [14]. Kappa statistic only measures agreement while Quadratic kappa also takes into account as the degree of disagreement between raters. Figure 2 shows that a moderately good agreement between the model-score with both the raters.

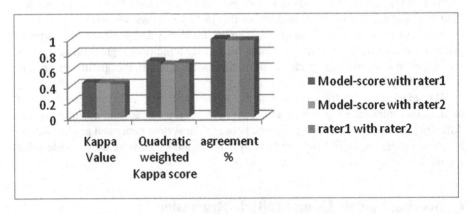

Fig. 2. Measurement of Kappa and quadratic kappa Scores

We also looked at the accuracy of adjacency agreement, when the two scores differ by one or less and have a 98 % agreement of the model with rater1. The agreement of the model with both the raters is similar to the agreement between the two manual raters. In A-TEST, content is the key parameter for the grading mechanism. Due to which the scoring technique is more relevant to any existing mechanism. Students would get the scores in a range approximately same as of manual evaluation which satisfies the criteria for coachability. This automated mechanism is must faster and cost-effective in terms of involvement of human resources at different levels of grading process. The human resources must be trained to a specific standard for achieving quality grading. Such training involves great amount of investments. A-TEST ignores the misconceptions from the pile of concepts and misconceptions considered for evaluation. Figure 3 does a graphical representation of improvement in kappa score thereby justifying the grading methodology which increases the defensibility.

The scoring accuracy of the model that includes both concepts and misconceptions is compared to the model that ignores the misconceptions. There is a small increase in kappa scores when taking into account the misconceptions showing that the scoring accuracy improved by considering misconceptions Fig. 3.

Though the percentage agreement and the kappa values were slightly better than the corresponding values between rater1 and rater2, these can be further improved by considering additional factors such as grammar, complexity of essay, parts of speech count, punctuations and more advanced NLP features.

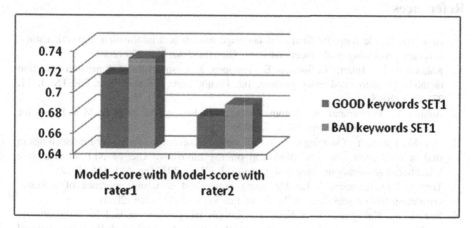

Fig. 3. Comparison of models with valid keywords to one that also includes misconceptions

8 Conclusions

In this paper, we design and develop an automatic essay scoring system that can learn from previously scored essays and training materials. A novel approach based on LSA to identify key concepts and present this to the educator for feedback. The system generates the summary of the learnt concepts with their corresponding weights and a scoring formula so that it can be used by the web based system to provide personalized feedback to text answers.

In addition to learning from a corpus and pre-scored text answers, the system can also learn additional keywords or bi-grams that are directly entered by an educator. The model is useful for large scale formative evaluation of science assessments where learning the significant keyword related to science concepts is important. Performance on essays can be improved by incorporating content and advance features that can contribute towards a good prediction.

The performance of A-TEST for a sample text answer using a dataset of pre-scored essays was comparable to the accuracy between two human evaluators. Though our prediction model worked as well as the manually evaluated teacher model, additional enhancements such as better pattern matching algorithms, correcting grammar specific errors, and comparing with other dimensionality methods such as PLSA may further improve the prediction model and are planned as further work. The current system is applicable for essay with raw text. In the future, proposed work will include the grading of essays containing tables and mathematical equation.

Acknowledgment. This work derives direction and inspiration from the Chancellor of Amrita University, Sri Mata Amritanandamayi Devi. We thank Dr. Ramachandra Kaimal for his valuable feedback.

References

1. Hiemstra, D., de Jong, F.: Statistical language models and information retrieval: natural language processing really meets retrieval. Glot Int. **5**(8), 288–293 (2001)
2. Kakkonen, T., Myller, N., Sutinen, E., Timonen, J.: Comparison of dimension reduction methods for automated essay grading. Int. Forum Educ. Technol. Soc. (IFETS) J. **11**, 275–288 (2008)
3. Adhitia, R., Purwarianti, A.: Automated essay grading system using SVM and LSA for essay answers in Indonesian. JSI 5(1) (2009)
4. Flor, M., Futagi, Y.: On using context for automatic correction of non-word misspellings in student essays. In: The 7th Workshop on the Innovative Use of NLP for Building Educational Applications, Montreal, Canada, 3–8 June 2012, pp. 105–115 (2012)
5. Turney, P.D., Littman, M.L.: Measuring praise and criticism: inference of semantic orientation from association. ACM Trans. Inf. Syst. **21**, 315–346 (2003)
6. Nagata, R., Kakegawa, J., Yabuta, Y.: A topic-independent method for automatically scoring essay content rivaling topic-dependent methods. In: 2009 Ninth IEEE International Conference on Advanced Learning Technologies (2009)
7. Liu, C.-L., Hsiao, W.-H., Lee, C.-H., Chi, H.-C.: An HMM-based algorithm for content ranking and coherence-feature extraction. IEEE Trans. Syst. Man Cybern. **42**, 397–407 (2012)
8. Miller, T.: Essay assessment with latent semantic analysis. Department of Computer Science, University of Toronto, Toronto, ON M5S 3G4, Canada (2002)
9. Loraksa, C., Peachavanish, R.: Automatic Thai language essay scoring using neural network and latent semantic analysis. In: Proceedings of the First Asia International Conference on Modeling & Simulation (AMS'07), pp. 400–402 (2007)
10. Haley, D.T., Thomas, P., Roeck, A.D., Petre, M.: Measuring improvement in latent semantic analysis based marking systems: using a computer to mark questions about HTML. In: Proceedings of the Ninth Australasian Computing Education Conference (ACE), pp. 35–52 (2007)
11. Monjurul Islam, M., Latiful Hoque, A.S.M.: Automated essay scoring using generalized latent semantic analysis. J. Comput. **7**(3), (2012)

12. Berry, M.W., Dumais, S.T., O'Brien, G.W.: Using linear algebra for intelligent information retrieval. National Science Foundation under grant Nos. NSF-CDA-9115428 and NSF-ASC-92-03004
13. Kakkonen, T., Myller, N., Sutinen, E.: Applying part of speech enhanced LSA to automated essay grading. Automated Assessment Technologies for Free Text and Programming Assignments by Academy of Finland (2006)
14. Warrens, M.J.: Weighted kappa is higher than Cohen's kappa for tridiagonal agreement tables. Stat. Methodol. **8**, 268–272 (2011)
15. The William and Flora Hewlett Foundation (Hewlett Foundation), Automated Student Assessment Prize (ASAP) designed by The Common Pool, LLC, managed by Open Education Solutions, Inc., 12 April 2012

E-education – Using the Simplest Technologies to Empower Local Communities for Development in Malawi

Alexander Mtembenuzeni[1] and Chomora Mikeka[2(✉)]

[1] Faculty of Education, University of Malawi, P.O. Box 280, Zomba, Malawi
exprinm@gmail.com
[2] Department of Physics, University of Malawi, P.O. Box 280, Zomba, Malawi
chomora@gmail.com

Abstract. Community empowerment through the transfer of knowledge and skills has the potential to build capacity of people in communities to enhance their lives by engaging in activities that will develop their lives. This paper demonstrates that the use of two very simple technological innovations: pre-recorded video training sessions and automated mobile help-line service, coupled with the establishment of community learning centers can ensure that people learn anywhere, anytime, at their own pace, in their native language over the most accessible devices and with little or no cost.

Keywords: E-education · Community empowerment · ICT4D · Community learning centers

1 Introduction

All over Africa, the common talk is "community empowerment for national development". It has been proved that the most sustainable way of bringing about development is through empowering local communities through skills building. Such empowerment would be through vocational training, business skills training, agricultural skills training or health training among others. As the saying goes, "it is better to give a man a fishing line rather than fish". Hence it is of bigger benefit to equip communities with skills to work more and produce more rather than providing them with handouts.

Given the level of development of these African countries, the biggest challenge is that of devising mass educational programs that are efficient and cost-effective. So far, governments and charitable organizations have resorted to community training workshops, deployment of advisors, using community clubs or Community Based Organizations (CBOs) as well as using radio and Television Programs. Although these media have brought about quite a number of benefits, they have also proved falling short of the desired outcome. This paper will show that community training workshops, supporting full-time advisors and training community clubs or CBOs are expensive ways of going about community skills building and provision of knowledge to locals. Considering the high population in developing countries like Malawi, mass

© Institute for Computer Sciences, Social Informatics and Telecommunications Engineering 2014
T.F. Bissyandé and G. van Stam (Eds.): AFRICOMM 2013, LNICST 135, pp. 282–286, 2014.
DOI: 10.1007/978-3-319-08368-1_32

training that covers all local communities is only a dream. Most of these programs have targeted a few selected communities and hence can be regarded as experimental. Radio and Television programs, although cost-effective and covering wide areas with the same standardized message, have also fallen short considering the fact that they do not give room for communities to learn at their own pace and in their convenience. Most of the content in radio and television programs are also compressed to cover the available air time.

As a solution to these problems, this paper suggests employing ICT4D (Information and Communication Technology for Development). African Ministers of Education, meeting at the first African ministerial round table on ICT for education, training, and development in Nairobi on June 1, 2007, stated in their communiqué that: "ICTs are seen as one key solution that will allow African countries to meet the needs in rural and under-served areas and bring education to their citizens rapidly and cost efficiently." [1].

This paper has been organized as follows: Sect. 2 describes the proposed innovations; Sect. 3 provides a summary of case studies where the innovations or their variants have been used; and Sect. 4 provides the conclusion to this paper.

2 Proposed Solutions

As regards to the above stated premises, this paper suggests two simple technologies: using training sessions pre-recorded on video that would be transmitted through Digital Video Discs (DVD) playable through ordinary DVD players, DVD ROMs to be played interactively on computer and through a web library service; and using an automated mobile phone helpline service. The paper also suggests the introduction of Community Learning Centers that are going to facilitate and aid in access to these materials and other new technologies that would be developed later.

2.1 Pre-recorded Video Training Sessions

The last five years has seen quite a sharp rise of the number of families owning Television sets and DVD players in Malawi. This can be accounted to the influx of cheap electronics manufactured by the Chinese. This paper will show how this can be utilized for mass education. Carefully planned and recorded training sessions in indigenous languages and on a given topic, for instance, "Growing Tomatoes for Maximum Profits" would be distributed on DVD. The DVDs would contain chaptered instructions and information on how to go about such an agro-business. Farmers would then access the DVDs through outlets such as Agro-dealers, community libraries or Community Learning Centers. In addition, these videos could also be distributed through interactive DVD ROMs and through the internet. Such an arrangement would allow farmers to form clubs or use the already existing farmers clubs or CBOs to follow the instructions together and help each other out when one is in need of clarification, for instance.

Justification. This innovation is beneficial for many reasons. In short, it would allow the local people to learn anywhere, anytime, at their own pace, in their native language, over the cheapest gadget and at the cheapest fees in the history of learning! The innovation would put the latest, easy to follow information at their fingertips. As the saying goes, "a picture is worth a thousand words", such an audio-visual way of training communities in their convenience and in the language they understand the most would only give them unprecedented opportunities to venture into developmental activities that would lift their lives in the end. Scientific research has shown that the human eyes have exceptionally refined nerve endings linked directly to the brain, hence 80 percent of what we learn is through the eyes [2]; this points to the effectiveness of this audio-visual way of learning. Having those DVDs in one's house would be equated to owning a powerful library of information where you would refer in the best time of need. Not only would this innovation be cost-effective since it would only need one time of recording material that would be used by a wider population for quite a long time, but it wouldn't also need too much expertise to go about it. In addition, communities would also contribute towards the innovation by buying the materials, hence contributing to the sustainability of the innovation.

2.2   Automated Mobile Phone Help-Line Service

The rise in the number of mobile phone owners over the past five years could only be described as a revolution. The influx of cheap handsets made by the Chinese as well as others traded by mobile phone operating companies has made it possible for even the poorest Malawian to own a handset. The survey of ICT and education in Africa by infoDEV [2] remarked that, "The availability of mobile phone technology is increasing at a remarkable rate." If only this medium was utilized to equip skills to local communities, development would leap several steps. This paper will show how an automated mobile phone help-line service set up would help provide information to local communities helpful in empowering them for development. In this innovation, categorized instructions of different topics would be pre-recorded and fed into a server which would serve up such information to phone users upon selecting the desired topic by a set of instructions.

Justification. Such an innovation would also allow local people to learn anywhere, anytime, at their own pace, in their native language, on the gadgets they already own, and free of charge. Although falling short of visual capabilities, the audio instructions would ensure portability, ease of use and ever-readiness.

In this information age, strides have to be made to ensure that such information that is vital for development is available to the grassroots through the most efficient and cost-effective media. It is of great belief of this researcher that the two innovations presented above represent the best examples of the simplest technologies that would empower local masses for development.

2.3   Community Learning Centers

To enhance service, reach over those who would not be able to own multimedia players and also to allow for the utilization of other technologies, the authors suggest developing Community Learning Centers (CLCs) also known as Community Multimedia Centers (CMCs) which would make available all tools and resources needed to provide viewing of the pre-recorded Video Sessions as well as tutorials on how they would use these innovations. The tools and resources would include a TV set, a DVD player, and several sets of computers with internet connection. It should be mentioned that these have been tried and have been very successful in providing useful knowledge that empower local communities. For instance, the United Nations Educations, Scientific and Cultural Organization (UNESCO) through its Communication and Information sector has implemented as the sector's flagship program, the Community Multimedia Center program where they have built Community Multimedia Centers in countries like Mali, Benin, Mozambique and Tanzania among others. In its evaluation report, UNESCO reports that

> "Across all regions, the CMC pilots are demonstrating an important role in community development and community resilience: strengthening cultural roots and values; breaking through social isolation for marginalized groups; connecting communities to the diaspora and to national and international trends and events; supporting education, health, skills development and other important social and economic development efforts [3]."

3   Case Studies

A number of case studies exist that demonstrate the importance of the two innovations explained above.

The best applied case of the video approach is the Digital Green, a project by Microsoft Research India and the GREEN Foundation aimed at disseminating locally relevant agricultural information to small and marginal farmers in India using participatory video and mediated instruction [4]. The project is reported to have achieved an adoption rate of good agricultural practices of 85 % compared to the traditional training and visit by extension workers. The project is also reported to have been resource-efficient to the effect that the cost per adoption was $3.70 compared to $38.18 of the traditional training and visit through extension workers.

In a program led by the International Institute for Communication and Development (IICD) in Burkina Faso, it is reported of how a community of 11, 000 got empowered through watching a video that was filmed by trained women on how to prepare a sauce called "Sumbala". It is also reported of how rapidly the communities accepted this technology [5].

Several organizations in Africa have already been on the forefront creating video educational content on DVD, DVD ROM, through TV and websites. These include Learnthings Africa, CurriculumNet in Uganda, and Mindset (South Africa) [6]. These organizations have however dwelled much on creating content to compliment instruction in schools and not for non-formal education for locals.

In a study by Granfeld and Hoon Ng to establish the effectiveness of multimedia non-formal Open Distance Learning for farmers in Cambodia over face to face training, it is reported that quite a big number farmers who were taught using the Multimedia methods (self-instructional material on DVD) adopted the new methods of farming that those trained through face to face instruction [6].

4 Conclusion

In this era of information and knowledge-based economies, there is a growing need to make knowledge available to citizens if individual, community and consequently national development is to be achieved. An example of this is the rate at which people have been empowered to voice out their concerns over African leadership through social networks like YouTube and Facebook. This can be attributed to the availability of rapid information technologies which are making it possible for locals to acquire information and knowledge that empower them. In the same respect, simple technologies that would cut costs, provide learning anywhere, anytime, at leaners' own pace, in their native language and over the cheapest gadgets can be employed to serve the millions of locals in communities in Malawi, providing to them knowledge useful in aspects like business, agriculture, governance, justice and health. This paper has suggested two simple and cost-effective technologies: pre-recorded video training sessions that would be transmitted through Digital Video Discs (DVD) playable through ordinary DVD players, DVD ROMs to be played interactively on computer and through a web library service; and using an automated mobile phone helpline service. The paper has also suggested the introduction of Community Learning Centers that would facilitate and aid access to these materials and other new technologies that would be developed later.

References

1. Farrell, G., Isaacs, S.: Survey of ICT and Education in Africa: A Summary Report, Based on 53 Country Surveys. Washington, DC: infoDev/World Bank, p. 16 (2007)
2. Seiderman, A.S., Marcus, S.E.: 20/20 is Not Enough: The New World of Vision. Knopf, New York (1989)
3. Creech, H., et al.: Evaluation of UNESCO's Community Multimedia Centers - Final Report, UNESCO. p. 9 (2006)
4. Ghandi, R., Veeraraghavan, R., Toyama, K., Ramprasad, V.: Digital green: participatory video for agricultural extension
5. Laureys, F.: ICTs and Rural Development - a Case from Burkina Faso, May 2010. www.iicd. org/articles/icts-and-rural-development-a-case-from-burkina-faso
6. Grunfeld, H., Hoon Ng, M.L.: A multimedia approach to ODL for agricultural training in cambodia. Int. Rev. Res. Open Distance Learn. (2013). www.rrodl.org/index.php/irrodl/aricle/view/1275-2440

Author Index